Practical Guide in
# Assisted Reproductive Technology

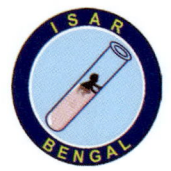

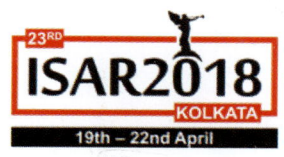

To commemorate the occasion of 23rd ISAR National Conference
**ISAR Bengal** published monogram titled **"Practical Guide in 4 volumes"**.
- Infertility
- Assisted Reproductive Technology
- Reproductive Surgery
- Andrology and Embryology

# Practical Guide in
# Assisted Reproductive Technology

*Editors*

**Gita Ganguly Mukherjee** DGO MD FICOG FICMCH FRCOG
*Formerly,* Professor and Head
Department of Obstetrics and Gynecology
RG Kar Medical College and Hospital
Kolkata, West Bengal, India

**Gautam Khastgir** MD (Cal) FRCS (Edin) FRCOG (Lond) FICOG
Medical Director and Subspecialist
Department of Reproductive Medicine and Surgery
Bengal Infertility and Reproductive Therapy Hospital (BIRTH)
Kolkata, West Bengal, India

**Siddhartha Chatterjee** DGO DNB MRCOG FICOG FRCOG
Director, Calcutta Fertility Mission
Vice-President, ISAR Bengal
Kolkata, West Bengal, India

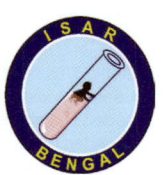

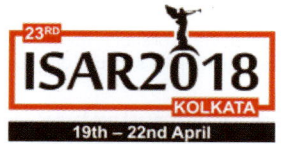

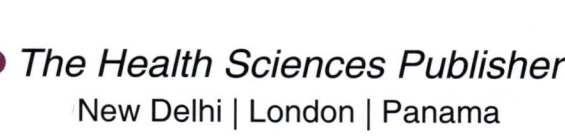

*The Health Sciences Publisher*
New Delhi | London | Panama

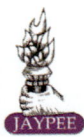 **Jaypee Brothers Medical Publishers (P) Ltd**

### Headquarters
Jaypee Brothers Medical Publishers (P) Ltd
4838/24, Ansari Road, Daryaganj
New Delhi 110 002, India
Phone: +91-11-43574357
Fax: +91-11-43574314
Email: jaypee@jaypeebrothers.com

### Overseas Offices

J.P. Medical Ltd
83 Victoria Street, London
SW1H 0HW (UK)
Phone: +44 20 3170 8910
Fax: +44 (0)20 3008 6180
Email: info@jpmedpub.com

Jaypee-Highlights Medical Publishers Inc
City of Knowledge, Bld. 235, 2nd Floor,
Clayton, Panama City, Panama
Phone: +1 507-301-0496
Fax: +1 507-301-0499
Email: cservice@jphmedical.com

Jaypee Brothers Medical Publishers (P) Ltd
17/1-B Babar Road, Block-B, Shyamoli
Mohammadpur, Dhaka-1207
Bangladesh
Mobile: +08801912003485
Email: jaypeedhaka@gmail.com

Jaypee Brothers Medical Publishers (P) Ltd
Bhotahity, Kathmandu, Nepal
Phone: +977-9741283608
Email: kathmandu@jaypeebrothers.com

Website: www.jaypeebrothers.com
Website: www.jaypeedigital.com

© 2018, Jaypee Brothers Medical Publishers

The views and opinions expressed in this book are solely those of the original contributor(s)/author(s) and do not necessarily represent those of editor(s) of the book.

All rights reserved. No part of this publication may be reproduced, stored or transmitted in any form or by any means, electronic, mechanical, photocopying, recording or otherwise, without the prior permission in writing of the publishers.

All brand names and product names used in this book are trade names, service marks, trademarks or registered trademarks of their respective owners. The publisher is not associated with any product or vendor mentioned in this book.

Medical knowledge and practice change constantly. This book is designed to provide accurate, authoritative information about the subject matter in question. However, readers are advised to check the most current information available on procedures included and check information from the manufacturer of each product to be administered, to verify the recommended dose, formula, method and duration of administration, adverse effects and contraindications. It is the responsibility of the practitioner to take all appropriate safety precautions. Neither the publisher nor the author(s)/editor(s) assume any liability for any injury and/or damage to persons or property arising from or related to use of material in this book.

This book is sold on the understanding that the publisher is not engaged in providing professional medical services. If such advice or services are required, the services of a competent medical professional should be sought.

Every effort has been made where necessary to contact holders of copyright to obtain permission to reproduce copyright material. If any have been inadvertently overlooked, the publisher will be pleased to make the necessary arrangements at the first opportunity. The **CD/DVD-ROM** (if any) provided in the sealed envelope with this book is complimentary and free of cost. **Not meant for sale.**

Inquiries for bulk sales may be solicited at: jaypee@jaypeebrothers.com

*Practical Guide in Assisted Reproductive Technology*

First Edition: **2018**

ISBN 978-93-5270-483-5

*Printed at* Rajkamal Electric Press, Kundli, Haryana.

## Dedicated to

*"All the infertile couples and those who are devoted to alleviate their agony"*

# Contributors

**Abhimanyu Tejrao Shinde**
Clinical Fellow and Fertility Associates
Mumbai, Maharashtra, India

**Ameet Patki**
Medical Director
Fertility Associates Mumbai
General Secretary–ISAR
Chair, West Zone–RCOG
Mumbai, Maharashtra, India

**Antima Rathore**
Senior Resident
Institute of Human Reproduction
Guwahati, Assam, India

**Anuradha Chaudhary**
Consultant
Genome–The Fertility Centre
Raipur, Chhattisgarh, India

**Arti Gupta**
Clinical Embryologist
Ajanta Hospital and IVF Centre
Lucknow, Uttar Pradesh, India

**Arup Kumar Majhi**
Professor
Department of Obstetrics and Gynecology
RG Kar Medical College
Kolkata, West Bengal, India

**Astha Chakravarty**
Consultant IVF and Reproductive Medicine
Milann Fertility Centre
New Delhi, India

**Bharti Jain**
Consultant Sinologist and ART Specialist
KJIVF and Laparoscopy Centre
New Delhi, India

**Bhushan Shrikhande**
Resident
Department of Obstetrics and Gynecology
Government Medical College
Nagpur, Maharashtra, India

**Biman Kumar Chakraborty**
Head
Department of Obstetrics and Gynecology
Saroj Gupta Cancer Centre and Research Institute
Kolkata, West Bengal, India

**BN Chakravarty**
Director
Institute of Reproductive Medicine
Kolkata, West Bengal, India

**Deepak Goenka**
Consultant
Institute of Human Reproduction
Guwahati, Assam, India

**Dibyendu Banerjee**
Consultant, Gynecologist
Kolkata, West Bengal, India

**Diksha Goswami**
Consultant Infertility Specialist
ART Rainbow IVF
Global Rainbow Healthcare
Agra, Uttar Pradesh, India

**Duru Shah**
Director, Gynaecworld–The Center for Women's Health and Fertility
President, Indian Society of Assisted Reproduction (ISAR)
Founder President, The PCOS Society (India)
Consultant, Obstetrician and Gynecologist
Breach Candy Hospital/Jaslok Hospital/Global Hospital
Mumbai, Maharashtra, India

**Farhat Kazim**
Consultant
Ajanta Hospital and IVF Centre
Lucknow, Uttar Pradesh, India

**Fessy Louis T**
Senior Consultant
Department of Reproductive Medicine
and Surgery
Amrita Fertility Centre
Amrita Institute of Medical Sciences
Kochi, Kerala, India

**GA Ramaraju**
Director
Krishna IVF Clinic
Visakhapatnam, Andhra Pradesh, India

**Gautam Khastgir**
Medical Director and Subspecialist
Department of Reproductive Medicine
and Surgery
Bengal Infertility and Reproductive
Therapy Hospital (BIRTH)
Kolkata, West Bengal, India

**Gita Ganguly Mukherjee**
*Formerly*, Professor and Head
Department of Obstetrics and
Gynecology
RG Kar Medical College and Hospital
Kolkata, West Bengal, India

**Gita Khanna**
Scientific Director–ART Unit
Ajanta Hospital and IVF Centre
Lucknow, Uttar Pradesh, India

**Indranil Saha**
Consultant IVF and Reproductive Medicine
Institute of Reproductive Medicine
Kolkata, West Bengal, India

**Jaideep Malhotra**
President, FOGSI–2018
Managing Director, ART Rainbow-IVF
Agra, Uttar Pradesh, India

**J Tan**
Department of Obstetrics and Gynecology
University of British Columbia, Canada
Vancouver, BC, Canada

**Kakoli Acharyya**
Consultant Pediatrician
Calcutta Medical Research Institute (CMRI)
Kolkata, West Bengal, India

**Kalika Dubey**
Consultant
Ajanta Hospital and IVF Centre
Lucknow, Uttar Pradesh, India

**Kamini A Rao**
Medical Director
Milann (A Unit of BACC
Healthcare Pvt Ltd)
Bengaluru, Karnataka, India

**Kamini Patel**
Infertility Specialist
The VANI IVF and Surrogacy Center
Ahmedabad, Gujarat, India

**Kanthi Bansal**
Director
Safal Fertility Foundation
Ahmedabad, Gujarat, India

**Kattera S**
Asia Pacific Institute of Embryology
(ASPIER)
Mysore, Karnataka, India

**Keshav Malhotra**
Laboratory Director (Chief Embryologist)
ART Rainbow-IVF
Agra, Uttar Pradesh, India

**K Jayakrishnan**
Managing Director and Chief Consultant
Department of Reproductive Medicine
KJK Hospital, Fertility Research and
Gynec Centre, Nalanchira
KJK Well Woman Centre
Thiruvananthapuram, Kerala, India

# Contributors

**Kuldeep Jain**
Director
KJIVF and Laparoscopy Centre
New Delhi, India

**Laxmi Shrikhande**
Consultant Gynecologist and IVF Specialist
Shrikhande IVF and Surrogacy Centre
Nagpur, Maharashtra, India

**Maansi Jain**
Senior Resident
Department of Obstetrics and Gynecology
Kasturba Gandhi Hospital
New Delhi, India

**Manjusree Chakraoarty**
Consultant Obstetrician and Gynecologist
Institute of Reproductive Medicine
Kolkata, West Bengal, India

**MH Dahan**
Assistant Professor
Division of REI
Department of Obstetrics and Gynecology and Reproductive Endcrinology and Infertility (REI)
McGill University
Origin Elle Fertility Clinic and Women Health Centre
Montreal, Canada

**ML Goenka**
Consultant
Institute of Human Reproduction
Guwahati, Assam, India

**Monica Chetani**
Consultant ART Specialist
Mumbai, Maharashtra, India

**Moumita Naha**
Consultant
Department of Reproductive Medicine and Surgery
Bengal Infertility and Reproductive Therapy Hospital (BIRTH)
Kolkata, West Bengal, India

**Mumtaz Sanghamita**
*Formerly*, Professor and Head
Department of Obstetrics and Gynecology
Medical College
Kolkata, West Bengal, India

**Namrata Biswas**
Consultant Anesthesiologist
Columbia Asia Hospital
Kolkata, West Bengal, India

**Narendra Malhotra**
Professor, Dubrovnik International University, Croatia
Director, Global Rainbow Healthcare
Agra, Uttar Pradesh, India

**Nayana Patel**
Medical and Managing Director
Akanksha Hospital and Research Institute
A Unit of Sat Kaival Hospital Pvt Ltd
Anand, Gujarat, India

**Neharika Malhotra Bora**
Assistant Professor
Bharati Vidyapeeth University
Pune, Maharashtra, India
Consultant, ART Rainbow-IVF
Agra, Uttar Pradesh, India

**Niranjana Jayakrishnan**
Consultant
Department of Gynecology and Reproductive Medicine
KJK Hospital, Fertility Research and Gynec Centre, Nalanchira
KJK Well Woman Centre
Thiruvananthapuram, Kerala, India

**Nitin Gupta**
Consultant Radiologist
Mumbai, Maharashtra, India

**NR Mondal**
In-Charge
Department of Obstetrics and Gynecology
Saroj Gupta Cancer Centre and Research Institute
Kolkata, West Bengal, India

**N Sanjeeva Reddy**
Professor and Head
Department of Reproductive Medicine
and Surgery
Sri Ramachandra Medical College and
Research Institute
Chennai, Tamil Nadu, India

**Paramita Hazari**
Consultant, Department of Reproductive
Medicine and Surgery
Bengal Infertility and Reproductive
Therapy Hospital (BIRTH)
Kolkata, West Bengal, India

**P Chan**
Origin Elle Fertility Clinic and
Women Health Centre
Department of Urology and
Male reproductive Medicine
McGill University
Montreal, Canada

**Pratap Kumar**
Professor, Manipal Assisted Reproductive
Centre (MARC)
Department of Obstetrics and Gynecology
Kasturba Medical College
Manipal Academy of Higher Education
(MAHE)
Mangalore, Karnataka, India

**Praveena Pai**
Consultant–Reproductive Medicine
Manipal Fertility
Mangalore, Karnataka, India

**Radhika L Kundul**
FNB–Reproductive Medicine, Infertility
Specialist, Gynecologist, Obstetrician,
Reproductive Health Specialist
Institute of Women Health and Fertility
Hyderabad, Telangana, India

**Rahul Roy Chowdhury**
Consultant, Department of Obstetrics
and Gynecology
Saroj Gupta Cancer Centre and
Research Institute
Kolkata, West Bengal, India

**Rajan S Vaidya**
Professor and Head
Department of Assisted Reproduction
Nowrosjee Wadia Maternity Hospital and
IVF Centre
Mumbai, Maharashtra, India

**Ramesh**
Senior Resident
Department of Reproductive Medicine
and Surgery
Amrita Institute of Medical Sciences
Kochi, Kerala, India

**Rashmi Goenka**
Lab Director
Institute of Human Reproduction
Guwahati, Assam, India

**Ratna Chattopadhyay**
Head (Embryology and Andrology)
Institute of Reproductive Medicine
Kolkata, west Bengal, India

**Ritika Rajan**
Consultant
Fertility Clinic and IVF Centre
Mumbai, Maharashtra, India

**Sadhana Gupta**
Consultant (Obs and Gyne), and
Advanced Infertility Specialist
Jeevan Jyoti Hospital and Medical
Research Centre
Gorakhpur, Uttar Pradesh, India

**Sadhana K Desai**
Founder Director
Fertility Clinic and IVF Centre
Mumbai, Maharashtra, India

**Saeeda Wasim**
Institute of Reproductive Medicine
Kolkata, West Bengal, India

**Sanghamitra Ghosh**
ART Specialist
Institute of Reproductive Medicine
Kolkata, West Bengal, India

# Contributors

**Sankalp Singh**
Director
Reproductive Medicine Unit
Craft Hospital
Kodungallur, Kerala, India

**Saugata Acharyya**
Consultant Pediatrician
Calcutta Medical Research Institute (CMRI)
Kolkata, West Bengal, India

**Seema Pandey**
Seema Hospital and Eva Fertility Clinic and IVF Center
Azamgarh, Uttar Pradesh, India

**Shally Gupta**
Consultant Infertility Specialist
ART Rainbow-IVF
Global Rainbow Healthcare
Agra, Uttar Pradesh, India

**Shaweez**
Fellow, Craft Hospital
Kodungallur, Kerala, India

**Shilpa Pawar**
Consultant and Head
Department of Obstetrics and Gynaecology
We Care Hospital
Raipur, Chhattisgarh, India

**Shiuli Mukherjee**
Founder
Mukherjee Fertility Centre
Howrah, West Bengal, India

**Shivani Sachdev**
Founder and Director
SCI Healthcare
New Delhi, India

**Siddhartha Chatterjee**
Director
Calcutta Fertility Mission
Vice-President, ISAR–Bengal
Kolkata, West Bengal, India

**Simi Mohandas**
Craft Hospital
Kodungallur, Kerala, India

**SK Goswami**
Consultant, ART Specialist
Institute of Reproductive Medicine
Kolkata, West Bengal, India

**SL Tan**
Division of REI
Department of Obstetrics and Gynecology and REI, McGill University
Origin Elle Fertility Clinic and Women Health Centre
Montreal, Canada

**Soma Singh**
Consultant IVF and Reproductive Medicine
BL Kapur Super Speciality Hospital
New Delhi, India

**Sonali Kusum**
Assistant Professor
Tata Institute of Social Sciences
Mumbai, Maharashtra, India

**S Tannus**
Division of Reproductive Endocrinology and Infertility (REI)
Department of Obstetrics and Gynecology and REI
McGill University
Montreal, Canada

**Sujata Kar**
Consultant Obstetrics and Gynecology
Kar Clinic and Hospital (P) Ltd
Bhubaneswar, Odisha, India

**Swarup Chakravarty**
Scientist
Institute of Reproductive Medicine
Kolkata, West Bengal, India

**Tanmoy Chatterjee**
Consultant
Department of Obstetrics and Gynecology
Saroj Gupta Cancer Centre and Research Institute
Kolkata, West Bengal, India

**V Radha**
Associate Professor
Department of Reproductive
Medicine and Surgery
Sri Ramachandra Medical College
and Research Institute
Chennai, Tamil Nadu, India

**Youcef Khoudja R**
Origin Elle Fertility Clinic and Women
Health Centre, Montreal, Canada

**ZF Naz**
Origin Elle Fertility Clinic and Women
Health Centre, Montreal, Canada

# Preface

The advent of *Assisted Reproductive Technology (ART)* has enabled millions of infertile couples around the world to have their biological children. Dr Patrick Steptoe and Prof Robert Edwards were the pioneers of modern in-vitro fertilization (IVF) leading to the birth of the first IVF baby, Louise Brown. This was followed shortly by the birth of Durga in Kolkata, the second IVF baby and the first in India by Prof Subhash Mukherjee. He used the unique technique of vaginal collection of oocytes after gonadotropin stimulation followed by cryopreservation and transferred in the subsequent cycle. Since the birth of Louise Brown born from natural cycle IVF, remarkable advances have been made in the field of ART over the last few decades. There has been improvement in ovarian stimulation protocols, laboratory procedures and introduction of genetic analysis. Clinicians, embryologists and scientists are working together to develop more effective and safer ART procedures. Though it is difficult to adequately cover the diverse field of ART in a single book, this volume highlights many aspects of human reproduction like individualization of ovarian stimulation protocols, embryo transfer techniques and third party reproduction. To make IVF procedures safe and efficacious, there has been a recent interest in mild stimulation, single embryo transfer and all freeze strategies. This book also provides evidence-based information on these aspects of ART.

This book is a result of collaborative efforts of many eminent professionals who have invested their time and effort in contributing to the advancement of knowledge of the readers. We thankfully acknowledge their sincere efforts. We are also thankful to Dr Sunita Sharma and Dr Chaitali Dutta Roy, for their special help in compiling this book.

We thank Shri Jitendar P Vij (Group Chairman) and Mr Ankit Vij (Managing Director) of M/s Jaypee Brothers Medical Publishers (P) Ltd., New Delhi, India, for their never ending support in making this book a reality.

Hope that this volume satisfies the curiosity of the clinicians in the field of ART.

**Gita Ganguly Mukherjee**
**Gautam Khastgir**
**Siddhartha Chatterjee**

# Contents

| | | |
|---|---|---|
| Chapter 1. | **Mild Ovarian Stimulation: Recent Status in Assisted Reproductive Technology**<br>*Gita Ganguly Mukherjee, Siddhartha Chatterjee* | 1 |
| Chapter 2. | **When to Refer IUI Cases for IVF?**<br>*Shilpa Pawar* | 12 |
| Chapter 3. | **Merits and Demerits of In Vitro Fertilization in Batches**<br>*Narendra Malhotra, Shally Gupta, Jaideep Malhotra, Diksha Goswami, Neharika Malhotra Bora, Keshav Malhotra* | 21 |
| Chapter 4. | **Agonist in ART Cycle**<br>*Fessy Louis T, Ramesh* | 33 |
| Chapter 5. | **Ovarian Hyperstimulation Syndrome in ART**<br>*Ameet Patki, Abhimanyu Tejrao Shinde* | 42 |
| Chapter 6. | **Difficulties during Embryo Transfer**<br>*ML Goenka, Deepak Goenka, Rashmi Goenka, Antima Rathore* | 54 |
| Chapter 7. | **Optimizing Embryo Transfer Technique**<br>*Shiuli Mukherjee* | 62 |
| Chapter 8. | **How to Improve Poor Endometrium in ART**<br>*Paramita Hazari, Gautam Khastgir* | 72 |
| Chapter 9. | **Personalized Luteal Phase Support in Assisted Reproductive Technology**<br>*Seema Pandey, Sujata Kar* | 81 |
| Chapter 10. | **Endometrial Preparation for Frozen Embryo Transfer**<br>*Kuldeep Jain, Bharti Jain, Maansi Jain* | 91 |
| Chapter 11. | **Role of Hormone Analysis in ART**<br>*SK Goswami, Radhika L Kundul, Manjusree Chakrabarty* | 100 |
| Chapter 12. | **Role of Transvaginal Sonography in Assisted Reproductive Technology**<br>*Sanghamitra Ghosh, Nitin Gupta, Monica Chetani, Mumtaz Sanghamita* | 108 |
| Chapter 13. | **Tests for Endometrial Receptivity**<br>*Moumita Naha, Gautam Khastgir* | 121 |
| Chapter 14. | **Endometrial Markers of Receptivity**<br>*Simi Mohandas, Shaweez, Sankalp Singh* | 127 |

| | | |
|---|---|---|
| Chapter 15. | **Challenges during Assisted Reproductive Technology in Polycystic Ovary Syndrome**<br>*Duru Shah* | 135 |
| Chapter 16. | **The Assisted Reproductive Technology in Endometriosis: Is it Different?**<br>*Kamini A Rao* | 145 |
| Chapter 17. | **Adenomyosis: A Biggest Challenge in Assisted Reproductive Technology**<br>*Sadhana K Desai, Ritika Rajan* | 155 |
| Chapter 18. | **Prevention of Complications in ART**<br>*Praveena Pai, Pratap Kumar* | 164 |
| Chapter 19. | **Assisted Reproductive Technology in Elderly Women: Risks and Outcome**<br>*Soma Singh, Astha Chakravarty, Indranil Saha* | 173 |
| Chapter 20. | **OHSS and its Management**<br>*Anuradha Chaudhary* | 183 |
| Chapter 21. | **AMH-based Stimulation Protocols: Can it Prevent OHSS and Predict ART Outcome**<br>*V Radha, N Sanjeeva Reddy* | 188 |
| Chapter 22. | **Endometrial Scratch: Does it Work?**<br>*Kamini Patel* | 196 |
| Chapter 23. | **Near-miss Situations in Assisted Reproductive Technology**<br>*Sadhana Gupta* | 199 |
| Chapter 24. | **Anesthesia in Assisted Reproductive Technology**<br>*Namrata Biswas* | 204 |
| Chapter 25. | **Surgery before ART: Does it Improve Outcomes?**<br>*Laxmi Shrikhande, Bhushan Shrikhande* | 213 |
| Chapter 26. | **Recurrent Implantation Failure**<br>*Kanthi Bansal* | 221 |
| Chapter 27. | **Empty Follicle Syndrome: Myth or Reality?**<br>*K Jayakrishnan, Niranjana Jayakrishnan* | 235 |
| Chapter 28. | **Luteinized Unruptured Follicle Syndrome: A Mystery**<br>*Gita Khanna, Kalika Dubey, Farhat Kazim, Arti Gupta* | 240 |
| Chapter 29. | **Poor Responders**<br>*GA Ramaraju* | 249 |

| | | |
|---|---|---|
| Chapter 30. | **Poseidon Criteria**<br>*Anuradha Chaudhary* | 255 |
| Chapter 31. | **Ovum and Embryo Donation: First or Final Choice in Poor Responders?**<br>*Nayana Patel* | 259 |
| Chapter 32. | **Third Party Reproduction for ART**<br>*Kanthi Bansal* | 267 |
| Chapter 33. | **Comparison of Growth of Newborn Babies Conceived Naturally with those Born following Assisted Reproduction Technology**<br>*Saugata Acharyya, Kakoli Acharyya* | 275 |
| Chapter 34. | **Fertility Preservation in the Present Era**<br>*J Tan, S Tannus, MH Dahan, R Youcef Khoudja, ZF Naz, S Kattera, P Chan, SL Tan* | 280 |
| Chapter 35. | **Fertility Following Gynecological Cancer**<br>*Biman Kumar Chakraborty, NR Mondal, Rahul Roy Chowdhury, Tanmoy Chatterjee* | 293 |
| Chapter 36. | **Fertility Preservation in Oncological Patients (Oncofertility)**<br>*Rajan S Vaidya* | 302 |
| Chapter 37. | **Surrogacy: Present Position in India**<br>*Shivani Sachdev, Sonali Kusum* | 318 |
| Chapter 38. | **Stem Cell Therapy in Reproductive Medicine**<br>*BN Chakravarty, Saeeda Wasim, Swarup Chakravarty* | 330 |
| Chapter 39. | **Past, Present and Future of ART**<br>*BN Chakravarty, Ratna Chattopadhyay, Arup Kumar Majhi, Dibyendu Banerjee* | 338 |
| *Index* | | *351* |

CHAPTER 1

# Mild Ovarian Stimulation: Recent Status in Assisted Reproductive Technology

*Gita Ganguly Mukherjee, Siddhartha Chatterjee*

## ■ INTRODUCTION

In vitro fertilization (IVF) has generally been used for years with idea for retrieving many eggs, created by ovarian stimulation, to enable production of many embryos, such that multiple embryos can be transferred, cryopreserved for future cycles, to find best embryos by allowing natural selection through blastocyst culture. Ovarian stimulation is utilized to increase the number of oocytes which might compensate the drawbacks of IVF procedure, enabling the selection of one or more embryos for transfer.[1] In recent past, long protocol (agonist suppression) along with gonadotropin (Gn) stimulation was the most frequently used stimulation protocol.[2,3] Such high dose of Gn (up to 450 IU per day) failed to demonstrate improvement in the outcome.[4,5] Even in recent days, the antagonist protocol where Gn use is less than Long protocol, has proved to be of comparable success as the previous protocol, but with less complications. Long protocol always associates with the risk of complication like ovarian hyperstimulation syndrome (OHSS),[6,7] and so also can lead to high dropout, emotional stress, as well as abdominal discomfort.[1] Whether such a long stimulation cycle raises the long-term health risk like ovarian cancer, is still uncertain. Some authorities opine that there is increased incidence of low birth rate and birth defect following IVF treatment.[8,9] Edwards et al. as far back in 1996 called for the use of milder stimulation protocols which they thought to be safer, more patient friendly, and with minimized risk of treatment, as compared to standard stimulation protocols.[10]

The problem of use of milder stimulation protocol in practice is availability of diminished number of eggs which may lead to diminished pregnancy rate. However, improved culture condition and instrumentation in many IVF laboratories and recent trend of diminishing the number of embryo transfer (ET) together reduce the need of large quantities of oocytes. The supportive evidence regarding potential negative effect of supra-physiological estradiol (E2) level on endometrial receptivity,[11,12] corpus luteal function,[13,14] oocyte and embryo qualities,[15,16] impress that mild ovarian stimulation might lead to beneficial effect on implantation potential as well as corpus luteal function.

## CLINICAL INDICATION OF MILD OVARIAN STIMULATION

1. Normogonadotrophic women with—(a) repeated failure of conventional stimulation, (b) repeated implantation failure with standard protocol
2. Poor responders and hypergonadotrophic women
3. Hyper-responders—polycystic ovarian (PCO) disease and high anti-Mullerian hormone (AMH).

Normogonadotrophic women may face recurrent IVF failure. Embryos those develop from high stimulation may present with high degree of chromosomal anomalies. There may be mitochondrial defects in eggs which may be inherent or age related leading to recurrent failure, after high stimulation (conventional stimulation). This may also lead to defect in endometrial receptivity.

Poor responders may be normogonadotrophic or hypergonadotrophic, with or without diminished ovarian reserve. Normo-Gn poor responders may face downregulation of follicle-stimulating hormone (FSH) receptors due to higher FSH dose received in conventional stimulation, leading to poor number of follicular growth. Women with diminished ovarian reserve (DOR) may have poor number of antral follicles available to be stimulated for ovulation.

Women with PCOD as well as high AMH level in serum are hyper-responders. With conventional stimulation, there is every possibility of development of OHSS. Moreover, such a large number of follicles often contain eggs of lower quality; even they may be empty follicles.

## DIFFERENT PROCEDURES OF MILD OVARIAN STIMULATION

1. Natural cycle
2. Natural cycle with FSH boost/add-back
3. Minimal Gn stimulation (low dose), alone or with adjuvants like oral ovulation-inducing (OI) agents.

### Development of Milder Stimulation Protocols

The introduction of gonadotropin-releasing hormone (GnRH) antagonist for downregulation of pituitary, brought into clinical practice of controlled ovarian stimulation (COS), has made planning of milder stimulation protocol possible.[17] Unlike GnRH agonist, GnRH antagonist does not cause initial flare of endogenous Gn release, instead cause reversible suppression of Gn secretion. The administration of GnRH antagonist in mid and late stimulation/follicular phase prevents any premature luteinizing hormone (LH) surge. This has made planned ovum pick-up (OPU) possible even in a natural menstrual cycle. This approach utilizes the endogenous intercycle FSH rise rather than suppressing it, resulting in reduction in the medication needed. The use of GnRH antagonist had made the stimulation period shorter (number of day of Gn stimulation) and diminished number of Gn ampoules required for stimulation and does not cause cyst formation. Though the initial studies suggested a detrimental effect on pregnancy rate following antagonist use, as compared to agonist,[18,19] a recent meta-analysis comprising of 22 randomized controlled trials (RCTs) showed no significant difference in probability of live birth.[20]

## Natural Cycle Stimulation for IVF

The first IVF baby was born out is a natural cycle oocyte recovery.[21] Thereafter, ovarian stimulation was used instead of natural cycle to improve success rate per cycle.[3,22] Natural cycle IVF requires simple monitoring of spontaneous cycle and retrieval of single oocyte prior to spontaneous LH surge or following attenuated LH surge by antagonist along with human chorionic gonadotropin (hCG) trigger. This excludes the possibilities of OHSS and multiple pregnancies. The cost per cycle becomes almost one-fourth as compared to a stimulated cycle.[23,24] Ongoing pregnancy rate was found to be quite low, for which it has not become popular. Repeated collection of oocytes in multiple natural cycles followed by multiple frozen embryo transfer (FET) might increase the success rate, particularly in elderly poor responders. The most drawback of natural cycle, IVF is premature LH surge leading to premature ovulation, and reduced chance of successful oocyte pick-up (OPU).[25] It is safe and less stressful method of stimulation and in selected cases, the cumulative pregnancy rate and live birth rate may be 45% and 32% respectively.[24] The use of antagonist in a natural cycle can be called to be a modified natural cycle. Modified natural cycle is quite useful in patients having previous poor ovarian response to conventional ovarian stimulation.

## Natural Cycle with FSH Add-back/Boost

The ongoing growth of dominant follicle is supported by addition of exogenous Gn (FSH add back) and use of antagonist to prevent premature LH surge. In most of the centers, GnRH antagonist and Gn (75–300 IU per day) initiated a follicular diameter of 12–14 mm. This protocol is also popular in patients with poor response with conventional stimulation or poor responders with poor ovarian reserve test (ORT). This protocol yields best success rate in young couple with severe male infertility, as an only fertility compromising factor. Modified natural cycle IVF in consecutive cycles in selected population may result in improved effectiveness.

## EXOGENOUS GONADOTROPIN FOR MILD OVARIAN STIMULATION

Mild ovarian stimulation in which low-dose gonadotropin (FSH/hMG–human menopausal gonadotropin) administration is delayed until the mid-follicular phase is based on the FSH window concept.[26] Exogenous FSH administration is limited to the mid to late follicular phase with the aim of preventing a decrease of FSH levels and thus inducing multifollicular development.[27] The use of GnRH antagonists for suppression of premature LH rise enabled this concept to be introduced into IVF.[28] A pilot study showed that multiple dominant follicles could even be induced when the initiation of FSH was postponed until CD 7.[29] However, there was a tendency toward a lower percentage of women presenting with multiple dominant follicle development compared with patients started on CD 3 or 5.[30] A fixed daily dose of 150 IU rFSH compared with 100 IU/day was found to be more effective in consistently inducing multiple follicular growths when ovarian stimulation was initiated on CD 5.[29]

A large randomized study to compare the efficacy of mild strategy (mild ovarian stimulation with antagonist) as compared to conventional stimulation protocol with agonist showed comparable live birth rate at the end of 1 year along with reduction in Gn requirement multiple pregnancy and overall cost involved.[31]

## Gonadotropin with Clomiphene Citrate or Aromatase Inhibitors

The antiestrogen clomiphene citrate (CC) was the first preparation used for ovarian stimulation in IVF.[22,32] Important advantages of CC compared with gonadotropins remain including its oral administration, low price and widespread availability. CC acts to increase pituitary FSH secretion by reducing negative estrogen feedback. An ovarian stimulation protocol combining CC with gonadotropins could lead to a reduction in the amount of gonadotropins required due to the combined synergistic effects. Additionally, because gonadotropins may counterbalance the undesired antiestrogenic effects of CC on the endometrium, it may be counterbalanced with Gn addition.[33,34] This combination might lead to improved pregnancy rates compared with CC alone. CC has now been largely replaced by more effective hMG/FSH protocols in combination with GnRH analog (GnRH-a) cotreatment.[3,35]

The available clinical data available for aromatase inhibitors (AI) in IVF treatment is limited. One uncontrolled study with 22 good responders with limited financial means, where Letrozole was used for first 5 days of cycle (CD 3–7), followed by hMG from CD-7 yielded 27% pregnancy rate. In other RCTs, AI did not show any significant benefit when used in IVF program.[36,37] A third RCT[38] showed more number of available oocytes following AI used.

## Late Follicular Phase hCG or LH

Human chorionic gonadotropin or LH administration in low doses may replace FSH administration in late follicular phase, as mild stimulation approach. This is based on acquired LH responsiveness of granulosa cells in dominant follicles in late follicular phase.[39] The administration of recombinant LH was found to be sufficient to maintain follicular growth in late follicular phase after initial stimulation with FSH.[40] Though this approach has been postulated to reduce OHSS,[41] this has not been substantiated till date.

## ■ CONVENTIONAL STIMULATION VERSUS MILD OVARIAN STIMULATION

The pros and cons of standard and mild ovarian stimulations are given in Table 1.

| Table 1: Pros and cons of standard and mild ovarian stimulations. | | |
| --- | --- | --- |
| Parameters | Standard Ovarian Stimulation | Mild Ovarian Stimulation |
| Stimulation | Complex | Less complex |
| Number of oocyte retrieved | Maximum | Less |
| Time counseled for stimulation | More | Less |
| Cost | High | Low |
| Patient discomfort | More | Less |
| Dropout | More | Less |
| Short-term complications (OHSS) | More | Less |
| Long-term health consequences, e.g. ovarian cancer | Uncertain, may be more | Probably less |
| Embryo quality and endometrial receptivity | Impaired due to supraphysiological E2 | Not affected |
| Available embryo for freezing | Yes | Mostly no |

## Embryo Quality

Some observations indicated relation between degree of ovarian stimulation and embryo quality, either morphologically or by chromosomal constitution,[16,42] by disrupting natural selection of good quality oocytes.

In mouse oocytes, high dose of Gn stimulation during in vitro maturation increased incidence of chromosomal abnormality had been observed.[43,44] High E2 level following conventional ovarian stimulation has negative impact on implantation potential,[45,46] as well as chromosomal constitution of human embryos.[47] One study indicated that high stimulation may disrupt the chromosomal segregation mechanism of embryo.[48,49]

The retrieval of modest number of oocytes following mild stimulation leads to distinctly higher implantation rate compared to conventional stimulation.[50] This may be due to retrieval of more homogenous group of good quality oocytes instead of pathological reduction of ovarian response. The fear of getting low number of oocytes following mild stimulation thus may be compensated in getting increased oocyte number, but lower pregnancy rate with high dose stimulation.[51,52]

It is true that with mild stimulation, cryopreservable embryos are less, leading to unavailability of subsequent FET. However, lesser number of good quality embryos leads to similar results as compared to conventional stimulation protocol, so far as the number of pregnancy is concerned.[16]

## Luteal Function and Endometrial Receptivity

Supraphysiological steroid levels are widely held responsible[53] for poor endometrial receptivity with high dose of Gn in COS. This results in impaired embryo implantation when compared with natural cycle with oocyte donation.[54] E2 level of more than 3,000 pg/mL on hCG day has been shown to reduce implantation rate, independent of embryo quality.[55] In contrary, improved implantation rate has been observed with mild stimulation approached[12] due to more physiological response. Increased pregnancy rate has been observed following FSH step down in high responders due to decrease in E2 in preimplantation period.[56]

## Economic Consideration

It is obvious that the cost involved in mild stimulation is much less as compared to conventional group. Moreover, mild stimulation carries negligible chance of OHSS which otherwise can impart more cost in treatment. Less chances of multiple pregnancies and preterm birth in mild strategy[57] leads to reduced cost involvement.

## Psychological Aspects

Mild stimulation which is a more shorter and patient-friendly protocol with little complication might decrease the treatment-related stress. In natural cycle, excess chance of cycle cancellation is not also that stressful, if patient is counseled properly. Furthermore, mild stimulation has been found to reduce significant dropout rate per cycle. A mild IVF treatment strategy was found to be associated with fewer symptoms of depression after overall treatment failure, than a standard IVF treatment.[31,58] As there is less psychological burden in mild stimulation, even a failure as accepted by the patient positively with a hope of having success in the following cycles, which compensates the low pregnancy rate per cycle.[59]

## ■ FUTURE DEVELOPMENT

It will be not far when ovarian stimulation will be replaced by in vitro maturation of the oocytes, after retrieval of immature eggs from unstimulated or minimally stimulated cycles, avoiding requirement of Gn stimulation for invivo follicular growth and oocyte maturation.[60,61] Till date, this procedure has not produced increased pregnancy rates due to poor implantation. Moreover, safety of this technique for the offsprings has not been identified.[62,63]

## CONCLUSION

Since the mid-90s, the long agonist stimulation protocol has been widely used worldwide. This was lengthy, expensive protocol, with advantages of more programmed IVF, less cycle cancellation and more number of oocytes of available with better pregnancy rate.[64] When compared against complications and disadvantages, long protocol showed more OHSS, more short- and long-term risks, more physical and emotional burden along with increased dropouts. It involved long continued repeated injections, multiple blood sample tests, and repeated ovarian ultrasound scan, requiring more attendance to the clinic.

The mild stimulation on the other hand, was devoid of more disadvantages of the long protocol, requiring shortened stimulation period. Though the retrieved oocytes were less in number, the pregnancy rate per ET seems to be comparable between two approaches (P-679–outlook–Hohmann). The embryo quality of mild regime was much better.[16,65]

Another aspect is very important as in many countries like Italy, there are IVF legislations which do not allow embryo banking. Hence, availability of excess number of oocytes is of no use.

Mild ovarian stimulation for IVF is gaining ground gradually, as evidenced in recent literature. It is very useful for selected group of patients like good responders of young age, some having polycystic ovarian disease (PCOD), but the drawback being reduction in pregnancy rate per cycle. The best part is less chance of complication, increased patient compliance and economic benefit, which is making it more popular day by day. It is difficult to draw a conclusion about the best agents for mild stimulation till date. A better understanding of physiology of follicular dynamics may lead to individual approaches.[66] It should be the aim to develop at least 3 follicles in mild stimulation to produce competitive IVF treatment outcomes. Reduction in dose of medication becomes highly beneficial so far embryo quality and implantation rate is concerned.

## REFERENCES

1. Fauser BC, Devroey P, Macklon NS. Multiple birth resulting from ovarian stimulation for subfertility treatment. Lancet. 2005;365:1807-16.
2. FIVNAT 1996 report. French National Register on In Vitro Fertilization. Contracept Fertil Sex. 1997;25:499-502.
3. Macklon NS, Stouffer RL, Giudice LC, et al. The science behind 25 years of ovarian stimulation for in vitro fertilization. Endocr Rev. 2006;27:170-207.
4. Wikland M, Bergh C, Borg K, et al. A prospective, randomized comparison of two starting doses of recombinant FSH in combination with cetrorelix in women undergoing ovarian stimulation for IVF/ICSI. Hum Reprod. 2001;16:1676-81.
5. Yong PY, Brett S, Baird DT, et al. A prospective randomized clinical trial comparing 150 IU and 225 IU of recombinant follicle-stimulating hormone (Gonal-F) in

a fixed-dose regimen for controlled ovarian stimulation in in vitro fertilization treatment. Fertil Steril. 2003;79:308-15.
6. Delvigne A, Rozenberg S. Epidemiology and prevention of ovarian hyperstimulation syndrome (OHSS): a review. Hum Reprod Update. 2002;8:559-77.
7. Aboulghar MA, Mansour RT. Ovarian hyperstimulation syndrome: classifications and critical analysis of preventive measures. Hum Reprod Update. 2003;9:275-89.
8. Wang YA, Sullivan EA, Black D, et al. Preterm birth and low birth weight after assisted reproductive technology-related pregnancy in Australia between 1996 and 2000. Fertil Steril. 2005;83:1650-8.
9. Kapiteijn K, de Bruijn CS, de Boer E, et al. Does subfertility explain the risk of poor perinatal outcome after IVF and ovarian hyperstimulation? Hum Reprod. 2006;21:3228-34.
10. Edwards RG, Lobo R, Bouchard P. Time to revolutionize ovarian stimulation. Hum Reprod. 1996;11:917-9.
11. Simon C, Cano F, Valbuena D, et al. Clinical evidence for a detrimental effect on uterine receptivity of high serum oestradiol concentrations in high and normal responder patients. Hum Repro. 1995;10:2432-7.
12. Devroey P, Bourgain C, Macklon NS, et al. Reproductive biology and IVF: ovarian stimulation and endometrial receptivity. Trends Endocrinol Metab. 2004;15:84-90.
13. Fauser BC, Devroey P. Reproductive biology and IVF: ovarian stimulation and luteal phase consequences. Trends Endocrinol Metab. 2003;14:236-42.
14. Beckers NG, Platteau P, Eijkemans MJ, et al. The early luteal phase administration of oestrogen and progesterone does not induce premature luteolysis in normo-ovulatory women. Eur J Endocrinol. 2006;155:355-63.
15. Valbuena D, Martin J, de Pablo JL, et al. Increasing levels of estradiol are deleterious to embryonic implantation because they directly affect the embryo. Fertil Steril. 2001;76:962-8.
16. Baart EB, Martini E, Eijkemans MJ, et al. Milder ovarian stimulation for in-vitro fertilization reduces aneuploidy in the human preimplantation embryo: a randomized controlled trial. Hum Reprod. 2007;22:980-8.
17. Tarlatzis BC, Fauser BC, Kolibianakis EM, et al. GnRH antagonists in ovarian stimulation for IVF. Hum Reprod Update. 2006;12:333-40.
18. Ludwig M, Katalinic A, Diedrich K. Use of GnRH antagonists in ovarian stimulation for assisted reproductive technologies compared to the long protocol meta-analysis. Arch Gynecol Obstet. 2001;265:175-82.
19. Al-Inany HG, Abou-Setta AM, Aboulghar M. Gonadotrophin-releasing hormone antagonists for assisted conception. Cochrane Database Syst Rev. 2006:19:CD001750.
20. Kolibianakis EM, Collins J, Tarlatzis BC, et al. Among patients treated for IVF with gonadotrophins and GnRH analogues, is the probability of live birth dependent on the type of analogue used? A systematic review and meta-analysis. Hum Reprod Update. 2006;12:51-71.
21. Steptoe PC, Edwards RG. Birth after the preimplantation of a human embryo. Lancet. 1978;2:366.

22. Cohen J, Trounson A, Dawson K, et al. The early days of IVF outside the UK. Hum Reprod Update. 2005;11:439-9.
23. Aboulghar MA, Mansour RT, Serour GA, et al. In vitro fertilization in a spontaneous cycle: a successful simple protocol. J Obstet Gynaecol. 1995;21:337-40.
24. Nargund G, Waterstone J, Bland J, et al. Cumulative conception and live birth rates in natural (unstimulated) IVF cycles. Hum Reprod. 2001;16:259-62.
25. Pelinck MJ, Hoek A, Simons AH, et al. Efficacy of natural cycle IVF: a review of the literature. Hum Reprod Update. 2002;8:129-39.
26. Fauser BC, van Heusden AM. Manipulation of human ovarian function: physiological concepts and clinical consequences. Endocr Rev. 1997;18:71-106.
27. Schipper I, Hop WC, Fauser BC. The follicle-stimulating hormone (FSH) threshold/window concept examined by different interventions with exogenous FSH during the follicular phase of the normal menstrual cycle: duration, rather than magnitude, of FSH increase affects follicle development. J Clin Endocrinol Metab. 1998;83:1292-8.
28. Macklon NS, Fauser BC. Regulation of follicle development and novel approaches to ovarian stimulation for IVF. Hum Reprod Update. 2000;6:307-12.
29. Jong D, Macklon NS, Fauser BC. A pilot study involving minimal ovarian stimulation for in vitro fertilization: extending the 'follicle-stimulating hormone window' combined with the gonadotropin-releasing hormone antagonist cetrorelix. Fertil Steril. 2000;73:1051-4.
30. Hohmann FP, Laven JS, de Jong FH, et al. Low-dose exogenous FSH initiated during the early, mid or late follicular phase can induce multiple dominant follicle development. Hum Reprod. 2001;16:846-54.
31. Heijnen EM, Eijkemans MJ, De Klerk C, et al. A mild treatment strategy for in-vitro fertilisation: a randomised non-inferiority trial randomized trial. Lancet. 2007;369:743-9.
32. Quigley MM, Schmidt CL, Beauchamp PJ, et al. Enhanced follicular recruitment in an in vitro fertilization program: clomiphene alone versus a clomiphene/human menopausal gonadotropin combination. Fertil Steril. 1984;42:25-33.
33. Markiewicz L, Laufer N, Gurpide E. In vitro effects of clomiphene citrate on human endometrium. Fertil Steril. 1988;50:772-6.
34. Nelson LM, Hershlag A, Kurl RS, et al. Clomiphene citrate directly impairs endometrial receptivity in the mouse. Fertil Steril. 1990;53:727-31.
35. Fraser HM, Baird DT. Clinical applications of LHRH analogues. Baillieres Clin Endocrinol Metab. 1987;1:43-70.
36. Goswami SK, Das T, Chattopadhyay R, et al. A randomized single-blind controlled trial of letrozole as a low-cost IVF protocol in women with poor ovarian response: a preliminary report. Hum Reprod. 2004;19:2031-5.
37. Kahraman K, Ozmen B, Satirogly H, et al. A comparison of aromatase inhibitor plus recombinant-FSH/GnRH antagonist versus recombinant-FSH microdose co-flare analog protocols in poor responders undergoing ICSI/ET. Hum Reprod. 2005;20:i124.

38. Verpoest WM, Kolibianakis E, Papanikolaou E, et al. Aromatase inhibitors in ovarian stimulation for IVF/ICSI: a pilot study. Reprod Biomed Online. 2006;13:166-72.
39. Hillier SG. Current concepts of the roles of follicle stimulating hormone and luteinizing hormone in folliculogenesis. Hum Reprod. 1994;9:188-91.
40. Sullivan MW, Stewart-Akers A, Krasnow JS, et al. Ovarian responses in women to recombinant follicle-stimulating hormone and luteinizing hormone (LH): a role for LH in the final stages of follicular maturation. J Clin Endocrinol Metab. 1999;84:228-32.
41. Filicori M, Cognigni GE, Taraborrelli S, et al. Luteinizing hormone activity supplementation enhances follicle-stimulating hormone efficacy and improves ovulation induction outcome. J Clin Endocrinol Metab. 1999;84:2659-63.
42. Katz-Jaffe MG, Trounson AO, Cram DS. Chromosome 21 mosaic human preimplantation embryos predominantly arise from diploid conceptions. Fertil Steril. 2005;84:634-43.
43. Van Blerkom J, Davis P. Differential effects of repeated ovarian stimulation on cytoplasmic and spindle organization in metaphase II mouse oocytes matured in vivo and in vitro. Hum Reprod. 2001;16:757-64.
44. Roberts R, Iatropoulou A, Ciantar D, et al. Follicle-stimulating hormone affects metaphase I chromosome alignment and increases aneuploidy in mouse oocytes matured in vitro. Biol Reprod. 2005;72:107-18.
45. Ertzeid G, Storeng R. The impact of ovarian stimulation on implantation and fetal development in mice. Hum Reprod. 2001;16:221-5.
46. Van der Auwera I, D'Hooghe T. Superovulation of female mice delays embryonic and fetal development. Hum Reprod. 2001;16:1237-43.
47. Katz-Jaffe MG, Trounson AO, Cram DS. Chromosome 21 mosaic human preimplantation embryos predominantly arise from diploid conceptions. Fertil Steril. 2005;84:634-43.
48. Munne S, Magli C, Adler A, et al. Treatment-related chromosome abnormalities in human embryos. Hum Reprod. 1997;12:780-4.
49. Hodges CA, Ilagan A, Jennings D, et al. Experimental evidence that changes in oocyte growth influence meiotic chromosome segregation. Hum Reprod. 2002;17:1171-80.
50. Gougeon A. Regulation of ovarian follicular development in primates: facts and hypotheses. Endocr Rev. 1996;17:121-55.
51. Melie NA, Adeniyi OA, Igbineweka OM, et al. Predictive value of the number of oocytes retrieved at ultrasound-directed follicular aspiration with regard to fertilization rates and pregnancy outcome in intracytoplasmic sperm injection treatment cycles. Fertil Steril. 2003;80:1376-9.
52. Kok JD, Looman CW, Weima SM, et al. A high number of oocytes obtained after ovarian hyperstimulation for in vitro fertilization or intracytoplasmic sperm injection is not associated with decreased pregnancy outcome. Fertil Steril. 2006;85:918-24.
53. Beckers NG, Macklon NS, Eijkemans MJ, et al. Nonsupplemented luteal phase characteristics after the administration of recombinant human chorionic

gonadotropin, recombinant luteinizing hormone, or gonadotropin-releasing hormone (GnRH) agonist to induce final oocyte maturation in in vitro fertilization patients after ovarian stimulation with recombinant follicle-stimulating hormone and GnRH antagonist cotreatment. J Clin Endocrinol Metab. 2003;88:4186-92.
54. Paulson RJ, Sauer MV, Lobo RA. Embryo implantation after human in vitro fertilization: importance of endometrial receptivity. Fertil Steril. 1990;53:870-4.
55. Simon C, Cano F, Valbuena D, et al. Clinical evidence for a detrimental effect on uterine receptivity of high serum oestradiol concentrations in high and normal responder patients. Hum Reprod. 1995;10:2432-7.
56. Simon C, Garcia Velasco JJ, Valbuena D, et al. Increasing uterine receptivity by decreasing estradiol levels during the preimplantation period in high responders with the use of a follicle-stimulating hormone step-down regimen. Fertil Steril. 1998;70:234-9.
57. Polinder S, Heijnen EM, Macklon NS, et al. Cost-effectiveness of a mild compared with a standard strategy for IVF: a randomized comparison using cumulative term live birth as the primary endpoint. Hum Reprod. 2008;23:316-23.
58. de Klerk C, Heijnen EM, Macklon NS, et al. The psychological impact of mild ovarian stimulation combined with single embryo transfer compared with conventional IVF. Hum Reprod. 2006;21:721-7.
59. Verberg MF, Eijkemans MJ, Heijnen EM, et al. Why do couples drop-out from IVF treatment? A prospective cohort study. Hum Reprod. 2008;23:2050-5.
60. Barnes FL, Kausche A, Tiglias J, et al. Production of embryos from in vitro-matured primary human oocytes. Fertil Steril. 1996;65:1151-6.
61. Oktay K, Newton H, Aubard Y, et al. Cryopreservation of immature human oocytes and ovarian tissue: an emerging technology? Fertil Steril. 1998;69:1-7.
62. Chian RC, Buckett WM, Tulandi T, et al. Prospective randomized study of human chorionic gonadotrophin priming before immature oocyte retrieval from unstimulated women with polycystic ovarian syndrome. Hum Reprod. 2000;15:165-70.
63. Rao GD, Tan SL. In vitro maturation of oocytes. Semin Reprod Med. 2005;23:242-7.
64. Hughes EG, Fedorkow DM, Daya S, et al. The routine use of gonadotropin-releasing hormone agonists prior to in-vitro fertilization and gamete intrafallopian transfer: a meta-analysis of randomized controlled trials. Fertil Steril. 1992;58:888-96.
65. Hohmann FP, Macklon NS, Fauser BC. A randomized comparison of two ovarian stimulation protocols with gonadotropin-releasing hormone (GnRH) antagonist cotreatment for in-vitro fertilization commencing recombinant follicle stimulating hormone on cycle day 2 or 5 with the standard long GnRH agonist protocol. J Clin Endocrinol Metab. 2003;88:166-73.
66. Fauser BC, Diedrich K, Devroey P. Evian Annual Reproduction (EVAR) Workshop Group. Predictors of ovarian response: progress towards individualized treatment in ovulation induction and ovarian stimulation. Hum Reprod Update. 2008;14:1-14.

# CHAPTER 2

# When to Refer IUI Cases for IVF?

*Shilpa Pawar*

## ■ INTRODUCTION

Intrauterine insemination (IUI) and in vitro fertilization (IVF) are the most popular infertility treatment available today. There is no one size fits all solution to infertility and the path you will take will be unique to your specific case, but there is some common cause. Understanding what they are who they are intending for and what the success rates are for these two options will guide you to begin your treatment.

## ■ WHAT IS AN IUI?

Intrauterine insemination is an assisted conception technique that involves the deposition of processed semen sample in upper uterine cavity, overcoming natural barriers to sperm ascent in the female reproductive tract. IUI is cost-effective, noninvasive, first-line therapy for selected patients with functionally normal tube, cervical factor, anovulation, moderate male factor, immunological, unexplained and ejaculatory disorders with clinical pregnancy rates per cycle ranging from 10% to 20%. Despite popularity of IUI its effectiveness is not consistent and when used with fertility medications carry significant risk of multiple pregnancies including higher order (triplets or more) and ovarian hyperstimulation syndrome (OHSS).

Intrauterine insemination is not ideal for all cases of fertility issues especially in cases of women age above 35 years, severe male factor infertility, bilateral tube block, decrease ovarian reserve, advance endometriosis, use of donor eggs and genetic screening should directly go to IVF. IUI may be performed with or without ovarian stimulation. Controlled ovarian stimulation, particularly with low dose gonadotropins, with IUI offers significant benefit in terms of pregnancy outcomes compared with natural cycle or timed intercourse, while reducing associated COH complications such as multiple pregnancies including higher order (triplets or more) and OHSS (Table 1).

# When to Refer IUI Cases for IVF?

**Table 1:** Indications of intrauterine insemination (IUI)

| Male factor | Female factor | Cryopreserved semen IUI |
|---|---|---|
| Ejaculatory dysfunction | Cervical factor | Absentee husband |
| Retrograde ejaculation | Tubal factor atleast one patent tube | Surgery |
| Anatomical problems like hypospadias | Unexplained infertility | Cancer therapy |
| Subnormal sperm parameters | Minimal and mild endometriosis | Poor semen parameters |
| Immunological factor | Ovulatory dysfunction | HIV infection |
|  | Immunological factor | Donor semen |
|  | Anatomical defects of vagina or cervix |  |

## Prognostic Indicators

Prognostic indicators of success with IUI depends on
- Age of patient <35 years
- Duration of infertility
- Stimulation protocol
- Infertility etiology
- Number of cycles
- Timing of insemination
- Number of preovulatory follicles on the day of hCG
- Processed total motile sperm >10 million
- Insemination count $> 1 \times 10^6$ with > 4% normal spermatozoa.

## Prerequisites

A complete couple work up that includes patient history, clinical examination, clinical and laboratory investigations is mandatory to justify the choice in favor of IUI and guide alternative patient management, while individualizing the treatment protocol according to the patient characteristics with a strict cancellation policy to limit multifollicular development may help optimize IUI pregnancy outcomes.

## ■ WHAT IS AN IVF?

In vitro fertilization is the most successful method to fertility treatment utilized today help couples to conceive. The basic components of the IVF process include stimulation of the ovaries to produce multiple eggs at a time, removal of eggs from the ovary (egg retrieval), fertilization of the eggs in the laboratory and subsequent placement of the resulting embryos into the uterus (embryo transfer). The chances of pregnancy from IVF depend primarily on the age of the woman, the cause of infertility, and factors related to the quality of the IVF laboratory.

## When to Attempt IUI First?
- At least one unblocked fallopian tube
- Able to ovulate, perhaps with the help of fertility medications
- Healthy ovarian reserve, good amount of healthy eggs
- Normal uterine cavity
- Cervical issue scarring/hostile cervix may block fertilization
- Mild ovulation issue like polycystic ovarian syndrome (PCOS)
- Donor sperm
- Mild to moderate male factor
- After male fertility preservation before cancer treatment or surgery
- Same sex couple.

## Go Straight to IVF
- Age >38 years
- Both fallopian tubes block
- Decrease ovarian reserve [in women > 35 years with total antral follicle count (AFC)< 5]
- Use of donor eggs
- Minimal or mild endometriosis (stage I or II) with documented failure in tubal transport
- Advance endometriosis (stage III or IV)
- Abnormal pelvic anatomy not amenable to microsurgical repair
- Severe male factor infertility which may require use of advanced ICSI
- High levels of sperm immobilizing antibodies[13]
- Genetic screening [preimplantation genetic screening (PGS) or preimplantation genetic diagnosis (PGD)].

## ■ IUI VERSUS IVF

1. *Complexity:* IUI refers to one step procedure while IVF needs multiple steps more complex.
2. *Multiple pregnancy:* The high multiple pregnancies is still a major problem with IUI in cycles stimulated with classical doses of FSH. Multiple PRs range from 10% to 40% and have not changed in more recent reports. In IVF and ICSI cycles, one embryo or even two embryo transfer are safer than IUI in superstimulated cycles.
3. *Success rate:* It is never easy to be specific about success rates of a given treatment as there are so many variables that affect individual case but statistically IUI has lower success rates than IVF, the gap widens as woman age:

A. IUI with fertility medications success rate 8–15% per cycle below 35 years and 2–5% above 40 years of age. While success of IVF using woman's own eggs is 40–45% below 35 years and <15% above 40 years of age.[1]
4. *Cost-effectiveness:* Local conditions are the most practical source of cost information on IUI and IVF. Studies on cost-effectiveness of infertility treatment mainly involve IVF treatment.[2] Although there are no recent patient based studies, starting treatment with IUI rather than IVF was either cheaper or more cost-effective in unexplained and persistent infertility.

## WHEN TO REFER IUI CASES FOR IVF?

1. *Cervical factor infertility:* In couples with cervical factor diagnosed by a well timed, nonprogressive postcoital test with normal semen parameters, higher pregnancy rates (PRs) have been reported following IUI compared to expectant management (51% vs 33%) respectively,[3] with acceptable pregnancy rates even without COH. High levels of antibodies need to be direct refer to IVF.
2. *Ovulatory factor infertility:* It is a major contributory factor in 15–20% of infertility. First-line management is weight reduction. Second line is ovulation induction with clomiphene citrate or letrozole with or without metformin. IUI with COH carries high risk of multiple pregnancy and OHSS. IVF provides a suitable, more complex alternative, with careful monitoring of IVF stimulation protocols in women with PCOS can avoid excess follicular development and high risk of OHSS.
3. *Tubal factor:* IUI with COH can be suggested as initial treatment of choice in patients with unilateral proximal tubal occlusion, while patients with mid distal or distal tubal occlusion on hysterosalpingography (HSG) should be referred for IVF with or without surgery. Pandian et al. (2008) in his Cochrane review concluded that tubal surgery offer no added advantages over IVF.[4] In practice IVF is considered first-line treatment in severe tubal damage. Success rate (live births rates) of IVF by age <35 years 32.9%; 35–40 years: 19–27%; >40 years: 2–13%, risk of ectopic pregnancy is very less 1–2% as compared to tubal surgery.[4]
4. *Endometriosis:* It is a leading cause of infertility with a prevalence of 0.5–5% in fertile and 25–40% in infertile women.[5] IUI with COH is recommended in early stage and surgically corrected endometriosis when pelvic anatomy is normal. IUI yields poor pregnancy rates despite normal semen parameters and patent fallopian tubes, necessitating resources to IVF/ICSI. In patients with stage IV endometriosis and in women >38 years of age, significantly higher PR, fecundity and cumulative fecundity have been reported following IVF-ET should be first-line approach in management of infertility in such patients.[6] Certainly, IVF is appropriate for couples with 2 years or more of infertility with minimal or mild endometriosis. Women with moderate or severe endometriosis may benefit from earlier access to IVF.

5. *Unexplained infertility:* Initial treatment for unexplained infertility is IUI.[7] Pashayan et al. (2006) pregnancy rate per cycle was higher in the IVF group than in IUI group (12.2% vs 7.4%) spontaneous cycle and 8.7% COH–IUI respectively: p-0.09. IVF may be more cost effective primary treatment option compared to IUI in lieu of low success rate with IUI and subsequent requirement for IVF in the event of failure.[8]

   **IUI versus IVF**
   In a trial comparing IVF with IUI, differences in live birth rates between IVF (41%) and IUI (26%) were not statistically significant, with an OR of 1.96 (95% CI 0.88–4.36). The wide confidence interval reflects the relative lack of precision of this estimate due to small sample size.

   **SO + IUI versus IVF**
   A Cochrane review by Pandian et al. compared three cycles of SO + IUI with one cycle of IVF did not show a clear difference in outcomes between two treatments (OR 1.09, 95% CI 0.7–1.59). The multiple pregnancy rates were also comparable (OR 0.64; 95% CI 0.31–1.29).[9]

   Results of Cochrane reviews on the effectiveness of various treatments for unexplained infertility in achieving live birth are summarized in Table 2.[10]

   British study used a mathematical model to compare cost effectiveness of primary IVF with IUI and IVF as treatment option and concluded that a primary strategy of IVF was more cost effective than IUI or SO+IUI followed by IVF in these who did not become pregnant following initial treatment.[9]

6. *Male factor infertility:* IUI is considered the best first-line treatment and cost-effective procedure for mild to moderate male factor subfertility.[11] Severe male factor infertility with significant deterioration in sperm parameters or function may necessitate direct referral to IVF or ICSI, depending on degree of severity.

## Semen Parameters

The following semen parameters guide us to directly refer to IVF:
- Processed total motile sperm (PTMS) <10 million[12]
- Sperm survival <70%
- Normal morphology 5%
- Inseminating motile count (IMC) $<1 \times 10^6$
- Prewash IUI semen pregnancy score (IUI-SPS) <150.

| Table 2: Effectiveness of treatments for unexplained infertility (odds ratio (OR) of live birth) | | |
|---|---|---|
| Treatment | OR | 95% CI |
| IVF versus IUI | 1.96 | 0.88–4.36 |
| IVF versus stimulated IUI | 1.09 | 0.74–1.59 |

## Ejaculatory Problem

When drugs fail, alternatives include external vibratory massage, direct aspiration of sperm from epididymis or testes and electroejaculation. All methods produce poor quality sperm samples. The results of IVF/ICSI are better than IUI and rest methods.

## Immunological Infertility

It refers to presence of antisperm antibodies in the seminal fluid or bound to sperm. The current practice to refer patients with high levels of IgA or IgG antibodies directly to IVF/ICSI.[13]

## Obstructive Azoospermia

It may be due to vas duct obstruction due to infection or vasectomy. The first line of management for these cases is sperm retrieval by testicular biopsy followed by ICSI. No role of IUI in these cases.

## ■ NUMBER OF CYCLES OF IUI

The National Institute for Health and Care Excellence (NICE) fertility guidelines 2013[1] advocate for upto six IUI cycles for patients with unexplained infertility, male subfertility, cervical factor and minimal to mild endometriosis.[1] Khali et al. showed CPR were highest in first treatment cycle and cumulative birth rate rose only slightly after fourth treatment cycle.[14] Dickey et al. showed that after four cycles, CPR were 46% for ovulatory, 38% for cervical factor, male factor and unexplained infertility; 34% for endometriosis and 26% for tubal factor.[15]

If no pregnancy achieved by end of fourth to sixth cycle, patients should be offered IVF. Aboulghar et al. showed that in women who were offered IVF after their third IUI cycles, the cycle fecundity increased to 36.6% per cycle compared to 5.6%, if they were offered another three IUI cycles.[16]

## ■ NICE GUIDELINES 2013[1]

In women aged under 40 years who have not conceived after 2 years of regular unprotected intercourse or 12 cycles of artificial insemination (where 6 or more are by IUI), offer 3 full cycles of IVF, with or without ICSI. If women reach by age of 40 during treatment, complete the current full cycle but do not offer further full cycles.

In women aged 40–42 years who have not conceived after 2 years of regular unprotected intercourse or 12 cycles of artificial insemination (where 6 or more by IUI), offer 1 full cycle of IVF with or without ICSI, provided the following three criteria are fulfilled:
1. They have never previously had IVF
2. There is no evidence of low ovarian reserve

3. There has been a discussion of additional implications of IVF and pregnancy at this age.

Where investigations show there is no chance of pregnancy with expectant or IUI treatment, where IVF is the only effective treatment, refer the woman directly to IVF.

## ■ DISCUSSION

Four infertility management RCTs compared IVF treatment and standard management including IUI with ovarian stimulation, with inconsistent results because of differences in patients and definition of the control intervention.[17,18] The results of these trials are no longer relevant to practice because IVF success rates are much higher than they were before 2000, while success rates with stimulated IUI have not changed.

One management trial, reported so far only in abstract form, addresses the comparison of IVF and IUI in stimulated cycles.[2] The trial involved couples with unexplained infertility who had had no previous treatment. The standard protocol was three cycles of CC/IUI, no FSH/IUI and up to six cycles of IVF. In the accelerated arm 167 (65%) of 256 couples had a clinical pregnancy compared with 157 (64%) of 247 in the standard arm. The median time to pregnancy was shorter in the accelerated arm. The numbers in the abstract imply that the average number of IVF cycles was 1.1 and 1.4 in the standard and accelerated arm respectively. These results indicate where IVF is affordable, IUI is unnecessary. Otherwise potentially IVF may be premature choice in woman aged less than 35 with unexplained infertility less than 3 years duration.

## ■ COUNSELING COUPLES

Information for couples should include the beneficial effects of a good prognosis. In the Steures et al.[19] trial for example, the enrolled couples were selected to have a good prognosis without treatment. In these couples, IUI with ovarian stimulation did not improve the PR compared with no treatment. For severe male infertility, however neither unstimualted nor stimulated IUI is effective (ESHRE Capri workshop group, 2007).[20]

## ■ CONCLUSION

Despite the extensive literature on the subject, controversies remain about the order of treatment and effectiveness of stimulated IUI cycles in relation to IVF and ICSI. Management trials are needed to address these questions. Such trials should evaluate not only success rate but also other important outcomes such as availability of the methods, adverse effects, satisfaction, likelihood of resolution and cost, together with an analysis of the invasiveness of the techniques and likelihood of couple compliance.

## KEY POINTS

- IUI is simple, cost effective, noninvasive first-line therapy for cervical factor, anovulatory, moderate male factor, unexplained and immunological infertility.
- Three to six cycles of IUI may be offered before considering alternate therapy.
- Couples should be informed about risk of IUI and COH as well as alternative treatment options.
- Patients with advance maternal age, severe male factor, tubal pathology and severe endometriosis will benefit from a direct referral to IVF/ICSI.
- Although IUI treatment is cheaper and less demanding on the patient, IVF is the most effective treatment for infertility.

## REFERENCES

1. National Collaborating Centre for Women and Children's Health, National Institute for Health and Clinical Excellence. Fertility: assessment and treatment for people with fertility problems, 2nd edition. London: Royal College of Obstetricians and Gynaecolgists; 2013.
2. Ombelet W. IUI and evidence based medicine: an urgent need for translation into our clinical practice. Gynecol Obstet Invest. 2005;59(1):1-2.
3. SteuresP, Vander Steeg JW, Hompes PG, et al. Effectiveness of intrauterine insemination for subfertile couples with isolated cervical factor, a randomized control trial. Fertil Steril. 2007;88(6):1692-6.
4. Pandian Z, Akande VA, Harrid K, et al. Surgery for tubal infertility .Cochrane Database Syst Rev. 2008;(3):CD006415.
5. Ozkan S, Arici A. Advances in treatment options of endometriosis. Gynecol Obstet Invest. 2009:67(2):81-91.
6. Dmowski WP, Pry M, Ding J, Rana N. Cycle specific and cumulative fecundity in patients with endometriosis who are undergoing COH–IUI or IVF–ET. Fertil Steril. 2002;78(4):750-6.
7. Homburg R. The case for initial treatment with intrauterine insemination as opposed to in vitro fertilization for idiopathic infertility. Hum Fertil (Camb). 2003;6(3):122-4.
8. Pashayan N, Lyratzopoulos G, Mathur R. Cost effectiveness of primary offer of IVF vs primary offer of IUI followed by IVF (for IUI failures) in couples with unexplained or mild male factor subfertility. BMC Health Serv Res. 2006;6:80.
9. Pandian Z, Bhattacharya S, Vale L, et al. In vitro fertilization for unexplained subfertility. Cochrane Database Syst Rev. 2012;(4):CD003357.
10. Veltman-Verhulst SM, Cohlen BJ, Hugesh G, et al. Intrauterine insemination for unexplained subfertility. Cochrane Database Syst Rev. 2012;(9):CD001838.
11. Ombelet W, Deblaere K, Cox A, et al. Semen quality and intrauterine insemination. Reprod Biomed Online. 2003,7(4):485-92.
12. Van Voorhis BJ, Barnett M, Sparks AE, et al. Effects of the total motile sperm count on the efficacy and cost effectiveness of intrauterine insemination and in vitro fertilization. Fertil Steril. 2001;75 (4):661-8.

13. Shibahara H, Koriyama J, Shiraishi Y, et al. Diagnosis and treatment of immunologically infertile women with sperm immobilizing antibodies in their sera. J Reprod Immunol. 2009;83(1-2):139-44.
14. Khali MR, Rasmussen PE, Erb K, et al. IUI with donor semen. An evaluation of prognostic factors based on areview of 1131 cycles. Acta Obstet Gynecol Scand. 2001;80(4):342-8.
15. Dickey RP, Taylor SN, Lu PY, et al. Effect of diagnosis, age, sperm quality and number of preovulatory follicles on the outcome of multiple cycles of clomiphene citrate in IUI. Fertil Steril. 2002;78(5):1088-95.
16. Aboulghar M, Mansour R, Serour G, et al. Controlled ovarian stimulation and intrauterine insemination for treatment of unexplained infertility should be limited to maximum of three trials. Fertil Steril. 2001;75(1):88-91.
17. Goverde AJ, McDonnell J, VermeidenJP, et al. Intrauterine insemination or in vitro fertilization in idiopathic subfertility and male subfertility, a randomized trial and cost effectiveness analysis. Lancet. 2000;343(1):2-7.
18. Bahadur G, Homburg R, Ilahibuccus A, et al. IVF and intrauterine insemination cannot be compared. Reprod Biomed Online. 2015;31:246-7.
19. Steures P, Vander Steeg JW, Hompes PG, et al. Controlled ovarian stimulation and intrauterine insemination versus expectant treatment for couples with unexplained infertility and intermediate prognosis: a randomized clinical trial. Lancet. 2006;368(9531):216-21.
20. Aboulghar M, Baird DT, Collins J, et al. ESHRE Capri workshop Group. Intrauterine insemination. Hum Reprod Update. 2009;15(3):265-77.

# CHAPTER 3

# Merits and Demerits of In Vitro Fertilization in Batches

*Narendra Malhotra, Shally Gupta, Jaideep Malhotra, Diksha Goswami, Neharika Malhotra Bora, Keshav Malhotra*

## ■ INTRODUCTION

Batching of in vitro fertilization (IVF) cycles is a technique of recruiting of patients for assisted reproductive technology (ART) so that all can have IVF or intracytoplasmic sperm injection (ICSI) and embryo transfer within a limited span of days. It is more commonly practiced in developing countries or new IVF facilities or beginners in IVF practice in low resource settings. Practitioners who have a busy obstetric and gynecological practice and do not want to invest too much time and money into setting up a large unit, but want to upgrade themselves with less money can do so by doing batch IVF.[1,2] Facilities that have less number of patients can also benefit by it as they do pooling. Another reason for doing batch IVF is bringing highly skilled infertility specialists to peripheral centers, so benefitting larger population by providing quality treatment to patients who otherwise would not be able to access them. Busy Centers do batch IVF to coordinate high footfall. Selection and management of patients for batch IVF is same as in patients not in batches.

## ■ ADVANTAGES OF BATCH IVF

### Benefits for Patients

1. Batch IVF makes it more cost-effective and affordable for poorer patients, bringing IVF within reach of masses and not just classes.
2. It involves less travel and less loss of time away from work for these patients and their family members so less financial crunch indirectly.
3. Peripheral centers and remote hospitals can do IVF, so make it more accessible and convenient for patients.
4. Support of copatients, by discussing their fears and hence relieves stress.

## Benefits for Clinicians

1. It is upgradation in technology for a clinician remotely placed without going for long training themselves to leave their private practice unattended at a stretch.
2. It makes it cost-effective for the clinician as one can order multidose vials of media, drugs, and multiple numbers pack of disposables which reduces costs for the center and with less wastage of short half-life media.[3]
3. The staff can be focused only for IVF in the days of batch, making it less need for trained staff all the time and hence less chance of mistakes by untrained staff.
4. The laboratory need not be functional all the time, so decreasing running costs.[3]
5. The cleaning and calibration of laboratory needs work free days. So doing in batches gives one some batch free days for this.
6. It gives time to the center to audit results.

## Benefit for Visiting IVF Specialist Team

1. The IVF team gets to practice more and become experienced by working in all kinds of setups, building their confidence and enhancing their skills.
2. They can spread their name and fame.
3. It is financially beneficial for them too.

## ■ LIMITATIONS OF BATCH IVF (TABLE 1)

### Patient

1. Sometimes the remote doctor with less experience in infertility practice, who is guided by distant specialist on phone, gives less than optimum care to the patients and affecting results.
2. There is inflexibility in timings of batch. So accommodating all patients within limited time can lead to compromising of treatment for these patients. It may lead to cancellation of cycles or suboptimum treatment cycles for some patients due to either less oocytes retrieved, postmature oocytes or endometrial asynchrony.
3. It is difficult to prepare antagonist protocols for hyper-responders in batch IVF.
4. Any mistake affects entire batch.
5. There are problems associated with workload and tiredness of staff, embryologists, surgeons, etc.
6. It is difficult to modify or change treatment protocols based on individual needs like doing blastocyst transfer, sequential transfer, blastocyst transfer or need for embryo freezing.
7. Embryo vitrification program can be compromised due to unavailability of embryologist for more days for freezing.
8. Regular auditing and accountability of work is not possible simultaneously due to time constraints of visiting doctors.

**Table 1:** Pros and cons of batch IVF.

| Pros | Cons |
|---|---|
| *Patients:* <br>• Convenient <br>• Economical <br>• Less travel/loss of work <br>• Support of copatients <br><br> *Clinician:* <br>• Economical <br>• Work gets focused in limited number of days <br>• Time to clean and calibrate lab <br>• Time free to audit results <br><br> *Visiting IVF team:* <br>• Increased experience <br>• Profitable | *Patients:* <br>• Suboptional care due to inexperience of resident clinicians <br>• Inflexibility of patient protocols <br>• Less antagonist protocol/so more chance of OHSS <br>• Any mistake can affect adversely entire batch <br>• Overwork/tiredness of team <br><br> *Clinician:* <br>• Larger infrastructure and setup, more number of incubators, etc. <br>• High dependence on team members <br><br> *Visiting IVF team:* <br>• Having to see the patient first time and not knowing important details before hand <br>• Loss of time in travel |

(OHSS, ovarian hyperstimulation syndrome)

9. There are problems in maintenance of quality control of laboratory associated with batch IVF due to frequent opening of incubators, too much movement of personnel in the laboratory.

# Clinicians

1. A bigger setup or infrastructure is needed like more beds, more incubators, bigger staff and larger waiting area.
2. Stress of any team member being unavailable or incapacitated due to sudden sickness can affect the entire batch.

# For Visiting Team

1. The visiting doctor is not aware about minor details of patients and to see the patients first time in the operation theater can be a disadvantage.
2. Lot of time is wasted in travel.

## ■ HOW TO PREPARE A BATCH FOR IVF?

Key steps in preparing for a batch are preparing patients, getting the unit ready which should include ordering of drugs and consumables cleaning of IVF lab and calibration of instruments. Preparing checklists for every procedure and having easy access to it everywhere.

Having the embryologist or IVF specialist to come a day before or even few hours before can help streamline many things during the batch.

Sometimes the engineer or the company who installed the machine or lab can be asked to stay for at least the first day of the batch to ensure smooth functioning.

Having meeting of your core team including junior doctors, nurses, other staff planning everything in advance, assign duties and roles.

## Ordering Drugs and Consumables and Disposables for Laboratory

Dose of drugs like gonadotropins and gonadotropin-releasing hormone (GnRH) agonists and antagonists, hCG, needed should be calculated beforehand and ordered according to the number of patients recruited, their response and expected oocyte yield. One should keep in mind some 10–15% extra as backup and keep it available timely (at least 1 week) before batch.

A trained staff should be designated to administer injections to prevent wastage and inappropriate administration.

There should be adequate biopsy guide, ovum pick-up (OPU) needles, ICSI dishes, test tubes and petri dishes. The brands used should be standard and the one visiting team is accustomed to. The culture media should be ordered based on the embryologists and their way of working.

## IVF Lab Preparation

Apart from disposables and consumables uninterrupted power supply should be ensured for lab during batch days.

The calibration and cleaning of lab should be performed before every batch (7–10 days). Operation theater (OT) equipment like suction pump, mobile nest, warmers, anesthetic drugs and gas cylinders and lab equipment like laminar, microscope, micromanipulator, incubators, MINC, etc. are in good working condition. Liquid nitrogen and cryocans should be ready available. Lab cultures should be sent 2 weeks before scheduled batch. Incubator contracon should be done 1 week before batch. An engineer from the lab can be asked to be present during the days of the batch to ensure smooth running.

## Patient Preparation

The workup of couple including history, blood investigations, radiological investigations, cultures and semen analysis should be done timely before batch and an individualized treatment protocol planned. Those requiring hysteroscopy (polyp, septum, adhesions) or laparoscopic management of tubo-ovarian masses like endometrioma or hydrosalpinx should be recruited only after it is done. Problems in male partner such as fear or anxiety in collecting semen sample in the hospital facility should be discussed and picked up before hand and adequate time given to manage that. Freezing of semen sample prior to ovum pick-up if possible or preparation for any unplanned testicular sperm aspiration should be done, in case of any unexpected difficulty in semen sample collection. Doing mock embryo transfer and doing dilatation for those with difficult or stenosed cervical canal prevents many last minute cancellations of embryo transfers. Check number of patients recruited and plan media and drugs accordingly. One should be in touch with visiting team and keep them informed about everything including special need patients. The preprocedure counseling of couple should be done before hand and any doubts cleared.

Synchronization of menstrual cycles and targeted individualized ovarian stimulation has to be performed carefully to optimize the success in batch IVF program. For timing of menstrual cycles pretreatment with oral contraceptive pills (OCP) can be done.[4,5,6] It should be withdrawn 6 days before expected date of ovarian stimulation if we are planning a GnRH antagonist cycle.[7] But more centers prefer GnRH agonist or long protocol as it gives more flexibility in batching and less cycle cancellations. OCP should be started from previous menstrual cycle and should be given for a minimum of 12–16 days. GnRH agonist should be started 3–4 days before stopping OCP. Progesterone alone or in combination with estrogen can also be used for cycle regulation. Even then there will be a small percentage of patients who will not be ready by the time the ovarian stimulation will be started, leading to cycle cancellations or postponement, and that should be kept in mind while calculating logistics of batch.

If the batch (OPU) is planned for $X$ date then ovarian stimulation is started on X-11 or 12 days. Ovarian stimulation is done with gonadotropins (either recombinant FSH or hMG). The drugs used should be standard ensuring good cold chain maintenance and those with which the visiting team is accustomed too. The day 2 hormonal profile should be done and the labs should be instructed to give reports timely. Stimulation should be individualized and dose and drug adjusted according to protocol, age and ovarian reserve of patients. Some centers prefer to give daily injections at the center, whereas others allow the patients to take home for 2–5 days at a time. Either way one must ensure that they are given properly and no mistake happens in their administration.

The follicular development can be monitored using transvaginal sonography (TVS) and or serum estradiol levels. The timing of starting antagonist, and dose adjustment like stepping down or stepping up should be done based on the monitored values. The hCG trigger is planned 36 hours before scheduled OPU and time of OPU confirmed. If some patients seem to get ready a day early then delaying hCG by a day does not seem to affect the outcome adversely. The hCG injections should be given at interval of 30–45 minutes keeping in mind the interval between two OPUs. hCG injection can be administered at the center to avoid any delay or inaccurate injection.

All consent forms and documentation should be in order as the visiting team will have limited time to look into all minor details.

Culture media needs to be equilibrated day before of batch according to number and response of patients. Check with $CO_2$ analyzer, thermometer, pH analyzers and humidity that everything is in order.

## Ovum Pick-up Day

On ovum pick-up day patients are given proper instructions, time to report for OPU, keeping in mind unplanned delays. The anesthetist, staff, doctors all need to be on time. The operation theater, Boyle's machine, anesthesia drugs, gases, mobile nest and suction pressure pump, ultrasound machine, biopsy guide, OPU needles, transvaginal probe, etc. should be checked. Ensure adequate sterilized instruments for surgical procedures.

Backup equipment like ultrasound machine if needed, probes, ovum pick-up pressure pump be made available on OPU day. The collection of semen samples should be in properly marked and labeled containers so that there is no mix up, and only one embryologist or technician should be handed over this task. Partners with anxiety or difficulty in giving semen samples should be identified, and either sufficient be given to them for the same or a backup semen sample frozen few days before.

In the lab, the dishes with follicular fluid and oocyte-cumulus complexes (OCCs), culture dishes should be labeled correctly with at least triple identification mark, viz. patient's name, partner's name, patient Hospital ID (Fig. 1). Maximum 5–6 patients can be done in one incubator, to prevent temperature, $CO_2$ and pH changes. One should develop a system of witnessing and cross-checking every laboratory procedure like thawing, freezing, ICSI, denuding, etc. This can be done manually by a colleague/staff or electronically by digital witness system installed in the machines such as microscope and manipulator. Checklists should be prepared for every ART procedure to prevent human errors (inadvertent) (Figs. 2 to 4).

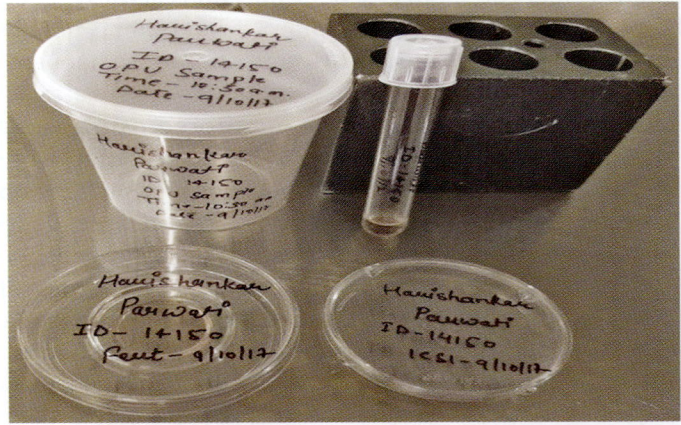

**Fig. 1:** Triple marker (Partner Name, Patient Name, Hospital ID).

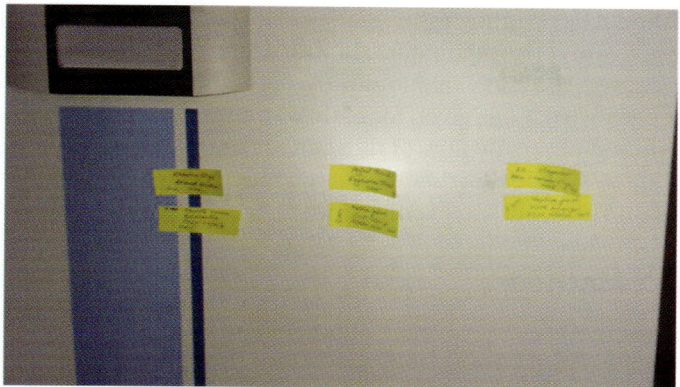

**Fig. 2:** Incubator showing post on it with name of dishes inside.

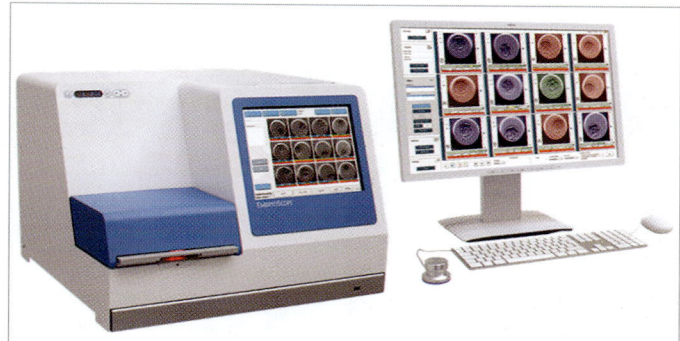

**Fig. 3:** Embryoscope.

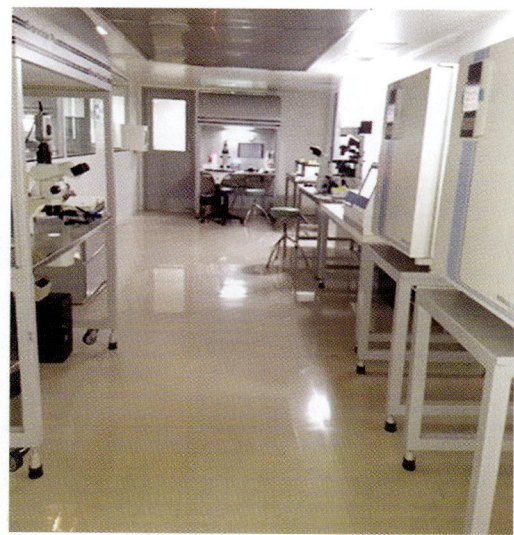

**Fig. 4:** Model assisted reproductive technology (ART) (Laboratory of Rainbow IVF, Agra).

There should be no unnecessary staff or extra person's movement in the lab to maintain quality. The incubators should be opened least number of times.

Postoperative care and vital monitoring should be done by trained nurses. Postoperative instructions given for embryo transfer (ET).

There should be steady flow of movements and timely discharges should be given side by side so that there is not too much crowding by patients, their attendants and staff, adding to confusion.

## Incorrect Method

The incorrect methods are given in Figures 5 and 6.

## Correct Method

The correct methods are given in Figures 7 and 8.

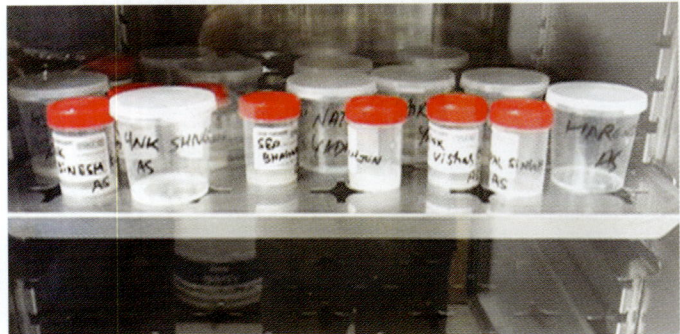

**Fig. 5:** Semen samples.

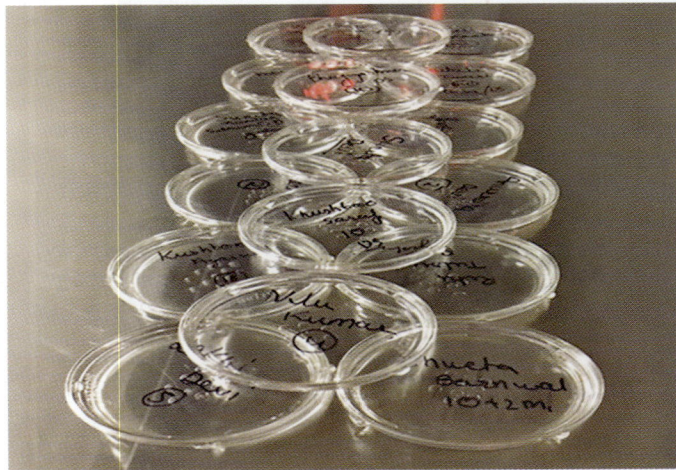

**Fig. 6:** Culture dishes.

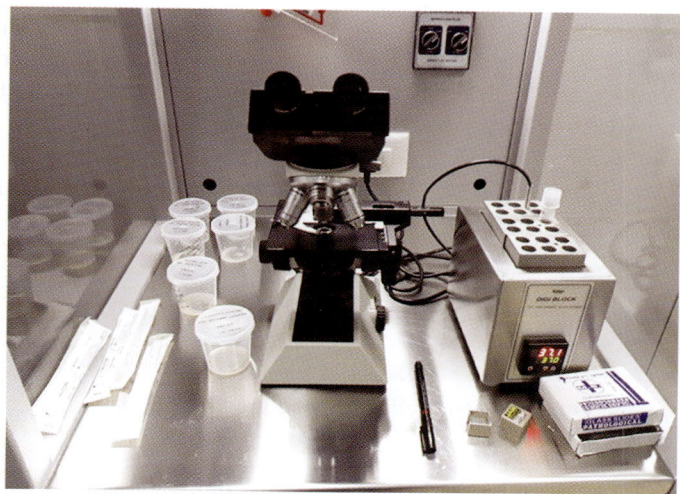

**Fig. 7:** Well-arranged semen samples.

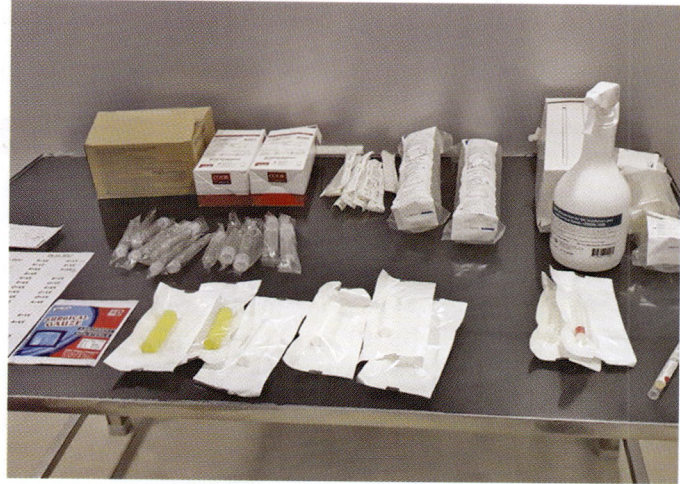

**Fig. 8:** Disposables arranged properly.

## Embryo Transfer Day

Similar to ovum pick-up day, proper instructions should be given. Patients are attended for any postoperative complaints and ET done with utmost care and calm.

## Beta hCG Day

This is the most stressful day of batch IVF (Fig. 9), it is like going back to school and facing your examination results. One is judged on every positive or negative

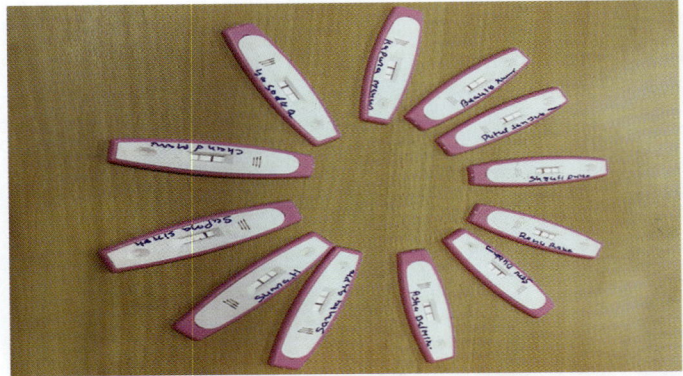

**Fig. 9:** Human chorionic gonadotropin (hCG) day.

result. Here one has to be ready for counseling of negative results and to be able to plan for next cycle.

## ■ MANAGEMENT OF TRICKY SITUATIONS/GOOF-UPS

The management of tricky situation of batch IVF has been given in Table 2.

| Table 2: Management of tricky situations/goof-ups. | |
|---|---|
| Problem | Management |
| Patients not taken injections properly.<br>GnRH Agonists | Do TVS. Check endometrium, and follicles, get blood tests E2, P4, levels and accordingly either increase the dose, or continue agonists longer or stop and restart next month |
| GnRH Antagonists | Do TVS, Check LH level. May need to give hCG early and schedule OPU before surge happens and all eggs ovulate |
| Gonadotropins | Do TVS, check follicular response. Stepup or down accordingly |
| hCG | Do TVS get LH and P4<br>Can plan OPU later after repeat trigger or dual trigger, if hCG not taken properly |
| OPU day<br>OPU pump not working | Check plug points, take out and reinsert, switch on and off, keep extra OPU pump handy |
| No follicular fluid aspirated | Check pump pressure—increase and check<br>See if needle or biopsy guide is blocked<br>Check if tube is cracked<br>Check for lose connections at joints |
| Mobile nest not maintaining normal temperature | Keep warmers and blocks handy |

*Contd...*

Contd...

| Problem | Management |
|---|---|
| TVS probe not working | Arrange from nearby radiology setup |
| USG machine not working | Have a backup, arrange from nearby center |
| Biopsy guide broken or not sterilized | Keep disposable as backup |
| Ovary not accessible | Deepen anesthesia with good relaxation, can use abdominal or vaginal manipulation |
| Eggs ovulated | Can try pelvic fluid aspiration but only by experienced specialist |
| Bleeding per vaginum | Manage puncture site. May need stitch or packing for a few hours |
| Injury to bladder or bowel | Catheterize, flush, consult urologist<br>Consult gastrosurgeon<br>Keep admitted and watch for progress of symptoms |
| Lab ICSI/micromanipulator | An engineer be present with preferably a spare part<br>Can get spare from nearby IVF centers, so have good relationships with them |
| Forgot to incubate media overnight | Atleast 4 hours incubation is needed in petri dishes and OPU can be delayed to maximum till 38 hours for the incubation to be complete |
| Bigger $CO_2$ incubator not working | Always have two incubators |
| Difficult embryo transfer | May need stillete, dilator set<br>May need general anesthesia or<br>Postpone and freeze embryos, plan later after hysteroscopy dilatation of cervix |

## ■ STATUS OF BATCH IVF IN MODERN DAY ART PRACTICE

There are both pros and cons of doing batch IVF and hence proponents as well as opponents. But we need to understand that in an era of individualization and tailor made protocols batching of IVF involves lot of care and management so that one gets best results without compromising patient care. One need to be prepared with adequate staff and junior doctors and embryologists so that pressure of working long hours in short time can be decreased. The infertility specialist should be able to differentiate cases that require tertiary care facilities like recurrent implantation failure, poor responders, polycystic ovaries, severe male factor, wanting oocyte freezing, seropositive patients such as hepatitis B and C and HIV and those requiring vitrification and advice early referral. Above all troubleshooting at needed hours with utmost vigilance plays the crucial role in batch IVF program because the problems during the batch IVF will affect the outcome in en masse. A fully equipped and dedicated cryopreservation unit will be of great use in batch IVF to optimize the success rates in batch IVF. Knowledge in reproductive endocrinology and hormonal manipulation, experience in laboratory science, precision in laboratory processes and dedicated team will help in achieving success in batch IVF.

## ■ KEY POINTS

- Batch IVF is a boon for clinicians practicing in smaller towns and cities having limited experience in IVF.
- Individualization of patient protocol cannot be done.
- Cryopreservation program not too well developed in batch IVF.
- Batch IVF makes IVF economical for clinician and hence more affordable and cost-effective for patients.
- It is very hectic for the team, and documentation and record keeping is not good.

## ■ REFERENCES

1. Ahemmed BP, Varghese AC. Batch IVF Programme in ART: Practical Considerations. In: Fleming S, Varghese A (Eds). Organization and Management of IVF Units. New York: Springer; 2016.
2. Das MC, Jayaprakasan K, Angras S, et al. Batch in vitro fertilization program. In: Verghese AC, Sjoblom P, Jayaprakasan K (Eds). A practical guide to setting up an IVF lab, embryo culture systems and running the unit. New Delhi: Jaypee Brothers Medical Publishers (P) Ltd.; 2013.
3. Chandrareddy A, Kutty BA, Pandey S. Batch IVF practical considerations. In: Rao KA, Carp H, Fischer R (Eds). Principles and Practice of Assisted Reproductive Technologies. New Delhi: Jaypee Brothers Medical Publications; 2014. pp. 827-33.
4. Ramsewak SS, Duffy S, Taylor J, et al. The oral contraceptive pill effectively permits cycle batching for an intermittent in vitro fertilization programme in Trinidad and Tobago. West Indian Med J. 2005;54(2):127-9.
5. Garcia-Velasco JA, Bermejo A, Ruiz F, et al. Cycle scheduling with oral contraceptive pills in the GnRH antagonist protocol vs the long protocol: a randomized, controlled trial. Fertil Steril. 2011;96:590-3.
6. Hauzman EE, Zapata A, Bermejo A, et al. Cycle scheduling for *in vitro* fertilization with oral contraceptive pills versus oral estradiol valerate: a randomized, controlled trial. Reprod Biol Endocrinol. 2013;11:96.
7. Basu S, Garcia-Velasco J, Gutgutia R, et al. Scheduling cycles with gonadotropin-releasing hormone antagonist protocol in in vitro fertilization: is there a scope in batch in vitro fertilization? J Hum Reprod Sci. 2014;7(4):230-5.

CHAPTER

4

# Agonist in ART Cycle

*Fessy Louis T, Ramesh*

## ■ GnRH PHYSIOLOGY

Gonadotropin-releasing hormone (GnRH) is a decapeptide secreted by the arcuate nucleus of hypothalamus.[1] It is having a very short half-life of about 2–4 minutes. It is rapidly degraded by the GnRH-degrading enzyme in the pituitary. The human specific GnRH molecule has a fairly conserved central amino acid sequence composed of Tyrosine-Glycine-Leucine-Arginine (TGLA).[1] The 6th position of the decapeptide is occupied by Glycine and the bonds at 5-6 (T-G), 6-7 (G-L) and 9-10 (P-G) are very weak. This accounts for the short half-life of endogenous GnRH (Fig. 1).[1]

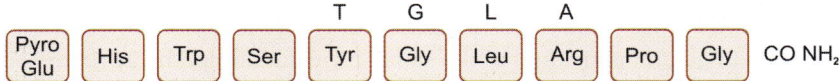

**Fig. 1:** GnRH structure.

The modifications in the amino acids are often employed to obtain GnRH analogs (agonist or antagonist) which have increased half-life and relatively more affinity to the receptor. Therefore these molecules stay in the receptor for more time resulting in a continuous action at the receptor level.

When GnRH binds to its receptor in pituitary gland (GnRH I receptor), the immediate event is a release of stored gonadotropins [follicle-stimulating hormone (FSH) or luteinizing hormone (LH) or both] which is described as a release effect or a flare effect. Then it also causes further storage of gonadotropins so that next pulse of GnRH can produce similar effect.[1] The physiologically important aspect is the pulsatile secretion of GnRH which can produce pulsatile release of gonadotropins too.

## ■ PULSE FREQUENCY AND AMPLITUDE

Gonadotropin-releasing hormone (GnRH) is secreted in a pulsatile fashion. The pulsatility is established after some periods of irregular secretion followed by nocturnal pulsatility and ultimately leading to the complete 24-hour pulsatile secretion. The pulse has both frequency (number of pulses per unit time) and amplitude (the actual magnitude or amount of hormone released). The amplitude changes in various days of the cycle are not very significantly different and hence no much importance is given to it. What we are concerned is the frequency of the pulses.[1]

Classically, high levels of E2 will increase the pulse frequency and is responsible for the preovulatory LH surge. Low levels of progesterone will decrease the frequency which is responsible for the FSH release in the preovulatory period (second peak of FSH) and also the late luteal rise of FSH from about day 24 of a 28 day cycle (responsible for FSH rise and final recruitment of the follicles for the next cycle).[1]

Hence, it may be concluded that increased frequency will cause LH release, decreased frequency will cause preferential FSH release and mixture of increased and decreased frequencies will cause release of both FSH and LH. The phenomenon is explained by the signal transduction pathways involved in the GnRH action. Pituitary gonadotropes have α subunit of FSH and LH as a common subunit. The β subunit is different. The rate limiting step in gonadotropin synthesis and release is the synthesis and storage of the β subunit.[1] If there is more of β FSH, the hormone released would be FSH and if there is more of β LH, the LH release will occur.

At low pulse frequencies, GnRH receptor concentrations on the gonadotrope cell surface are relatively low with activation of a single signal transduction pathway stimulating the expression of both βFSH and βLH but mainly FSH. Faster GnRH pulse frequencies increase the GnRH receptor concentrations resulting in greater activation of the signal transduction pathway (increase β FSH and β LH) and at the same time stimulating a second signal transduction pathway that specifically inhibits β FSH gene expression thereby causing preferential secretion of LH.[2]

## ■ RECEPTOR ACTION

When GnRH acts on the receptor on cell surface (G protein coupled receptor), the hormone receptor unit leads to formation of second messenger (cyclic AMP) which then acts on the effector system. Then it leads to transcription and translation leading to synthesis of relevant proteins culminating in the desired action. The hormone (GnRH) immediately is degraded, makes the receptor free so that it can combine with another GnRH molecule in the subsequent pulse (Receptor recycling).[3]

## ■ GnRH AGONISTS

These are molecules obtained from modification of GnRH molecule. Chief modification is at the position 6 amino acid (Glycine) which is replaced by other amino acids (Leucine/Histidine/Naphthylamine/Serine) thereby strengthening the bonds 5-6 and 6-7 giving rise to a GnRH agonist having longer half-life and therefore more affinity to the receptor (would not leave the receptor even if its action is completed). The available molecules are either nonapeptides (9 amino acids: Leuprorelin, Goserelin, Buserelin, Histrelin) or decapeptides (10 amino acids: Nafarelin and Triptorelin). The details are as shown in Table 1.

When we administer GnRH agonist to a subject, it will produce same effect as endogenous GnRH although in a greater magnitude (Flare effect). The action will however last longer than that of the endogenous molecule. The single dose may not have any further effect than just liberating all available stored gonadotropins in the pituitary gland at that point of time. This will virtually drain most of the stored gonadotropins (responsible for the triggering action when given in preovulatory period) and will also favor some amount of subsequent storage of gonadotropins (priming action). But since the molecule is not disintegrated rapidly, the receptor is not recycled.

Whenever an agonist molecule is continuously present in the receptor, there occurs desensitization of the receptors (phenomenon of tachyphylaxis). Also, the receptors are decreased (loss of receptors) mainly due to absent or reduced recycling of receptors. Added to this, there is no de novo synthesis of receptors as the body thinks it is having sufficient action of the molecule. Along with it, the effector system is saturated leading to an uncoupling of receptor-effector systems (receptor hormone complex can produce second messenger, but the effector system is saturated and hence no effects occur). These events culminate in down regulation (suppression) of hypothalamic–pituitary–gonadal (HPO) axis.

**Table 1:** GnRH and GnRH agonists.

| Molecule | 1 | 2 | 3 | 4 | 5 | 6 | 7 | 8 | 9 | 10 |
|---|---|---|---|---|---|---|---|---|---|---|
| GnRH (10) | pGlu | His | Trp | Ser | Tyr | Gly | Leu | Arg | Pro | Gly-NH$_2$ |
| Leuprolide (9) | | | | | | Leu | | | | NH-Ethylamide |
| Buserelin (9) | | | | | | D-Ser | | | | NH-Ethylamide |
| Goserelin (9) | | | | | | D-Ser | | | | Aza-Gly |
| Nafarelin (10) | | | | | | Naphthyl Alanine | | | | Gly-NH$_2$ |
| Histrelin (9) | | | | | | His | | | | NH-Ethylamide |
| Deslorelin (9) | | | | | | D-Trp | | | | NH-Ethylamide |
| Triptorelin (10) | | | | | | L-Trp | | | | Gly-NH$_2$ |

Therefore the factors bringing out suppression are [1]
1. Desensitization of receptors
2. Loss of receptors
3. Receptor-effector uncoupling.

The flare effect will be seen for about 3–4 days. This will be followed by decreased release and total suppression of HPO axis by about 7 days. However it may take variable periods and even up to 3 weeks[1] for some subjects depending on the pharmacogenic properties of individual subjects. This point is particularly important while considering some protocols.

## GnRH Agonist Preparations

There are preparations available which can be administered subcutaneously or intramuscularly or as nasal spray. Usually intramuscular preparations are depot preparations. These are available for administration in variable strengths, to be effective from one month and up to 3 months.

## Use of Agonist in Non-ART Cycles

Agonist can be used in non-ART cycles as a substitute to hCG in the final triggering of Ovulation. Here, when we administer agonist, it will cause an exaggerated flare effect leading to the release of gonadotropin especially LH to simulate a physiological LH surge. And ovulation ensues and further management can be done. This is routinely employed in cases who are likely to go for hyper-response. However agonist trigger is found to be having slightly decreased pregnancy rate as opposed to hCG trigger in most of the available studies.

Another possible use of agonist is in a case of severe polycystic ovary syndrome (PCOS), resistant to standard treatments. Here the HPO axis can be suppressed followed by stimulation with gonadotropins (FSH or HMG) and then can be combined with IUI if indicated. This is not a very commonly employed method as ART is a good option with increased pregnancy rates in these group of subjects. However, if the couple is not agreeing for ART or if all other factors are normal other than the resistant PCOS, the method may be employed.

## ■ AGONIST IN ART CYCLES

Agonist can be administered in assisted reproductive techniques (ART) cycles in a number of ways giving rise to a number of variable protocols. These are as follows.

## Long Protocol (Fig. 2)

Here the agonist is started in the previous cycle in and around third week or day 21 (long luteal protocol) or less commonly in the follicular phase of previous cycle (long follicular protocol). Then after confirming suppression, stimulation is started and folliculogenesis is monitored. hCG trigger is given when around 2–3 follicles reach around 17–18 mm and few other follicles around 14 mm. This protocol gives a very good control over the cycles and is very useful in batching. It also is useful in achieving a follicular synchrony on day 2 so that net follicular yield on stimulation is maximum. For the same reason, it do have higher incidence of OHSS. Also since the endogenous gonadotropins are totally not available due to suppression, it may be, at least theoretically, detrimental in poor responders.

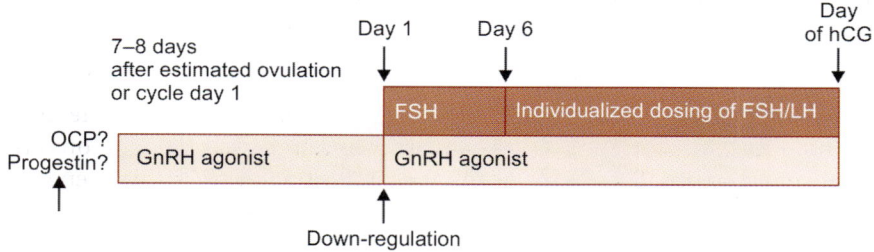

**Fig. 2:** Long protocol.[5]

## Ultra Long (Prolonged Suppression) Protocol

Here we administer agonists for a prolonged period of about 3 months to achieve a profound suppression. The depot preparations are commonly utilized here. The theoretical indications are endometriosis, adenomyosis, and severe PCOS (to manage the altered androgen levels and tonically elevated LH levels).

## Short/Flare Protocol (Fig. 3)

The agonist is started from day 2/day 3 which will give an FSH flare. The exogenous gonadotropin is also started soon. There will be an additive effect to bring out a good stimulation. But since there is absence of follicular synchrony on day 2, the net folliculogenesis is comparatively less than long protocol.

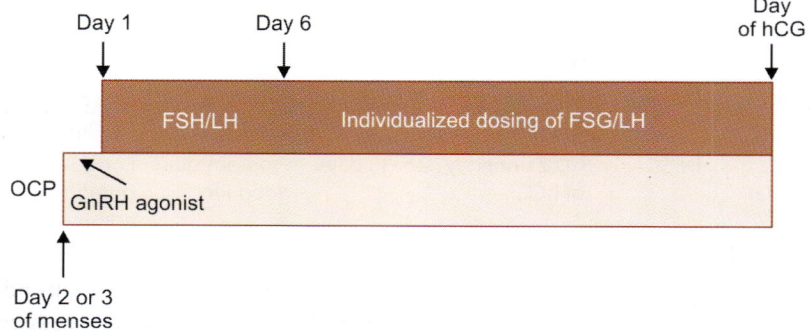

**Fig. 3:** Short/Flare protocol.[5]

## Ultrashort Flare Protocol

This is not much used now. Here agonist is administered only for 3 days to utilize the FSH flare. But there is no control over the ovulation like that in a natural cycle protocol.

## Microdose Flare Protocol (Fig. 4)

Especially useful in poor responders. The suppression is less profound so that stimulation is proposed to be more effective.

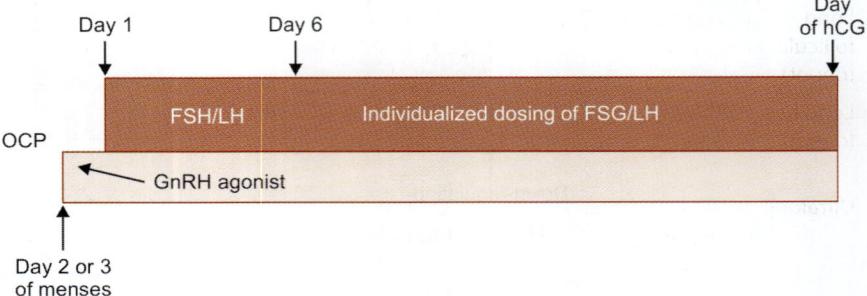

**Fig. 4:** Microdose Flare protocol.[5]

## Menstrual Early Cessation Protocol and Follicular Early Cessation Protocol (Table 2)

- Mainly of historical importance. Not much in use
- Minidose protocol (Fig. 5)
- This is recommended again in poor responders. Here the dose of suppression in a long protocol is reduced to half along with stimulation so that net ovarian suppression is reduced.

| Table 2: GnRH agonists in various protocols.[4] | | | | | |
|---|---|---|---|---|---|
| GnRH agonist protocol | Route of administration | Administration days of cycle (CD) | Duration of administration | Advantages | Disadvantages |
| Ultrashort protocol | IN/SC | CD 2, 3–4, 5 | 3 days | Patient's comfort | Low PR |
| Short protocol | IN/SC | CD 2, 3 until day of hCG | 8–12 days | Patient's comfort | No programming |
| Long follicular | IN/SC | CD 2 until day of hCG | 28–35 days | Programming, good PR | Long duration of administration |
| Long luteal | IN/SC | CD 21 until day of hCG | 21–28 days | Programming, good PR | Long duration of administration |

*Contd...*

*Contd...*

| GnRH agonist protocol | Route of administration | Administration days of cycle (CD) | Duration of administration | Advantages | Disadvantages |
|---|---|---|---|---|---|
| Menstrual early cessation | IN/SC | CD 21 until menses | 7–12 days | Inconclusive | Low estradiol levels |
| Follicular early cessation | IN/SC | CD 21 until stimulation day 6, 7 | 13–20 days | Inconclusive | Low estradiol levels |
| Long follicular (depot) | Depot | CD 2 | Once | Patient's comfort | (Too) long duration of action |
| Long luteal (depot) | Depot | CD 21 | Once | Patient's comfort | (Too) long duration of action |
| Ultralong | IN/SC/depot | CD 2 or 21 | 8–12 weeks, depot two or three times | Only for special cases | Side effects due to estrogen deficiency |

*Abbreviations:* CD, cycle day; hCG, human chorionic gonadotropin; IN, intranasal; PR, pregnancy rate; SC, subcutaneous.
*Source:* Gardner DK, Weissman A, Howles CM, et al. Text Book of Assisted Reproductive Techniques, 5th edition. Boca Raton, FL: CRC Press Taylor and Francis Group; 2018.

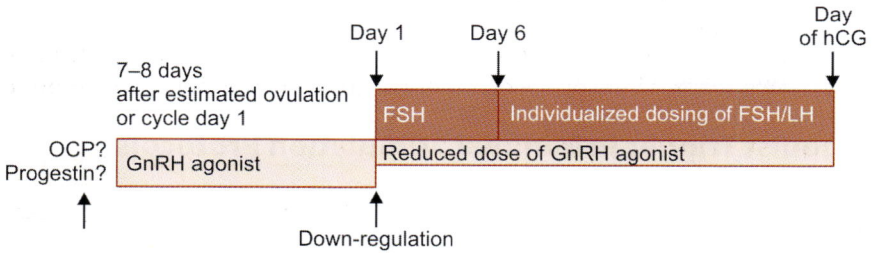

**Fig. 5:** Minidose protocol.[5]

## Agonist/Antagonist Conversion Protocol (Fig. 6)

Previous cycle luteal phase agonist is given. Once menstruation occurs, antagonist is started and cycle is continued as antagonist cycle.

## Agonist Antagonist Combination Protocol (Fig. 7)

This utilizes pretreatment with COC/estradiol/progestins to achieve follicular synchrony. Then from day 2, agonist is administered like that in ultrashort protocol for 3–4 days and stopped. Once the criteria of starting antagonist is

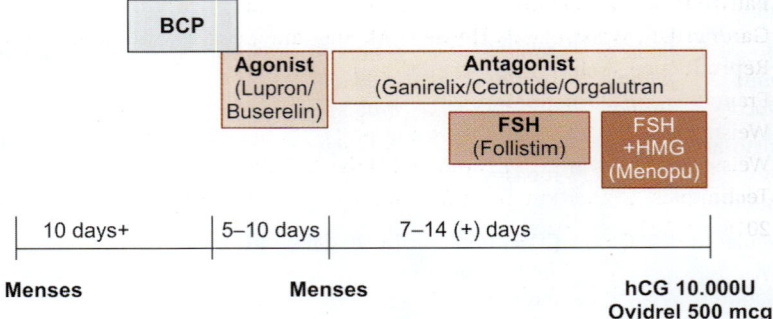

**Fig. 6:** Agonist/antagonist conversion protocol (A/ACP).

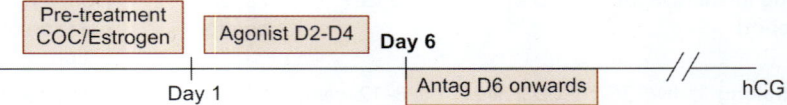

**Fig. 7:** Agonist-Antagonist combination protocol.

reached (lead follicle 13–14 mm and/or serum estradiol > 400–500 pg/mL), the cycle is continued as the standard antagonist protocol.

## Agonist Trigger in Antagonist Protocol

This is utilized in possible hyper-responders. It is the most important aspect of utilizing antagonist protocol in achieving an OHSS free clinic.

## Agonist Trigger in Minimal Stimulation Protocols

Agonist trigger in minimal stimulation is not much employed as there are less chances of hyper-response and also due to the fact that almost all studies support hCG trigger as opposed to agonist trigger whenever possible.

### ■ REFERENCES

1. Fritz MA, Speroff L. Clinical Gynecologic Endocrinology and Infertility, 8th edition. Philadelphia: Lippincott Williams & Wilkins; 2011. pp. 157-98.
2. Kaiser UB, Sabbagh E, Katzenellenbogen R, et al. A mechanism for the differential regulation of gonadotropin subunit gene expression by gonadotropin-releasing hormone. Proc Natl Acad Sci USA. 1995;92:12280-4.
3. Fritz MA, Speroff L. Clinical Gynecologic Endocrinology and Infertility, 8th edition. Philadelphia: Lippincott Williams & Wilkins; 2011. pp. 29-104.

4. Patrizo P, Ghazal S, Huirine JA, et al. Endocrine characteristics of ART cycles. In: Gardner DK, Weissman A, Howles CM, Shoham Z (Eds). Text Book of Assisted Reproductive Techniques, 5th edition. Boca Raton, FL: CRC Press/Taylor and Francis Group; 2018. pp. 547.
5. Weisman A, Howles CM, Sunkara SK. GnRH agonist triggering. In: Gardner DK, Weissman A, Howles CM, Shoham Z (Eds). Text Book of Assisted Reproductive Techniques, 5th edition. Boca Raton, FL: CRC Press/Taylor and Francis Group; 2018. pp. 623-6.

CHAPTER
5

# Ovarian Hyperstimulation Syndrome in ART

*Ameet Patki, Abhimanyu Tejrao Shinde*

## ■ INTRODUCTION

There has been increase in number of patients undergoing treatment of infertility with assisted reproductive technology (ART) in recent years.[1] Although there are many evidences supporting safety of ART but we should be aware of its complications too, most serious of it is ovarian hyperstimulation syndrome (OHSS). OHSS is a potentially fatal iatrogenic condition resulting from excessive stimulation of the ovaries.

The vast majority of OHSS occurs in the setting of injectables like gonadotropins in in vitro fertilization (IVF) although in the absence of proper monitoring oral clomiphene and other drugs can result in massive ovarian hyperstimulation. Anovulatory women treated with different preparations for ovulation induction the incidence of mild OHSS is 5–10%, moderate OHSS is 2–4% and severe forms of OHSS occur in 0.5–5.0% of IVF cycles.[2]

The risk of venous thromboembolism associated with OHSS is reported to be between 0.8% and 2.4%.[3] Pregnancies with fresh IVF cycles complicated by OHSS were at a 100-fold increased risk of venous thromboembolism in the first trimester if compared with the background population.[3] In addition to this, recent published data support a statistically significant increase in pregnancy-related complications among IVF pregnancies in women with OHSS compared to IVF controls.[4]

## ■ PATHOPHYSIOLOGY

Ovarian hyperstimulation syndrome is an exaggerated response to controlled ovarian stimulation (COS) characterized by the shift of protein-rich fluid from the intravascular space to the third space, mainly the abdominal cavity that occurs when the ovaries become enlarged due to follicular stimulation.[5] The pathophysiology of this condition is characterized by ovarian enlargement, massive extra, vascular exudates accumulation in combination with profound intravascular volume depletion and hemoconcentration. This shift in fluid is due to increased vascular permeability in response to stimulation with human chorionic gonadotropin (hCG).[5] Prostaglandins, inhibin, the renin-angiotensin-aldosterone system and inflammatory mediators have all been implicated in the etiology of OHSS.[6] However, vascular endothelial growth factor (VEGF) has been identified as the major mediator (Fig. 1).[5] The expression of VEGF and VEGF receptor 2 (VEGFR-2) mRNA increases significantly in response to hCG, and peak levels coincide with maximum vascular permeability.[7] The angiogenic properties of human follicular fluid combined with high prorenin, high plasma renin like activity, angiotensin II like immunoreactivity and angiotensinogen converting enzyme raised the hypothesis on possible involvement of renin-angiotensin system in pathogenesis of OHSS through new vessel formation and increased capillary permeability.[7]

The clinical manifestations of OHSS reflect the extent of the shift of fluid into the third space and the resulting hemoconcentration due to intravascular volume depletion. Symptoms range from mild abdominal distention due to enlarged ovaries alone or with an accompanying fluid shift into the abdomen, to renal failure and death as a result of hemoconcentration and reduced perfusion of organs such as the kidneys, heart and brain (Flowchart 1, Table 1).[5,8] Indeed, as the severity of OHSS increases, so does the number of organs affected.[8]

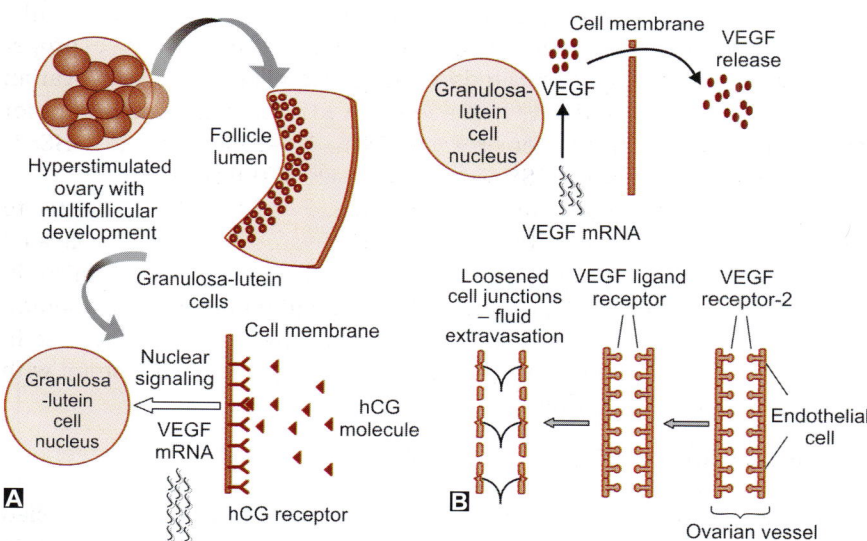

**Figs. 1A and B:** (A) The pathogenesis of ovarian hyperstimulation syndrome (OHSS). Human chorionic gonadotropin (hCG) stimulates a high number of granulosa-lutein cells leading to the increased production of vascular endothelial growth factor (VEGF) mRNA. (B) Downstream signaling augments vascular permeability.
*Source:* Adapted from Soares SR, Gómez R, Simón C, et al. Targeting the vascular endothelial growth factor system to prevent ovarian hyperstimulation syndrome. Hum Reprod Update. 2008;14:321-33.

**Flowchart 1:** Severe and critical ovarian hyperstimulation syndrome (OHSS).

```
                    Increased capillary permeability
                    /                              \
              Hypovolemia              Third space fluid accumulation (ascites,
                                          hydrothorax, pericardial effusion)
                                                    /        \
                                              Azotemia    Hypovolemic shock
              /         |              \
         Oliguria   Hemoconcentration   Electrolyte imbalance
                        |
                    Thrombosis
```

**Table 1:** Classification of ovarian hyperstimulation syndrome (OHSS).

| S. No. | Grade | Signs and Symptoms |
|---|---|---|
| 1. | Mild | • Abdominal bloating<br>• Mild abdominal pain<br>• Ovarian size < 8 cm |
| 2. | Moderate | • Moderate abdominal pain<br>• Nausea and vomiting<br>• Ovarian size 8–12 cm |
| 3. | Severe | • Ascites, pleural effusion<br>• Oliguria (< 30 mL/hr)<br>• Hematocrit (> 45%)<br>• Hypoproteinemia (Albumin < 3.5 mg/dL)<br>• Ovarian size > 12 cm |
| 4. | Critical | • Tense ascites or large pleural effusion<br>• Hematocrit (> 55 %)<br>• Oliguria/anuria<br>• Thromboembolism<br>• Respiratory distress |

The early form of OHSS is due to hCG and is related to an exaggerated ovarian response to gonadotropin stimulation whereas the late form is mainly related to secretion of placental hCG. The early form is within days after the ovulation triggering injection of hCG and the late form within 10 days after hCG. The early cases particularly constitute the serious and long lasting morbidity.

## ■ CLASSIFICATION OF OHSS

The scheme in Table 1 is based on the classification of OHSS severity proposed as per Royal College of Obstetricians and Gynaecologists (RCOG) guidelines combined with useful features from previous classifications.[10]

## ■ RISK FACTORS ASSOCIATED WITH OHSS

There are a number of well-established primary risk factors for the development of OHSS, including young age (<35 years of age), polycystic ovary syndrome (PCOS) and a history of an elevated response to gonadotropins, i.e. prior hyper-response/OHSS,[11] asthenic habitus, pregnancy and hCG-luteal supplementation. Studies investigating the impact of low body weight/body mass index (BMI) on the development of OHSS report contradictory results.[12]

Immunological sensitivity, i.e. hypersensitivity or allergies may also be predictive of OHSS. In a prospective cohort study, patients who developed severe OHSS (n = 18/428) had an increased prevalence of allergies (56% vs. 21% in the control group).[13] While a link between OHSS and allergy is plausible, as the pathophysiological changes in the ovaries during OHSS resemble an overactive inflammatory response, the influence of allergies on the development of OHSS requires further study.

Basal anti-Müllerian hormone (AMH) levels prior to COS have also been shown to be predictive for OHSS.[14] Two recent, prospective, randomized controlled trials (RCTs) in large cohorts demonstrated that basal AMH levels approximately more than or equal to 3.5 ng/mL were predictive of hyper-response/OHSS with high sensitivity and specificity.[12,15] Moreover, AMH may be a better predictive marker of excessive ovarian response to COS than age, basal follicle-stimulating hormone (FSH), and estradiol (E2) on the day of hCG administration and has been shown to be at least as good as antral follicle count (AFC).[12,14-16] Furthermore, AMH predicts ovarian response independently of age and PCOS.[15]

Activating mutations in the FSH receptor (FSHR) gene have been shown to confer a higher response to FSH and therefore FSHR genotype may predispose women to OHSS.[17] Although FSHR genotype cannot predict the risk of iatrogenic OHSS at present, it may be used to predict the severity of the condition. Furthermore, mutations in the bone morphogenic protein-15 (BMP-15) gene may predict ovarian hyper-response and OHSS, but further research is required.[17]

In a study by Kwee et al., an AFC more than 14 had the highest sensitivity (82%) and specificity (89%) to positively predict ovarian hyper-response.[18]

Risk of OHSS is observed in patients having higher number of immature follicles (<12 mm) and large follicles (> 18 mm) on the day of hCG administration, high E2 levels alone are poor predictors of OHSS.[19] The number of follicles in combination with serum E2 levels predicts OHSS with high sensitivity and specificity.[20] Despite E2 levels alone being poor predictors of OHSS, they are often closely monitored and used to drive secondary OHSS prevention strategies.

## ■ PREVENTION OF OHSS

This can be basically primary or secondary. Mechanism and management of OHSS has been described in Figure 2.

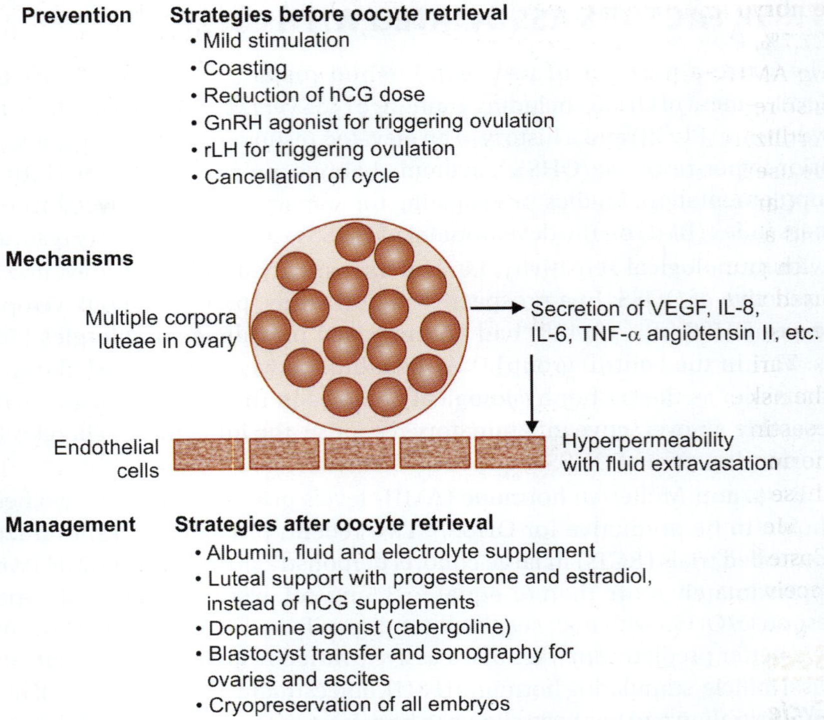

**Prevention** — **Strategies before oocyte retrieval**
- Mild stimulation
- Coasting
- Reduction of hCG dose
- GnRH agonist for triggering ovulation
- rLH for triggering ovulation
- Cancellation of cycle

**Mechanisms**

Multiple corpora luteae in ovary → Secretion of VEGF, IL-8, IL-6, TNF-α angiotensin II, etc.

Endothelial cells → Hyperpermeability with fluid extravasation

**Management** — **Strategies after oocyte retrieval**
- Albumin, fluid and electrolyte supplement
- Luteal support with progesterone and estradiol, instead of hCG supplements
- Dopamine agonist (cabergoline)
- Blastocyst transfer and sonography for ovaries and ascites
- Cryopreservation of all embryos

**Fig. 2:** Mechanisms and management of ovarian hyperstimulation syndrome.

# Primary Prevention

Prevention of OHSS is a multistage process. The key to the primary prevention of OHSS during COS is recognizing risk factors and individualizing the ovarian stimulation protocol appropriately using COS.[14,21]

Patients who have a primary risk of OHSS should be exposed to gonadotropins as little as possible. That means all other safer options like lifestyle changes to include diet and exercises, oral ovulation induction drugs, use of insulin sensitizers and laparoscopic ovarian drilling should be kept in mind. This holds true especially for young women and those with history of OHSS in the past.

Ovarian stimulation should aim to reduce the cycle cancellation rate and the iatrogenic complications of COS, including OHSS, and is key to improving ART outcomes.[15,21] Based on a retrospective study of 1,378 patients, basal FSH, BMI, age and number of follicles less than 11 mm at screening were reported to be the main predictive factors for ovarian response.[22]

The use of AMH, as a biomarker to individualize COS protocols, has been evaluated in a retrospective study of women undergoing ART.[23] The study compared 346 women using conventional COS with 423 women treated using COS protocols tailored to the level of AMH. The analysis reported increased embryo transfer rates (79–87%, P = 0.002), pregnancy rate per cycle (17.9–27.7%, P = 0.002) and live birth rate (15.9–23.9%, P = 0.007) in those women on AMH-tailored protocols compared with conventional COS. The study also reported a fall in the incidence of OHSS (96.9–2.3%, P = 0.002) and failed fertilization (7.8–4.5%, P = 0.066). In the future, pharmacogenetics could also be used to direct individualized COS.[17]

Careful history regarding thromboembolism in family, thrombophilia and antiphospholipid antibodies should be identified earlier to treatment with gonadotropins. Lowest possible doses of gonadotropins should be used with frequent monitoring with transvaginal scans and serum estradiol measurements. Prophylactic heparin can be used in selected cases.

Various preventative protocols have been proposed to reduce or minimize the risk of developing OHSS during COS, including in vitro oocyte maturation, coasting, decreasing the hCG trigger dose, and using a gonadotropin-releasing hormone agonist (GnRHa) trigger. However, despite the widespread use of these preventative techniques, supporting evidence is limited.

Metformin also has been used for prevention of OHSS. Study done by Costello MF et al., concluded that risk of OHSS significantly reduced in patients receiving metformin 2 months prior starting COC.[24]

## Secondary Prevention

### Cycle Cancellation

As OHSS is associated with hCG, terminating the ovulation cycle by cancelling the hCG trigger in the presence of several risk factors for OHSS is the most effective technique to prevent OHSS.[25] hCG induces the production of VEGF, the primary mediator of OHSS.[5] However, this course of action is costly and psychologically demanding for the participants. Therefore, it is usually reserved for patients at high risk of OHSS and those with total loss of cycle control.

### In Vitro Oocyte Maturation

Where immature oocytes are retrieved and matured in vitro before fresh embryo transfer, is also an option in these patients. In 56 patients with high risk of OHSS during the controlled ovarian hyperstimulation cycle, hCG was given when the leading follicle reached 12–14 mm in diameter.[26] Seventy-six percent of oocytes matured. All patients underwent fresh embryo transfers, resulting in a clinical pregnancy rate of 46%. There were no severe cases of OHSS. However, it is worth noting that in vitro maturation of oocytes remains an experimental procedure, used only in a small number of clinics around the world.

### Reducing hCG Dosage

Theoretically, decreasing the standard dose of hCG administered to trigger oocyte maturation (10,000 IU) might prevent OHSS. However, the benefit of low-dose hCG for the prevention of OHSS is not clear, as data are sparse and the studies that have been conducted comprised small sample sizes, involved a small number of cycles or were not powered to detect a difference in OHSS rate.[27]

### Coasting

In high risk patients with serum estradiol levels more than 3,000 pg/mL and/or more than 20 follicles per ovary, stimulation with gonadotropins can be stopped while continuing the GnRH agonist administration. The principle behind this management is that the larger follicles continue to grow while the intermediate and small follicles undergo atresia (FSH threshold theory).

Coasting also causes a downregulation of VEGF gene expression and protein production as a result of increased apoptosis in granulose cells of all, but mainly immature follicles, but does not influence oocyte quality and endometrial receptivity. Although, there are no clear guidelines when coasting should be started and stopped, this method is very popular with acceptable pregnancy rates. Based on studies coasting can be started when follicles are 14 mm in size and the estradiol levels are more than 3,000 IU. Coasting should not be more than 4 days since it can affect implantation rates.[28]

A recent Cochrane review concluded that there was no evidence to suggest a benefit of coasting to prevent OHSS compared with no coasting or other interventions, but only 4 of 16 studies included in the review met the RCT inclusion criteria.[29] Despite the lack of data from RCTs to support its use for the reduction of OHSS coasting has been widely adopted.

### Modification of the Ovulation Trigger Agent

An endogenous LH surge can be provoked by administration of a short acting GnRH agonist. This is only possible in cycles without pituitary desensitization by a GnRH agonist.

A single dose of recombinant LH can also be used. The development of recombinant LH (rLH) may offer an opportunity to replace hCG. The European rLH study performed a prospective and comparative study on the effective dose of rLH to induce oocyte maturation and luteinization in patients undergoing IVF. A dose of 15,000–30,000 IU rLH compares to 5,000 IU hCG resulting in similar number of oocytes, embryos and pregnancies.[30]

GnRH agonist (Triptorelin 0.2 mg) used as trigger agent in antagonist protocol significantly reduces chances of OHSS.

### Administration of Macromolecules

Prophylactic administration of 20% albumin is supposed to reduce the incidence of severe OHSS by preventing the fluid shift to the third space and binding factors responsible for the development of this syndrome.

The Cochrane review also shows that intravenous administration at the time of oocyte retrieval has a preventive effect in at-risk cycles. However, two studies have shown a reduced pregnancy rate after IV albumin. Albumin infusion has side effects like nausea, vomiting, and febrile reactions. Risk of viral transmission is also possible.

*Hydroxyethyl-starch solution (HES):* Works as effective as albumin, is cheaper and safer alternative. The recent Cochrane review of studies using IV albumin also analyzed the effects of HES at the time of oocyte retrieval in patients at high risk of OHSS in three RCTs. HES was associated with a significant reduction in the incidence of OHSS (OR 0.12, 95% CI 0.04–0.40), without affecting pregnancy rates.[31]

### Cryopreservation of all Embryos

Instead of cancelling the cycle, it is also possible to administer hCG as trigger, retrieve the oocytes and freeze all the resulting embryos. Although this can exclude late form of OHSS the early form can still occur and must be noted.

### Dopamine Agonists: Cabergoline

Most recent suggested strategy to prevent the development of OHSS is the use of low dose dopamine agonists such as cabergoline. It inhibits the phosphorylation of the VEGF receptor thereby preventing increased capillary permeability, the main action of VEGF.[9] In a study by Alvarez et al. 2007, cabergoline was given in the dose of 0.5 mg daily for 8 days starting from the day of hCG.[2] This was randomized with placebo. All patients underwent evaluation for OHSS. There was a statistically significant difference in the third space fluid collection in the cabergoline group. No difference was detected between groups in the fertilization, implantation, or pregnancy rates.

### GnRH Antagonist Administration

Studies, done by Lainas et al. (January 2009), showed that GnRH antagonist administration combined with cryopreservation of embryos for use in subsequent cycles might represent an effective approach for management of patients with severe OHSS. In the study the antagonist was administered daily for 1 week after retrieval.[32]

### Luteal Phase Support

A recent Cochrane review has shown that the choice of luteal phase support is related to the incidence of OHSS.[33] This review included a comparison of the use of progesterone versus hCG and progesterone, for luteal phase support, and showed an increased risk of OHSS in the groups taking hCG and progesterone (Peto OR 0.45, 95 % CI 0.26–0.79). The review concluded that the use of hCG should be avoided.

## TREATMENT OF OHSS

All patients of OHSS does not require inpatient management. Mild and moderate OHSS should be managed on outpatient basis.[34,10]

### Mild and Moderate OHSS

- Patient should be appropriately counseled and provided with information regarding fluid intake and output monitoring.
- Paracetamol and oral opiates including codeine can be offered to women for pain relief.
- Nonsteroidal anti-inflammatory drugs (NSAIDs) should be avoided as they may compromise renal function in women with OHSS.
- Clinicians and patients should be vigilant for signs that the severity of OHSS is worsening (RCOG guidelines, 2015).[10] These include:
  – Increasing abdominal distension and pain
  – Shortness of breath
  – Tachycardia or hypotension
  – Reduced urine output (< 1000 mL/24 hours) or positive fluid balance (more than 1,000 mL/24 hours)
  – Weight gain and increased abdominal girth
  – Increasing hematocrit (> 45%).

### Severe and Critical OHSS

- Patients with severe and critical OHSS must be hospitalized.
- Women with severe OHSS are at increased risk of thromboembolism. Although there are no trials on this subject, thromboprophylaxis should be provided for these women in view of the serious nature of this complication.
- GnRH antagonist administration and dopamine agonist help in quicker regression of established OHSS.[35]
- *Indications for paracentesis include the following:*[10]
  – Severe abdominal distension and abdominal pain secondary to ascites
  – Shortness of breath and respiratory compromise secondary to ascites and increased intra-abdominal pressure
  – Oliguria despite adequate volume replacement, secondary to increased abdominal pressure causing reduced renal perfusion.
- Paracentesis should be carried out under ultrasound guidance and can be performed abdominally or vaginally.
- Intravenous colloid therapy should be considered for women who have large volumes of fluid removed by paracentesis.

## KEY POINTS

- It is very important to identify high-risk patients prior to ART and choose appropriate therapy.
- Identification of all risk factors and its correlation with clinical features require more large randomized studies but can be the key to preventing and managing this rather dangerous condition.
- Patients who have a primary risk of OHSS should be exposed to gonadotropins as little as possible. That means all other safer options like lifestyle changes to include diet and exercises, oral ovulation induction drugs, use of insulin sensitizers and laparoscopic ovarian drilling should be kept in mind.
- Various preventative protocols have been proposed to reduce or minimize the risk of developing OHSS during COS, including in vitro oocyte maturation, coasting, decreasing the hCG trigger dose, and using a gonadotropin releasing hormone agonist (GnRHa) trigger.
- Using individualized protocols ovulation induction mostly using GnRH antagonist reduces chances of OHSS.

## REFERENCES

1. de Mouzon J, Goossens V, Bhattacharya S, et al. European IVF-monitoring (EIM) Consortium, for the European Society of Human Reproduction and Embryology (ESHRE): assisted reproductive technology in Europe, 2006: results generated from European registers by ESHRE. Hum Reprod. 2010;25:1851-62.
2. Alvarez C, Marti-Bonmati L, Maestre E, et al. Dopamine agonist cabergoline reduces hemoconcentration and ascites in hyperstimulated women undergoing assisted reproduction. J Clin Endocrinol Metab. 2007;92:2931-7.
3. Rova K, Passmark H, Lindqvist PG. Venous thromboembolism in relation to in vitro fertilization: an approach to determining the incidence and increase in risk in successful cycles. Fertil Steril. 2012;97(1):95-100.
4. Devroey P, Polyzos NP, Blockeel C. An OHSS-Free Clinic by segmentation of IVF treatment. Hum Reprod. 2011;26(10):2593-7.
5. Gómez R, Soares SR, Busso C, et al. Physiology and pathology of ovarian hyperstimulation syndrome. Semin Reprod Med. 2010;28:448-57.
6. Nastri CO, Ferriani RA, Rocha IA, et al. Ovarian hyperstimulation syndrome: pathophysiology and prevention. J Assist Reprod Genet. 2010;27:121-8.
7. Navot D, Bergh PA, Laufer N. Ovarian hyperstimulation syndrome in novel reproductive technologies: prevention and treatment. Fertil Steril. 1992;58:249-61.
8. Delvigne A, Rozenberg S. Review of clinical course and treatment of ovarian hyperstimulation syndrome (OHSS). Hum Reprod Update. 2003;9:77-96.
9. Soares SR, Gómez R, Simón C, et al. Targeting the vascular endothelial growth factor system to prevent ovarian hyperstimulation syndrome. Hum Reprod Update. 2008;14:321-33.

10. Royal College of Obstetricians and Gynaecologists. Reducing the Risk of Venous Thromboembolism during Pregnancy and the Puerperium. Green-top Guideline No. 37a. London: RCOG; 2015.
11. Humaidan P, Quartarolo J, Papanikolaou EG. Preventing ovarian hyperstimulation syndrome: guidance for the clinician. Fertil Steril. 2010;94:389-400.
12. Lee TH, Liu CH, Huang CC, et al. Serum anti-Müllerian hormone and estradiol levels as predictors of ovarian hyperstimulation syndrome in assisted reproduction technology cycles. Hum Reprod. 2008;23:160-7.
13. Enskog A, Henriksson M, Unander M, et al. Prospective study of the clinical and laboratory parameters of patients in whom ovarian hyperstimulation syndrome developed during controlled ovarian hyperstimulation for in vitro fertilization. Fertil Steril. 1999;71:808-14.
14. La Marca A, Sighinolfi G, Radi D, et al. Anti-Mullerian hormone (AMH) as a predictive marker in assisted reproductive technology (ART). Hum Reprod Update. 2010;16:113-30.
15. Nardo LG, Gelbaya TA, Wilkinson H, et al. Circulating basal anti-Müllerian hormone levels as predictor of ovarian response in women undergoing ovarian stimulation for in vitro fertilization. Fertil Steril. 2009;92:1586-93.
16. Broer SL, Dólleman M, Opmeer BC, et al. AMH and AFC as predictors of excessive response in controlled ovarian hyperstimulation: a meta-analysis. Hum Reprod Update. 2011;17:46-54.
17. Rizk B. Symposium: update on prediction and management of OHSS, genetics of ovarian hyperstimulation syndrome. Reprod Biomed Online. 2009;19:14-27.
18. Kwee J, Elting ME, Schats R, et al. Ovarian volume and antral follicle count for the prediction of low and hyperresponders with in vitro fertilization. Reprod Biol Endocrinol. 2007;5:9.
19. Papanikolaou EG, Humaidan P, Polyzos NP, et al. Identification of the high-risk patient for ovarian hyperstimulation syndrome. Semin Reprod Med. 2010;28:458-62.
20. Papanikolaou EG, Pozzobon C, Kolibianakis EM, et al. Incidence and prediction of ovarian hyperstimulation syndrome in women undergoing gonadotropin-releasing hormone antagonist in vitro fertilization cycles. Fertil Steril. 2006;85:112-20.
21. Bosch E, Ezcurra D. Individualised controlled ovarian stimulation (iCOS): maximising success rates for assisted reproductive technology patients. Reprod Biol Endocrinol. 2011;9:82.
22. Howles CM, Saunders H, Alam V, et al. Predictive factors and a corresponding treatment algorithm for controlled ovarian stimulation in patients treated with recombinant human follicle stimulating hormone (follitropin alfa) during assisted reproduction technology (ART) procedures. An analysis of 1378 patients. Curr Med Res Opin. 2006; 22:907-18.
23. Yates AP, Rustamov O, Roberts SA, et al. Anti-Mullerian hormone-tailored stimulation protocols improve outcomes whilst reducing adverse effects and costs of IVF. Obstet Gynecol Survey. 2011;66:760-76.

24. Costello MF, Chapman M. A systematic review and meta-analysis of randomised control trials on metformin co-administration during gonadotrophin ovulation induction or IVF in women with polycystic ovarian syndrome. Human Reprod. 2006;21:1387-99.
25. Delvigne A, Rozenberg S. Epidemiology and prevention of ovarian hyperstimulation syndrome (OHSS): a review. Hum Reprod. 2002;8:559-77.
26. Lim K, Lee W, Lim J. IVM after interruption of COH for the prevention of OHSS. Fertil Steril. 2005;84:S84-S85.
27. Kashyap S, Parker K, Cedars MI, et al. Ovarian hyperstimulation syndrome prevention strategies: reducing the human chorionic gonadotropin trigger dose. Semin Reprod Med. 2010;28:475-85.
28. Chen CD, Chao KH, Yang JH. Comparison of coasting and intravenous albumin in the prevention of ovarian stimulation syndrome. Fertil Steril. 2003;80:86-90.
29. D'Angelo A, Brown J, Amso NN. Coasting (withholding gonadotrophins) for preventing ovarian hyperstimulation syndrome. Cochrane Database Syst Rev. 2011;6:CD002811.
30. European Recombinant LH Study. Recombinant human luteinizing hormone is as effective as, but safer than, urinary human chorionic gonadotropin in inducing final follicular maturation and ovulation in vitro fertilization procedure: results of a multicentric double blind study. J Clin Endocrinol Metab. 2001;86:2607-18.
31. Youssef MA, Al-Inany HG, Evers JL, et al. Intravenous fluids for the prevention of severe ovarian hyperstimulation syndrome. Cochrane Database Syst Rev. 2011;2:CD001302.
32. Lainas TG, Sfontouris IA, Kolibianakis EM. Management of severe OHSS using GnRH antagonist and blastocyst cryopreservation in PCOS patients treated with long protocol. Reprod Biomed Online. 2009;18(1):15-20.
33. van der Linden M, Buckingham K, Farquhar C, et al. Luteal phase support for assisted reproduction cycles. Cochrane Database Syst Rev. 2011;10:CD009154.
34. Smith LP, Hacker MR, Alper MM. Patients with severe ovarian hyper stimulation syndrome can be managed safely with aggressive outpatient transvaginal paracentesis. Fertil Steril. 2009;92:1953-9.
35. Baumgarten M, Polanski L, Campbell B, et al. Do dopamine agonists prevent or reduce the severity of ovarian hyper stimulation syndrome in women undergoing assisted reproduction? A systematic review and meta-analysis. Hum Fertil (Camb). 2013;16:168-74.

CHAPTER

6

# Difficulties during Embryo Transfer

*ML Goenka, Deepak Goenka, Rashmi Goenka, Antima Rathore*

## ■ INTRODUCTION

Embryo transfer (ET) is the last, but one of the most important step in the process of in vitro fertilization (IVF). Although it is one of the most important factors that determine the outcome of IVF, yet it has been examined by only a few investigators.

The main objective of the ET is to deposit the embryos inside the uterine cavity, in a correct position, and more importantly, by an atraumatic method to maximize the chances of implantation.[1] The technique used for ET has a major impact on the IVF outcome. It has been observed that ET pregnancy rates differ depending upon the clinician performing the procedure even in the same IVF program. It is estimated that a poor ET technique may be responsible for 30% of all IVF failures.[2]

## ■ DEFINITION

A transfer is considered to be an "easy" transfer if it is performed smoothly without experiencing resistance on catheter while negotiating through cervical–uterine passage, with a complete and easy release of the embryos into the uterus. Examination of the catheter after "easy" ETs will reveal that it is usually devoid of mucus and blood.[1]

A "difficult transfer" is the one which requires uterine manipulation, multiple attempts, force, or rarely, dilatation, resulting into trauma to the endometrium. Difficult ETs have also been associated with increased uterine contractions, specially the junctional zone contractions which are capable of relocating the embryos and decreasing the implantation and pregnancy rates. Approximately 10% of all transfers can be classified as difficult.[3]

## ■ CLASSIFICATION OF EMBRYO TRANSFER DIFFICULTY

There is no universal definition of difficult ET. The difficulty experienced with ET may be categorized into slightly difficult, difficult, and very difficult.[4,5]

A *slightly difficult ET* is one where resistances is encountered using the soft catheter, but this is easily overcome by manipulation of the catheter alone or with the help of cervical tenaculum.

A *difficult ET* is one where the cervical os and/or the cervical canal require dilatation with the feeding tube or even with the uterine sound, use of rigid catheter or a soft catheter with stylet may be required. A speck of blood may be seen on the outer sheath of ET catheter.

A *very difficult ET* is one where the uterine sound as well as uterine dilator is used, in addition to the use of the cervical tenaculum to straighten the cervical canal. Most of these cases have cervical stenosis. Inner and outer catheter may have blood on their surfaces. Bleeding may be seen at external os.

## CAUSES

### Acute Anteflexion of Uterocervical Axis

An anteverted uterus is not an uncommon occurring.[1] However, the smooth introduction of the transfer catheter into the uterine cavity can be compromised by an acutely anteverted uterus. While introducing the catheter into the uterine cavity, the catheter strikes the anterior wall and stimulates the uterine contraction, and causes trauma. This can be prevented by straightening the uterocervical angle and thus, increasing the success of ETs. The uterocervical angle can be straightened by means of following techniques:

- *Distended bladder:* A distended bladder decreases the anteflexion of the uterus over the cervix, thereby straightening the uterocervical axis. On the contrary, posterior positions (retroverted) of uterus should not be further angulated posteriorly by a full bladder. This will result in an extremely difficult ET. In case of retroverted uterus, the uterocervical canal can be straightened by lifting the uterus anteriorly with the blade of the vaginal speculum.
- Holding the ectocervix with a tenaculum and gentle anterior traction would help in straightening of the uterocervical axis. However, holding the cervix with a vulsellum or tenaculum has been found to release oxytocin and to stimulate uterine junctional zone contractions.[6]
- Use of the metallic stylet can help to negotiate the internal cervical os and indicate the direction for insertion of the catheter. However, it can cause trauma to the endocervix and the endometrium, further compromising the results. It will also cause the discomfort to the patient.[7]
- Cervical stitch placement at the time of the ovum pickup. This will decrease the need for use of more traumatic tenaculum or vulsellum, for pulling the cervix.

## Cervical Stenosis

Presence of cervical stenosis produces hindrance to the passage of the ET catheter, resulting in difficulty in the catheter insertion, and increase in probability of manipulations, leading to kinking of the catheter or failure of the transfer.[4] In case of failure, the embryos had to be replaced using another more rigid catheter. This certainly exposes the embryos to the adverse environment for a longer duration. Ideally, embryos must be replaced in uterine cavity within 2 minutes of loading in ET catheter. ET in some cases may be extremely difficult or impossible even in the expert hands.

This problem can be tackled in the various ways. In case of prior failed attempt of ET due to cervical stenosis or anticipated stenosis, cervical dilatation before the attempt of the ET can be very useful. Cervical dilatation can be done using various methods, which includes:

### Cervical Dilatation

- *Metallic dilators:* Cervical dilatation using metallic dilators is done up to Hegar 9 under general anesthesia. However, it is associated with the trauma to the endocervix and the endometrium. It should be done at least 2 weeks before ET for healing of endocervix and endometrium.[8]
- *Hygroscopic cervical rods:* Cervical dilatation with hygroscopic cervical rods (Dilapan-S) has been suggested as an alternative to metallic dilators. The Dilapan-S rods are placed intracervically under general anesthesia and left for 4 hours and removed.[9]
- *Laminaria tents:* Slow dilatations of the cervical canal using laminaria tents have been tried. The tent is applied in the cervical canal under general anesthesia and removed after 24 hours.

Other methods such as transcervical placement of the "Malecot catheter" after hysteroscopic evaluation and use of stem pessaries have been suggested.

Most commonly used method of cervical dilatation is by Hegar's dilators. Cervical dilatation should be performed at the time of the initiation of gonadotropin administration in the cycles where fresh transfer has been planned. While in the frozen cycles, dilatation can be attempted during stimulation or one cycle prior to the one in which ET is done.

Dilatation performed at the time of oocyte retrieval may lead to an easier ET in patients with cervical stenosis but pregnancy rates are very low. The trauma and inflammation resulting from the dilatation procedure performed so close to ET will compromise the results.

Cervical dilatation frequently converts a difficult transfer to a moderate one but only rarely to an easy one. Despite of adequate dilatation, some form of difficulty may be encountered during the actual ET.

### Hysteroscopic Correction

Hysteroscopic correction of the cervical stenosis may be attempted in the cases where mechanical dilatation is inadequate or unsatisfactory. Hysteroscopic shaving of the cervical canal has been tried, but this technique itself may cause more harm to the cervical canal as it may initiate more fibrosis and may lead to cervical trauma or incompetence.

In some cases of difficult ET, despite all efforts, transcervical ET may not be possible. Some patients may have a history of surgery on the cervix, cervical fibroids, a history of diethylstilbestrol (DES) exposure or congenital anomalies that prevent the transcervical approach. In such cases, either transmyometrial embryo transfer (TMET) or tubal ETs are viable options.

## *Transmyometrial Embryo Transfer*

Transmyometrial approach can be used in the most difficult cases, where all the attempts of cervical dilatation have been futile. This is done using the transvaginal route under ultrasound guidance and general anesthesia. However, it is more invasive technique with myometrial trauma at the time of ET with lower pregnancy rate than transcervical approach. TMET is done with a special needle known as Towako Needle Set (Cook IVF, Queensland, Australia).[10] It consists of a needle, a matching stylet, and an inner catheter. The tip is echogenic to facilitate visualization by ultrasound. The matching stylet fits into the needle, with both bevels flushed. Needle is inserted with stylet to prevent blockage of needle by tissue debris. The 2 French polyethylene transfer catheter is used which is 1 mm longer than the needle. When its hub is pushed firmly into the Luer lock fitting of the needle, the catheter tip protrudes 1 mm beyond the needle tip.

## *Procedure*

1. Anesthesia is given.
2. The endometrial cavity is localized under transvaginal ultrasound guidance. The middle line in the case of a triple lined cavity may be easily visualized. In case of homogeneous echogenic endometrium, zoom-in on the endometrium to identify the central faint line depicting the endometrial cavity.
3. Towako needle with stylet is inserted through anterior vaginal fornix, and through the myometrium of the anterior uterine wall into the endometrium of the posterior uterine wall. In case of a retroverted uterus, needle is passed through posterior vaginal fornix via posterior myometrium into the endometrium of the anterior uterine wall.
4. Needle is then gently withdrawn into the uterine cavity and the stylet is removed.
5. The embryo loaded catheter is passed through the needle by the embryologist who then performs the embryo transfer.
6. Correct placement is confirmed by a flow of fluid seen inside the uterine cavity.
7. The needle and the catheter are then removed, and checked for retention of the embryo.

Approximate time taken (needle-in-uterus) is about 35 seconds (range: 31–47 seconds).

### Disadvantages
- The insertion of the Towako needle induces the junctional zone contraction, thereby reducing the clinical pregnancy rates.
- There is a risk of introduction of infection, while performing the procedure.

## Tubal Embryo Transfer

In patients with an impossible cervix but patent fallopian tubes, tubal embryo transfer (TET) can be employed with success. However, as the experience with gamete intrafallopian transfer (GIFT) has decreased over the years, the expertise with tubal transfers would have also declined. This must be taken into consideration when making this decision.

**Overcoming unanticipated difficult embryo transfer:**

On occasions, despite of adequate preparation, one may encounter a difficulty in transferring the embryo into the uterine cavity. In such cases, following steps can be useful:

1. Application of traction by tenaculum or vulsellum to straighten the uterocervical canal.
2. *After-loading technique:* Inner catheter with the loaded embryos can be returned to the embryologist, to be kept back in the incubator. Outer catheter alone is passed through the cervical canal. Once the tip of the outer catheter just crosses the internal os, inner catheter loaded with embryos can be introduced into the uterine cavity.
3. Wallace malleable stylet can be used to overcome the blockage at the internal os followed by subsequent passage of the inner catheter.
4. Switch to the hard catheter when all the maneuvers fail with the soft one.
5. Conscious sedation can be given to patient to allay her anxiety and increase cooperation during the procedure.
6. Finally, if all the attempts to transfer an embryo fail, it is better to cryopreserve the embryos and transfer them later on. Next attempt must be preceded by a trial ET and corrective measures.

## Removing the Mucus from Endocervical Canal

Cervical mucus interferes during ET procedure by blocking the passage of embryos through the tip of the catheter, dragging the embryos back from the releasing site, or contaminating the intrauterine environment with microorganisms. Therefore, it has been recommended that cervical mucus should be removed before ET to increase the pregnancy and live birth rates. One randomized control trial[11] and a prospective cohort study[11] demonstrated that removing mucus from the endocervical canal with sterile cotton swabs or aspiration with a catheter improves clinical outcomes.

## Trial Embryo Transfer

Dummy or mock or trial ET has been used to evaluate the exact passage of the ET catheter through the cervical canal, the length and the direction of the uterine cavity, and to determine the most suitable kind of ET catheter to be used for every patient. Such mock transfer not only detects the anatomically distorted cervical canals, but also an abnormally stenosed one. Therefore, dilatation can be attempted under anesthesia before the IVF treatment cycle, providing adequate time for the healing of the endometrium. In some patients, the pelvic adhesions pull the uterus acutely toward one side, and the dummy ET is useful to recognize the direction of the cervical canal. This will help to minimize the trauma at the time of the actual transfer.

## Transabdominal Ultrasound-guided Embryo Transfer

A difficult ET may result in the placement of embryos in nonideal locations. Ultrasound assistance can help in better visualization of catheter tip, as well as provide information of size, position and direction of uterus.[12,13] It also helps to avoid touching of uterine fundus and confirm the passage of catheter beyond the internal os. Ultrasound will also help to confirm the absence of fluid in endocavity after cervical mucus lavage. Visual confirmation of tip of catheter will also improve the participation of the patient, reduce the complication, and possibly decrease the couple's anxiety.

Ultrasound-guided ET has been found to increase implantation, pregnancy, and live-birth rates. Significantly higher pregnancy rates were observed when embryos were placed either 2 mm below the fundus or in the middle third of uterine cavity. Transabdominal ultrasound guided ET will help in proper positioning of the embryos.

## Selection of Catheter Type

Soft ET catheters are preferred over more rigid ones because the latter would be more likely to induce cervical and endometrial laceration. However, passing soft catheters through the cervical canal is often difficult and sometimes impossible. Failed ET and replacing the embryos using a different catheter is very frustrating and might have many adverse effects on the embryos. It has been suggested that every maneuver should be tried with a softer catheter before changing it to a firmer one, since it has a negative impact on the overall outcome due to the bleeding and uterine contraction.[14,15,16] However, too much maneuvering with the first catheter could produce trauma and introduction of blood, mucus, or bacteria, which is made worse by insertion of a second catheter.

## Use of Anesthesia in Difficult Embryo Transfer

General anesthesia can be utilized in difficult ET cases.[17] It serves to relax the sphincter of the internal cervical os, which is under voluntary control. Anesthesia allows the physician to use instruments such as a tenaculum, wider or longer speculum and multiple attempts which would otherwise be painful for the patient and result in uterine contractions. Conscious sedation is other preferred method of anesthesia compared to general anesthesia because of lesser morbidity and quicker recovery.

## Cryopreservation of Embryo during Difficult Embryo Transfer

In cases where negotiation of the catheter is expected to take prolong time, it is better to return the embryos to the IVF laboratory for cryopreservation, so that it can be transferred in the subsequent cycle after correction of the problem. Unnecessary prolong exposure of the embryos in the hostile environment will have a negative impact on the implantation and pregnancy rates.

### KEY POINTS

- Embryo transfer (ET) is considered a critical step in the IVF procedure. A difficult ET is the most frustrating clinical scenario at the end of an IVF cycle. Following steps will help in eliminating or overcoming most difficult ETs.
- A trial transfer performed will help in knowing the depth and shape of the uterus, selecting the optimal catheter type, and mapping the easiest and the least traumatic entry in the uterine cavity.
- ET should be done under transabdominal ultrasound guidance. This will help in proper guidance of catheter and placement of embryo in the uterine cavity at desired location.
- Use of soft catheter and removal of cervical mucus at the time of ET will improve clinical pregnancy and live birth rates.
- In anticipated difficult ET, patient should come empty stomach and anesthetist must be available, so that the anesthesia can be given, if needed.

### REFERENCES

1. Toth TL, Lee MS, Bendikson KA, et al. Embryo transfer techniques: an American Society for Reproductive Medicine survey of Current Society for Assisted Reproductive Technology practices. Fertil Steril. 2017;107:1003-11.
2. Madani T, Ashrafi M, Jahangiri N, et al. Improvement of pregnancy rate by modification of embryo transfer technique: a randomized clinical trial. Fertil Steril. 2010;94:2424-6.
3. Ghanem ME, Ragab AE, Alboghdady LA, et al. Difficult embryo transfer (ET) components and cycle outcome. Which is more harmful? Middle East Fertil Soc J. 2016;21:114-9.

4. Fiçicioglu C, Aksoy E, Dolgun N, et al. The difficulties encountered with embryo transfer and the role of catheter choice in clinical pregnancy success rates in an IVF cycle. Middle East Fertil Soc J. 2005;10(1):55-8.
5. Kava-Braverman A, Martíne F, Rodríguez I, et al. What is a difficult transfer? Analysis of 7,714 embryo transfers: the impact of maneuvers during embryo transfers on pregnancy rate and a proposal of objective assessment. Fertil Steril. 2017;107(3):657-63.
6. Lensy P, Killick SR, Robinson J, et al. Junctional zone contraction and embryo transfer: is it safe to use a tenaculum? Hum Reprod. 1999;14:2367-70.
7. Hagglund L, Ploman F, Sjoblom P. Characteristics of successful embryo transfer. Hum Reprod. 1999;14 (Suppl 3):29.
8. Abusheikha N, Lass A, Akagbosu F, et al. How useful is cervical dilatation in patients with cervical stenosis who are participating in an in vitro fertilization-embryo transfer program? The Bourn Hall experience. Fertil Steril. 1999;72(4):610-2.
9. Serhal P, Ranieri DM, Khadum I, et al. Cervical dilatation with hygroscopic rods prior to ovarian stimulation facilitates embryo transfer. Hum Reprod. 2003;18:2618-20.
10. Biervliet FP, Lesny P, Maguiness SD, et al. Transmyometrial embryo transfer and junctional zone contractions. Hum Reprod. 2002;17(2):347-50.
11. Practice Committee of the American Society for Reproductive Medicine. Performing the embryo transfer: a guideline. Fertil Steril. 2017;107:882-96.
12. Flisser E, Grifo JA, Krey LC, et al. Transabdominal ultrasound-assisted embryo transfer and pregnancy outcome. Fertil Steril. 2006;85:353-7.
13. Mirkin S, Jones EL, Mayer JF, et al. Impact of transabdominal ultrasound guidance on performance and outcome of transcervical uterine embryo transfer. J Assist Reprod Genet. 2003;20:318-22.
14. Munoz M, Meseguer M, Liza´n C, et al. Bleeding during transfer is the only parameter of patient anatomy and embryo quality that affects reproductive outcome: a prospective study. Fertil Steril. 2009;92(3):953-5.
15. Sallam HN, Agameya AF, Rahman AF, et al. Impact of technical difficulties, choice of catheter, and the presence of blood on the success of embryo transfer—experience from a single provider. J Assist Reprod Genet. 2003; 20(4):135-42.
16. Meriano J, Weissman A, Greenblatt EM, et al. The choice of embryo transfer catheter affects embryo implantation after IVF. Fertil Steril. 2000;74:678-82.
17. van der Ven H, Diedrich K, Al-Hasani S, et al. The effect of general anesthesia on the success of embryo transfer following human in vitro fertilization. Hum Reprod. 1988;3(Suppl 2):81-3.

CHAPTER
7

# Optimizing Embryo Transfer Technique

*Shiuli Mukherjee*

## ◼ INTRODUCTION

*Embryo transfer (ET)* refers to a necessary step in the process of assisted reproduction technology (ART) in which embryos are placed into the uterus of a female with the intent to establish a pregnancy. Nature chooses to implant one embryo for every intended pregnancy. The ultimate objective of any ART program is the birth of a healthy living baby. This outcome is based on multiple parameters which could be summarized under the following headings:

- Etiology of infertility.
- Efficient oocyte retrieval with adequate number of eggs.
- Proper laboratory techniques resulting in development of high quality embryos.
- A highly receptive endometrium.
- Efficient ET with minimum tissue injury.
- Skilled clinician to perform ET.
- Competent antenatal management.

The above-mentioned parameters are to be strictly maintained. The next step is under the control of in vitro fertilization (IVF) specialist. Successful outcome is dependent on the proper intrauterine transfer of high grade embryos. It has been estimated that poor ET technique may account for as much as 30% of all IVF failures,[1] and it has been seen that pregnancy rates differ significantly among different individuals performing ET with the same ART program.[2-4]

Generally, routine ET has been carried out on day 3, i.e. 72 hours after oocyte retrieval. However delaying ET till day 5 (blastocyst culture) has shown better pregnancy rates. Despite major advances in assisted reproductive techniques, the implantation rates remain low to allow the widespread use of single ET. Extra attention and time should be given to the procedure of ET so that it will be performed meticulously.[5]

## ■ TYPES OF EMBRYO USED

Embryos can be either "fresh" from fertilized egg cells of the same menstrual cycle, or "frozen", that is they have been generated in a preceding cycle and undergone embryo cryopreservation, and are thawed just prior to the transfer, which is then termed "frozen embryo transfer (FET)". The outcome from using cryopreserved embryos has uniformly been positive with no increase in birth defects or development abnormalities.[6] In fact, pregnancy rates are increased following FET, and perinatal outcomes are less affected, compared to embryo transfer in the same cycle as ovarian hyperstimulation was performed.[7]

In human, the uterine lining (endometrium) needs to be appropriately prepared so that the embryo(s) can implant. In a natural cycle the ET takes place in the luteal phase at a time where the lining is appropriately developed for nidation. In a stimulated or a cycle where a "frozen" embryo is transferred, the recipient woman could be given first estrogen preparations (about 2 weeks), then a combination of estrogen and progesterone so that the lining becomes receptive for the embryo.

## ■ PREEMBRYO TRANSFER PROCEDURE

### Trial or Sham Embryo Transfer

Different individuals have different cervical and uterine anatomy. Hence, a trial or practice ET is done. A higher pregnancy rate of 22.8% was seen with a previous trial transfer, as compared to no trial transfer group having a rate of 13.1%.[8] It is basically done to identify any discrepancies between perceived trial transfer depth and actual uterine cavity depth, and to describe which characteristics, if any, predispose patients to these differences. A dummy catheter is used in these transfers. The length and direction of the uterine cavity is measured which is noted for further use during the actual procedure. In case of difficult trial transfers patients are subjected to hysteroscopy. This can be done in both ways, under anesthesia or normally.

### Ultrasonographic Evaluation

The ultrasound (US) is a precise method to measure the length of uterine cavity and cervical canal. It is very important in evaluating the cervicouterine angle.[9,10] Ultrasonography is also essential in diagnosing the presence of fibroids and its encroachment on the uterine cavity or cervical canal. This condition can distort the uterine cavity and lengthen the cavity thus requiring the ET catheter to traverse large distances. Ultrasound also helps in evaluating the direction as well as degree of flexion of the uterus. Proper revision of the US findings prior to transfer, acts as an important guide to actual ET procedure. Ultrasound-guided transfer also helps the clinician to avoid hitting the fundus with the catheter and enables him/her to confirm that the catheter tip has just passed the internal OS atleast 1 cm prior to the injection of the embryos (Fig. 1).

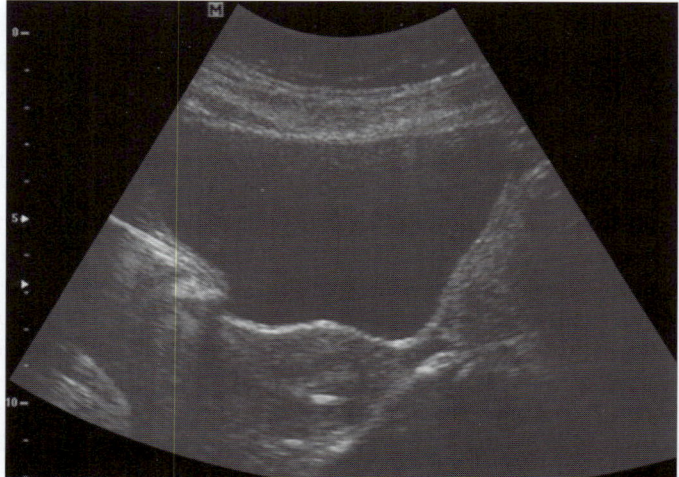

**Fig. 1:** Ultrasound image of embryo transfer.

## What is the Basic Target?

The atraumatic placement of the embryos 1.5 cm proximal to the fundus without pain, bleeding, trauma to the endometrium or embryos, and with the absence of uterine contraction. Ultrasound-guided transfer meets all the above-mentioned requirements thus serves as a visual treat to us, our parents and peers.

The Cochrane review reports that there are significantly higher clinical and ongoing pregnancies with ultrasound-guided embryo transfer than clinical touch (OR 1.38, 95%CI 1.16 to 1.64, P<0.0003).

## Hysteroscopy

It is the best method to detect the uterine cavity by endoscopy with access through the cervix. It allows for the diagnosis of intrauterine pathology and serves as a method for surgical intervention (operative hysteroscopy). It is usually done in cases where there is a high suspicion of uterine or cervical pathology and also in cases having history of repeated intrauterine inseminations (IUI) or ET. Hysteroscopy is useful in number of conditions:
- Endometrial polyp
- Abnormal uterine bleeding
- Adenomyosis
- Myomectomy or uterine fibroids.

It is seen that upto 45% of patients undergoing IVF had detectable uterine abnormalities like endometrial polyps, uterine malformations cervical stenosis.[11] The diameter of the hysteroscope is generally too large to conveniently pass the cervix directly, thereby necessitating cervical dilation to be performed prior to insertion. Cervical dilation can be performed by temporarily stretching the cervix with a series of dilators of increasing diameter.[12] Misoprostol prior to the hysteroscope with its sheath is inserted transvaginally guided into the uterine cavity, the cavity insufflated, and an inspection is performed. Hysteroscopy for cervical dilation appears to facilitate an easier and uncomplicated procedure only in premenopausal women.[13]

## ■ OPTIMUM CATHETERS USED FOR EMBRYO TRANSFER

Different types of catheters should be used for different patients. We can categorize Embryo Transfers into two categories—(1) easy embryo transfers, and (2) difficult embryo transfers.

### Soft Catheter

A soft catheter should be preferred for an easy ET. The value of soft ET catheters has been recognized since the beginning of IVF. The ideal catheter should be soft enough to avoid any trauma to the endometrium and malleable enough to find its way through the cervical canal into its uterine cavity.[14] Soft catheter is a combination of physical flexibility, malleability and smoothness of the tip. The soft catheter usually contains an outer sheath and a bulb like tip and a guard. The guard is adjusted according to the uterine cavity length. The outer sheath must be stopped at the internal cervical os (Figs. 2 and 3). Now under USG guidance the inner sheath is loaded with embryos and passed through the outer channel and lands upto the mid cavity of the uterus. However their extreme malleability makes them a liability in difficult ET.

### Soft Catheter with Stylette

In few cases or sometimes it happens that at the internal os of the cervix a spur remains. In these cases a stylette can surely negotiate the curvature of the endocervix. Catheter with stylette is especially useful in difficult embryo transfer for easy placement of the catheter. Using a malleable stylette to place

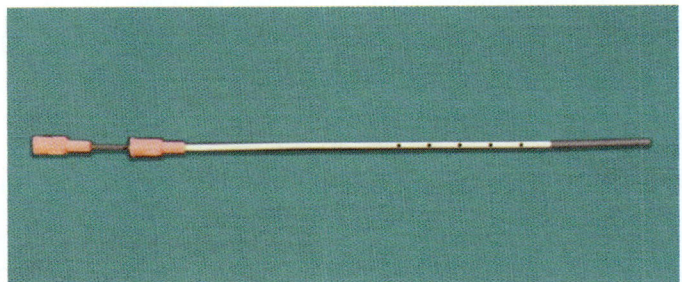

**Fig. 2:** Soft catheter used in embryo transfer (ET).

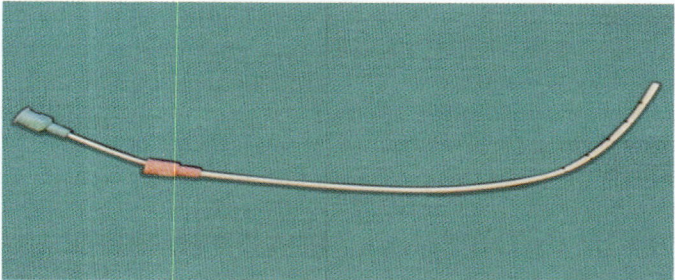

**Fig. 3:** Soft catheter with stylette.

the outer sheath correctly through the cervical canal before introducing the soft catheter did not have a negative impact on the implantation and the pregnancy rates. The embryologist loads the embryos into the inner sheath (under microscopic guidance) and then hands over this loaded catheter to the doctor. The doctor slowly withdraws the obturator out of outer sheath; after which the inner catheter (with its embryos) is slowly guided into the outer sheath. Once the tip of the inner catheter is beyond the other sheath (and safely within the uterine cavity), the embryos are placed gently into the uterine cavity by pushing the plunger of the syringe. The doctor then removes the inner and outer sheaths which are then checked by the embryologist to confirm that no embryos have been retained within them inadvertently.

## After-loading and Preloading Technique of Embryo Transfer

In after-loading technique the outer sheath is first inserted just on the internal os. Then internal sheath, carrying the embryos, is then supplied by the embryologist which is then inserted slowly by the clinician.

In the preloading technique the embryos are previously loaded into the inner sheath by the embryologist. This inner sheath loaded into the outer sheath is supplied by the embryologist to the clinician. This entire matter is then inserted into through the cervical canal by the clinician and the embryos are deposited in the mid cavity. This technique is usually not preferred as it involves high chances of loss of embryos as the inner sheath may kink inside the external os refusing to enter the internal os.

### ■ EMBRYO TRANSFER PROCEDURES

1. Confirmation of the name and identity of the patient who is made ready for the transfer.
2. Good embryos are selected by above-mentioned procedures. The selected embryos are washed and stored in 0.8 mL transfer media contained in Falcon™ Petri dish.

3. Patient is placed in lithotomy position. The ET procedure starts by placing a Cusco's speculum in the vagina to visualize the cervix. A soft[15] transfer catheter is loaded with the embryos and handed to the clinician. The catheter is inserted through the cervical canal and advanced into the uterine cavity.[16]
4. The catheter is passed under US-guidance control. The airtight syringe is opened and 10–15 μL of media is aspirated into the syringe. The syringe is attached to the catheter and media is expelled out till the piston of the syringe reaches the zero mark. In this way ET catheter is flushed with the medium and there is no air or dead space in the system.
5. After insertion of the catheter, the contents are expelled and the embryos are deposited. Mid cavity deposit of the embryos is made by advancing the piston of the syringe slowly.[17] After deposition there should be gentle pressure maintained on the syringe piston.
6. ET catheter can be withdrawn immediately or 30 seconds after the expulsion. A real time USG is done to confirm the proper placement of the embryos.
7. Following the ET, patient is made to stay supine on the ET table for 20–30 minutes. After this the patient is discharged with post-ET instructions.

## Postembryo Transfer Instructions

There are certain set of instructions which are to be followed by the patient during the posttransfer period. They are:
- The patient is advised an antibiotic course.
- The patient is provided with an adequate luteal support for a minimum period of 14 days till the beta-human chronic gonadotropin (β-hCG) test is carried out. The luteal support can be in form of—(1) tablet micronized progesterone (600 mg) pushed vaginally per day; (2) injection progesterone (50/100 mg) intramuscular per day; (3) Oral micronized progesterone (600 mg) per day; (4) progesterone gel 8% can be given.
- The patient is asked to report on any problem like abdomen pain, nausea, bleeding etc.

Standing shortly after ET does not plays a significant role in the final position of the embryo.[18] Many studies have shown that immediate getting up of the patient does not in in any way affect the result. Following the ET patient can easily walk home after 15–30 minutes of rest.[19]

## POTENTIAL NEGATIVE FACTORS ASSOCIATED WITH ET

Embryo transfer is routinely performed using the transcervical route, which is basically a blind technique associated with negative factors. They are:
- *Touching the uterine fundus:* It was seen that touching the uterine fundus with the catheter stimulated uterine contractions. Depositing the embryos in the mid fundal area of the uterus improved the pregnancy rates.[20,21]

- *Presence of cervical mucus:* Removal of the cervical mucus is advisable before ET to avoid any kind of adverse effects. It can be removed by repeated gentle aspirations using 1 cm$^3$ syringe with its tip placed at the external cervix os or using a soft catheter.
- *Uterine relaxing substances:* Serum progesterone levels on the day of ET correlate with the frequency of uterine contraction inversely.[22] Starting progesterone on the day of oocyte pick up to relax uterine contractility at the time of ET was suggested, although it did not improve the pregnancy rates as compared to starting it on the day of ET.[23]
- *Gentle manipulations:* Atraumatic delivery of embryos into the endometrial cavity is the prime goal of ET. Gentle manipulations should be observed even when introducing the vaginal speculum.

## PREVENTION OF EMBRYO EXPULSION

There are high chances of embryo expulsion after the ET process. So, after introducing the ET catheter in the uterine cavity the screw of the vaginal speculum is loosened so that its two valves press on the portio vaginalis of the cervix. After few minutes embryos are ejected and catheter withdrawn slowly. The speculum is kept in place pressing on the cervix for about 5–10 minutes and then removed.

## RETAINED EMBRYOS AFTER EMBRYO TRANSFER

The most important thing to do after the ET is to check the catheter for retained embryos. This problem occurs more frequently after difficult ET or when there is cervical mucus or blood. It decreases the implantation rates.[24,25] It is always advised to retransfer the retained embryos immediately.[26,27] The volume of the medium for ET is another cause for the embryos to be retained in the catheter. It is advisable to aspirate 10–15 μL of media first before aspirating the embryos to ensure the presence of enough media to push out the embryos. It is also advisable to withdraw the catheter slowly after ejecting the embryos to avoid creating any withdrawal of the embryos.

## EMBRYO TRANSFER TECHNIQUES AS A CAUSE OF ECTOPIC PREGNANCY

The risk of ectopic pregnancies following IVF was estimated to be 5% in a multicenter study undertaken on 1,163 pregnancies.[28] The authors reported a decrease in the ectopic rate associated with an increased distance between the fundus and the tip of the catheter. The midfundal deposition of the embryos reported in decreased rates of ectopic pregnancies. The size of the uterus also serves as a major cause for ectopic pregnancy. It was reported that the ectopic pregnancy rates were significantly higher in women with uterine cavity length less than 7 cm.[29]

## ADVANTAGES AND DISADVANTAGES OF EMBRYO TRANSFER[30]

A successful pregnancy and a healthy baby born are, of course, the biggest advantages of undertaking an ET procedure. Another advantage to ET is that it can be used to help bypass problems with a woman's fallopian tubes. ET was first pioneered for this very reason so women who had tubal damage or blockages could still have children of their own. Confirmation of fertilization is also an advantage of having ET treatment. As the embryo is formed outside artificially and then transferred to the uterus of the woman there are high chances of successful pregnancy.

A clear disadvantage with ET is that success is not guaranteed. In fact, less than 50% of all couples starting an IVF cycle will achieve a pregnancy. Of those who do become pregnant, not all of the pregnancies will result in a baby—a little over 25% of IVF cycles started, result in a live birth. Another disadvantage of ET is because the process involves an operative procedure, there are the associated risks of infection, anesthetic risks and hemorrhage. Ovarian hyperstimulation syndrome (OHSS) is also a risk that is only associated with treatment where the ovaries are stimulated through the use of medications, to make multiple eggs. Also despite all best efforts, embryos can implant in the wrong place (i.e. the fallopian tubes), which results in an ectopic pregnancy. This can quickly become a life-threatening situation requiring urgent surgery. In many cases an ET will not result in a successful implantation, despite everything being as optimal as possible.

## CONCLUSION

The main goal of ET is the skillful, gentle atraumatic, ultrasound-guided transfer of embryos near the fundus, without uterine contractions, pain bleeding or damage to the endometrium of the embryos. Trial, mock or dummy ET done in an office procedure in a cycle prior to the treatment cycle has its own advantages especially in cases suspected to present difficulty in negotiation of the cervical canal. If these goals can be attained it will result in a very successful ART program leading to the birth of a healthy and a living baby.

## REFERENCES

1. Madani T. Reply of the authors: improving of pregnancy rate by modifying embryo transfer technique. Fertil Steril. 2010;94(4):e69.
2. Fukuda A, Hakuri A, Matsuma H, et al. Performance of embryo transfer is critical to outcome of IVF especially in FET. Fertil Steril. 2012;98(3):S182.
3. Dessol L. Improving of pregnancy rate by modifying embryo transfer technique. Fertil Steril. 2010;94(4):e68.
4. Jungheim ES, Ryan GL. Embryo transfer techniques in the United States: a survey of clinics registered with the society of ART. Fertil Steril. 2010;94(4):1432-6.

5. Meldrum DR, Chetkwoski R. Evolution of a highly successful IVF embryo transfer programme. Fertil Steril. 1987;48:86-93.
6. Genetics and IVF Institute. Givf.com. [Accessed February, 2018].
7. Evans J, Hannan NJ, Edgell TA, et al. Fresh versus frozen embryo transfer: backing clinical decisions with scientific and clinical evidence. Hum Reprod Update. 2014;20(6):808-21.
8. Shamma FN, Lee G, Gutman JN. The role of office hysteroscopy in IVF. Fertil Steril. 1992;58(6):1237-9.
9. Mansour RT, Aboulgarh MA. Optimizing the embryo transfer technique. Hum Reprod. 2002;17:1149-53.
10. Sallam HN, Agameya AF, Rahman AF. Ultrasound measurement of the uterocervical angle before embryo transfer. Hum Reprod. 2002;17:1767-72.
11. H-Bar Yoseph, Levy A, Sonin Y. Morphological embryo assessment. Fertil Steril. 2011;95(5)1624-8.
12. ASRM. Laparoscopy and Hysteroscopy: A Guide for Patients. Washington, DC: American Society for Reproductive Medicine, Patient Education Committee; 2012.
13. Polyzos NP, Zavos A, Valachis A, et al. Misoprostol prior to hysteroscopy in premenopausal and post-menopausal women. A systematic review and meta-analysis. Hum Reprod Update. 2012;18(4):393-404.
14. Mansour RT, Aboulgarh MA. Optimizing the embryo transfer technique. Hum Reprod. 2002;17:1149-53.
15. Mains L, Van Voorhis BJ. Optimizing the technique of embryo transfer. Fertil Steril. 2010;94 (3):785-90.
16. Jain J. Embryo Transfer. [Video Accessed February, 2018].
17. Tiras B, Polar M. Impact of embryo placement depth on IVF and ET outcomes. Fertil Steril. 2010;94(4):1341-5.
18. Woolcott R, Stranger J. Ultrasound tracking of movement of embryo. Hum Reprod. 1998;13(8):2107-9.
19. Sharif K, Afnan M, Lenton W. The Birmingham experience of 103 in IVF cycles with no bed rest following embryo transfer. Hum Reprod .1995;10(60:1427-9.
20. Waterstone J, Curson R, Parson J. Embryo transfer to low uterine cavity. Lancet. 1991;3:1413.
21. Oliveria JB, Martins AM, Baruffi RL. Increased implantation and pregnancy rates obtained by placing the tip of the transfer catheter in the central area of the endometrial cavity. Reprod Biomed Online. 2004;17:341-6.
22. Fanchin R, Righini C Olivennes F. Uterine contraction at the time of ET alter pregnancy rates after IVF. Hum Reprod. 1998;13:1968-74.
23. Baruffi R, Mauri AL, Petersen CG. Effects of vaginal progesterone administration starting on the day of oocyte retrieval on pregnancy rates. J Assist Reprod Genet. 2003;20:517-20.
24. Visser DS, Fourie FL. Multiple attempts at embryo transfer. J Assist Reprod Genet. 1993;10:37-43.
25. Alvero R, Hearns Stokes RM, Seagers JH. The presence of blood in the transfer catheter negatively influences outcome at ET. Hum Reprod. 2003;18:1848-52.

26. Tur K, Yuval Y. Difficult or repeated sequential ET do not adversely affect IVF pregnancy rates or outcome. Hum Reprod. 1998;13:2452-5.
27. Leeton HC, Seifer DB. Impact of retained embryos on the outcome of ART. Fertil Steril. 2004;82:334-7.
28. Ohen J, Mayuax MJ. IVF and ET a collaborative study on 1163 pregnancies on the incidence and risk factors of ectopic pregnancies. Hum Reprod. 1986;14:255-8.
29. Egbase PE, Al Sharan M, al-Othman S, et al. Incidence of microbial growth from the tip of embryo transfer catheter after ET in relation to clinical pregnancy rate following IVF and ET. Hum Reprod. 1996;11:1687-9.
30. Fertilitysolutions. [2017]. Advantages and Disadvantages of IVF. [online] Available at: http://fertilitysolutions.com.au/advantages-and-disadvantages-of-ivf/. [Accessed February, 2018].

CHAPTER

8

# How to Improve Poor Endometrium in ART

*Paramita Hazari, Gautam Khastgir*

## ■ INTRODUCTION

Endometrium is a dynamic tissue which undergoes complex cyclical changes at morphological, biochemical and molecular stages governed by circulating estrogen and progesterone. Any deviation of these levels in luteal phase can cause implantation failure.[1] For a successful implantation and pregnancy outcome, the quality of embryo as well as the receptivity of endometrium both play a pivotal role. Various studies showed that endometrial receptivity is responsible for two-thirds of implantation failure.[2]

Poor endometrium is a frequent problem in assisted reproductive treatment leading to cycle cancellation, treatment delay and unplanned embryo cryopreservation. Thin endometrium is unable to support pregnancy development after implantation resulting in early miscarriages as well as it can lead to placenta accreta and postpartum hemorrhage. Though many theories are proposed, Casper et al. provided a revolutionary explanation stating that, when embryo is exposed to thin endometrium, it is closer to more vascularized stroma, thereby exposing the embryo to a much higher oxygen tension leading to implantation failure. Another explanation proposes dysfunction in estrogen receptor to be responsible for impaired endometrial proliferation and implantation.[3] In addition, controlled ovarian hyperstimulation has an adverse effect on endometrial receptivity and therefore, freezing of embryos and transfer in hormone replacement therapy (HRT)-frozen embryo transfer (FET) cycle is advocated to improve implantation rate. Thin endometrium is more likely seen in older patients with an incidence of 25% as compared to 5% in age group less than 40 years. This is mainly due to decreasing vascularity of endometrial tissue.[4,5]

Suboptimal endometrium is defined as endometrial thickness (ET) less than 7 mm or endometrial volume less than 2.5 cc or homogenous and non-multilayered endometrial pattern (in ultrasound) on the day of human chorionic gonadotropin (hCG) trigger or after 10–12 days of estrogen support. In a meta-analysis, endometrium less than or equal to 7 mm showed a correlation with decreasing chances of pregnancy in in vitro fertilization (IVF) patients although the cut off less than or equal to 7 mm was only seen in 2.4% patients. Thus, ET can only give us probability and is not predictive of pregnancy. Author suggested that ET cannot be used as a sole parameter to decide on cycle cancellation, freezing of all embryos or discontinuing IVF cycle.[6]

Endometrial thickness is widely used parameter to evaluate endometrial receptivity. In view of the fact that ET has poor sensitivity and predictive value, various other means of endometrial assessment are also being considered. These are endometrial pattern, endometrial volume, endometrial histologic dating, endometrial and subendometrial vascularity by 3D power Doppler, endometrial receptivity assay (ERA) and subendometrial contractility waves and matris.[4]

## ■ CAUSES OF THIN ENDOMETRIUM

Thinning of endometrium can be idiopathic or as a consequence of endometrial damage or impairment of vascular supply. Some of the factors responsible for thinning of endometrium are mentioned hereunder:
- *Drugs:* Clomiphene citrate, oral contraceptive pills, gonadotropin-releasing hormone (GnRh) analogs and progesterone contraceptives.
- *Surgical:* Dilation and curettage, postpartum curettage, following TCRF, ablation therapy, septoplasty, adhesiolysis, aggressive myomectomy, post-Strassman surgery.
- Radiotherapy
- *Infections*: *Streptococcus, Escherichia coli, Staphylococcus, Enterococcus, Ureaplasma urealyticum, Clamydia*, tuberculosis.
- Congenital Müllerian anomalies.

## ■ TREATMENT OF THIN ENDOMETRIUM

Various treatment modalities to improve thin endometrium are discussed below:

### Estrogen

It is the first approach by a clinician when encountered with a patient with thin ET. Exogenous estrogen alters serum and endometrial estrogen levels. E1 or estrone is the least potent estrogen and E2 is the potent estradiol. Estrogen helps in endometrial proliferation by spiral artery contraction and reducing oxygen tension of the functional layer in the proliferative phase which facilitates embryo implantation. This concept had been the basis of adding exogenous estrogen in patients with thin ET. Estrogen preferred is micronized estradiol or estradiol valerate.

Various routes of administration are oral, transdermal, vaginal and intramuscular. Oral estrogen undergoes first-pass metabolism and also metabolism in endometrium resulting in higher E1/E2 ratio. Nonoral routes bypass first-pass metabolism, and therefore, has a higher endometrial concentration leading to low E1/E2 ratio. However, parenteral route has the highest and most stable estradiol concentration with 2 injections per week (8 mg/week) but injections are painful and have a risk of abscess formation. Transvaginal estrogen administration is a very good alternative to parenteral route, but there runs a risk of vaginal estrogen and progesterone interaction leading to drop in serum estradiol levels. Vaginal estrogen also increases uterine contractility which may hamper embryo implantation. Transdermal application is thereby preferable when it comes to serum estradiol level and side effects.

In fresh stimulated cycles, endometrium develops due to endogenous estrogen secreted from growing follicles. Therefore, estrogen support is more significant in HRT-FET and ovum or embryo donated cycles. Estrogen can be given in escalating dose or at high dose (up to 16 mg) from D1 of the cycle. Some studies have mentioned the escalating dosage is not so beneficial as it can lead to decrease in endometrial receptors.[7] Endometrial response also depends on duration of estrogen treatment rather than serum estradiol concentration. Chen et al. in his study have shown extended estrogen support in HRT-FET cycles for 14–82 days improves mean ET from 6.7 mm to 8.6 mm with significant increase in pregnancy rates.[8]

## Gonadotropin-releasing Hormone Agonist

Luteal phase support with GnRH agonist is another method to improve endometrial lining.

In a study, 120 patients were evaluated, in which 60 patients received 0.1 mg of triptorelin on days of egg collection, embryo transfer and 3 days after embryo transfer whereas other 60 patients served as control. The study highlighted significant increase in ET and pregnancy rate.[8]

## Low Dose Human Chorionic Gonadotropin

Human chorionic gonadotropin upregulates various cytokines and growth factors in the endometrium promoting endometrial differentiation and receptivity. Papanikolau et al. in his pilot study studied 17 ovum and embryo recipient patients in whom 150 IU of hCG were given subcutaneously starting from D8/D9 of estrogen administration for 7 days. In 70.6% of patients, improvement in ET was noted and pregnancy rate was 52.9%.[9] In another nonrandomized clinical trial, 150 IU hCG was given intramuscularly to 28 patients from day 8 of FET cycle till ET achieved was 7 mm. Study demonstrated a significant improvement in ET and pregnancy rate with hCG administration.[8]

## Selective Estrogen Receptor Modulator

Tamoxifen is a selective estrogen receptor modulator (SERM) which has estrogen agonist effect. Tamoxifen given at a dose of 40 mg from D3–D9 in intrauterine insemination cycles has a thicker ET with a higher clinical pregnancy rate as compared to the group who was only given 100 mg CC on D3–D7 with alternating human menopausal gonadotropin (hMG) (150 IU).[1]

Recently Ke et al. stimulated endometrial growth in FET cycles by using tamoxifen. The group showed improvement in ET. However, tamoxifen offered greatest advantage in polycystic ovarian disease patients in terms of pregnancy rates.[10]

## Pentoxifylline and Tocopherol

Pentoxifylline induces vasodilatation and tocopherol acts as an antioxidant in treatment of thin endometrium. Studies have showed when pentoxifylline and tocopherol (800 mg and 1,000 IU, respectively) combination was given for 6–8 months in infertility patients who had inadequate endometrium with vaginal estrogen. There was marked improvement in ET, pregnancy and delivery rates at the end of the treatment. Though both drugs in combination worked well but there was no change in implantation and ongoing pregnancy rate with tocopherol only. Combination of pentoxifylline and tocopherol has also proven to improve ET in patients with radiation-induced thin endometrium.[8]

## Low Dose Aspirin

Aspirin increases endometrial blood flow by decreasing impedance across uterine artery. Some studies reported improved ET, pattern and blood flow but meta-analysis and Cochrane study revealed no benefit in clinical pregnancy or live birth rate with low dose aspirin.[8]

## Vaginal Sildenafil

It is a phosphodiesterase inhibitor which stops breakdown of cyclic guanosine monophosphate (cGMP) and enhances vascular muscle relaxation through nitric oxide (NO)-cGMP pathway. This vasodilatory effect of NO increases subendometrial blood flow. It is given vaginally at dosage of 25 mg 4 times per day x 8–12 days during fresh or HRT cycles. After this treatment, there is a marked increase in diastolic flow as indicated by reduced pulsatility index (PI) on color Doppler. Positive effect of sildenafil was noted in various trials, most recently shown by Eid et al. where vaginal sildenafil was inserted in 22 patients with thin ET and high PI for 7 days between ovulation trigger and embryo transfer. 68% patients had increased ET with 26% and 40% increase in implantation and pregnancy rates, respectively.[11]

## Nitroglycerin

Nitroglycerin releases nitric oxide which acts as a vasodilating agent. It helps in endometrial cycle control and uterine preparation for pregnancy. It is also a useful therapy in patients with thin endometrium due to vasodilatory effect. The effect of Nitroglycerin patches was evaluated in two studies in patients with RIF when used during D9-12 of menstrual cycle but no beneficial effect was observed. Therefore, there is no current evidence of its usage in thin endometrium.[8]

## L-arginine

It is an essential amino acid which is the main substrate for nitric oxide synthesis, thereby, playing an important role in uterine flow regulation. Takasaki et al. in 2010 used arginine at a dosage of 6 mg per day in 9 women with persistent thin endometrium. Author demonstrated increased blood flow in radial uterine arteries in 89% of their patients and endometrial growth of more than 8 mm in 67% patients. However, further studies are required to validate its use in clinical practice.[12]

## Granulocyte Colony-stimulating Factor

Granulocyte colony-stimulating factor (GCSF) is a glycoprotein which acts as a growth factor and cytokine. It is secreted from vascular endothelium, ovarian follicles, macrophages and other immunocytes. GCSF increases endometrial stromal cell decidualization via autocrine and paracrine route. In addition, GCSF stimulates endometrial stem cells and mobilizes bone marrow stem cells (BMSCs) to promote endometrial cellular differentiation and proliferation. It also plays a key role in implantation and pregnancy maintenance by inducing trophoblastic proliferation and invasion. It is also believed that GCSF helps in modulation of genes favoring adhesion of embryo, cell migration, tissue remodeling and angiogenesis.

Gleicher et al. in 2011 first introduced GCSF treatment to facilitate endometrial development. In this case study, four women with persistent thin endometrium (in spite of using estrogen and vaginal sildenafil) were given 300 mcg of GCSF in the uterine cavity 2-9 days before ET. In all the cases, endometrium measured was more than 7 mm and all four patients conceived but one had ectopic pregnancy.[13]

Intrauterine infusion of GCSF with endometrial scratch is another treatment option which can be explored in patients with thin endometrium as envisaged by Xu et al. In this study, higher embryo implantation rate and clinical pregnancy rate were observed. Endometrial scarification caused by scratching removes fibrous tissue, mucus and endometrium with proliferation disorder from endometrial surface, so that GCSF is absorbed easily.[14]

Meta-analysis of GCSF usage was conducted up to May 2016 which showed higher implantation and pregnancy rate, although not statistically significant. Study also showed GCSF administered subcutaneously had a better outcome than local uterine infusion.[2] GCSF can be given in one or two doses in the follicular phase of cycle, on the day of hCG trigger, on the day of ovulation or on the starting day of progesterone.[5]

Various studies thereafter similarly showed increase in ET, low cycle cancellation rate and better implantation rate but some studies failed to demonstrate any difference in ET and clinical pregnancy rate. The only randomized controlled trial conducted till date on GCSF was unable to show any favorable outcome with respect to endometrial growth or pregnancy rate. Limited data is available regarding GCSF in improving endometrial receptivity in patients of recurrent implantation failure and recurrent pregnancy loss.[7]

## Stem Cell

Stem cell therapy is a newer concept of improving endometrium especially in refractory cases. Endometrium or menstrual blood serves as a source of stromal fibroblast or clonogenic multipotent stem cell. These cells have multilineage potential. Basalis layer of endometrium contains 0.22% epithelial and 1.25% stromal or mesenchymal stem cells that differentiates to regenerate endometrium. Bone marrow derived hematopoietic and nonhematopoietic stem cells incorporate into the endometrium and transdifferentiate into endometrial, stromal and endothelial cells. CD45 cells arising from hematopoietic stem cells help in endometrial epithelial cell regeneration, endothelial progenitors help in neovascularization of endometrium, and stromal components help in healing especially after injury or inflammation. It is noted that ischemia or reperfusion or injury of uterus results in two-fold increase in BMSCs recruitment to the endometrium. Thus, BMSC helps in regeneration of endometrium and has been the basis of its therapeutic usage on thin and damaged endometrium.

First report of usage of BMSC to treat a damaged thin endometrium was by Nagori et al. in 2011. Bone marrow aspiration was done from patient's iliac crest. Endometrial curettage was done followed by ultrasound-guided transcervical uterine instillation of 0.7 mL of BMSC suspension on day 2 of menstrual cycle. Additionally, estrogen support and aspirin were given which resulted in ET more than 7 mm and it resulted in a live pregnancy.[15] Recently, Singh et al. reported a case series of six patients with secondary amenorrhea where 3 months of BMSC was implanted in subendometrial zone at 2–3 sites (fundus, anterior and posterior part of myometrium) using transmyometrial route. Mean ET achieved was 5.5 mm.[16] A human pilot trial was done infusing autologous CD133+ BMSC into spiral arterioles of 11 patients with refractory Asherman's syndrome and five patients with refractory endometrial atrophy. Increase in ET lasting up to 6 months was noted in patients with Asherman's syndrome (4.3 mm to 6.7 mm) and those in refractory atrophic endometrium

(4.2 mm to 5.7 mm) leading to three spontaneous conceptions and seven pregnancies after IVF-ET.[1]

Stem cell therapy is a promising option for patients with Asherman's syndrome, inadequate endometrium or in cases of severe endometrial damage where surgical and medical treatment has failed to improve ET and function. It is an invasive treatment option where bone marrow biopsy and interventional radiology to inject into the uterine arterioles is required. However, more research studies are needed to determine its safety, effectiveness and cost before incorporating this treatment in clinical practice.

## Autologous Platelet-rich Plasma

Intrauterine infusion of platelet-rich plasma (PRP) is a new arena of research in patients with poor endometrial growth.

Fresh whole blood is collected from peripheral vein which is then centrifuged. Clotting activates platelets which release cytokines and growth factors (vascular endothelial growth factor, transforming growth factor, platelet-derived growth factor and epidermal growth factor), thereby improving endometrial growth and receptivity. In comparison to GCSF, it is more accessible and affordable and there are less chances of immunogenic reaction.

Its first usage was reported by Chang et al. in 2015 where intrauterine injection of 0.5 mL PRP is instilled in 5 patients with thin ET on 10th day of HRT. If ET was still less than 7 mm after 72 hours, then a second infusion was made. All 5 patients had ET greater than 7 mm and each one of them conceived.[17]

Recently, in 2017, another case series was reported where intrauterine PRP was infused in 10 patients who had previous cancelled cycles due to poor endometrial growth. PRP was infused on D11–12 and repeated on D13–14. In all patients, ET achieved was more than 7 mm and 5 patients conceived, 4 patients of which had ongoing clinical pregnancy.[18] More research-oriented work still needs to be done to gather evidence in favor of this treatment.

## Hysteroscopy

Hysteroscopy is gold standard method of diagnosing previously unrecognized uterine pathology. It can be used to diagnose adhesions or fibrosis and at the same time, adhesiolysis can be done which might be a cause of recurrent thin endometrium. On the other hand, hysteroscopic manipulation or distension of the cavity can increase endometrial receptivity through immunological mechanism.[7]

## Acupuncture, Electroacupuncture and Neuromuscular Electrical Stimulation

Acupuncture is one of the oldest therapeutic intervention which can be incorporated in assisted reproductive technology (ART). Several randomized controlled trials show electroacupuncture reduces the resistance across uterine artery in infertility patients undergoing IVF but no significant difference in pregnancy rate was noted. It can be done twice weekly for 4 weeks.[1] Neuromuscular electrical stimulation (NMES) is used in patients with thin endometrium for 3–4 days starting from day 9 of stimulation. Endometrium thickness significantly increased in the treatment group, but no difference in clinical pregnancy rate was observed.[1]

## ■ CONCLUSION

Thin endometrium nonresponsive to standard treatment is still a challenge and clinical dilemma in ART. There is no single clinical approach to treat thin endometrium and no treatment has been validated so far. Transfer of embryos in HRT-FET cycles is a better option to yield better results. Additionally, hysteroscopic evaluation of uterine cavity is essential. If conventional treatment failed to increase endometrium then endometrial receptivity can be studied. Extended estrogen support may be the easiest treatment option, but is not the solution in every case. Sildenafil is the first line of treatment now followed by GCSF. GCSF is the potential and most popular treatment option but results are not consistent. Other treatment options like low dose aspirin, nitrates, hCG, tocopherol and arginine lacks evidence to support clinical application. Stem cell therapy is a promising new treatment modality that is undergoing clinical trials. Initial evaluation though is encouraging but still we need to wait before we incorporate in clinical practice. Thus, there is paucity of evidence to support one treatment over another. In spite of all these approaches, a subset of patients still remains nonresponsive to these remedies. We hope that in the near future we will be able to get clear-cut guidelines which may benefit pregnancy outcome in refractory cases.

## ■ KEY POINTS

- Endometrial receptivity is a complex process responsible for two-thirds of implantation failure.
- Endometrial thickness is a marker of endometrial receptivity.
- Estrogen and sildenafil are the first-line therapy.
- GCSF, stem cell therapy and PRP are new approaches which are being studied extensively in recent years.
- Treatment of thin endometrium is still a clinical enigma.

## ■ REFERENCES

1. Mouhayar Y, Sharara FI. Modern management of thin lining. Middle East Fertil Soc J. 2017; 22:1-12.
2. Zhao J, Xu B, Zhang Q, et al. Whether G-CSF administration has beneficial effect on the outcome after assisted reproductive technology? A systematic review and meta-analysis. Reprod Biol Endocrinol. 2016;14(62):1-9.

3. Casper RF. It's time to pay attention to the endometrium. Fertil Steril. 2011;96(3):519-21.
4. Samara N, Bentov Y. Current strategies to manage a thin endometrium. Scient Open Access J. 2016;2(4):1-6.
5. Mahajan N, Sharma S. The endometrium in assisted reproductive technology: How thin is thin? J Hum Reprod Sci. 2016;9(1):3-8.
6. Kasius A, Smit JG, Torrance HL, et al. Endometrial thickness and pregnancy rates after IVF: a systematic review and meta-analysis. Hum Reprod Update. 2014;20(4):530-41.
7. Garcia-Velasco JA, Acevedo B, Alvarez C, et al. Strategies to manage refractory endometrium: state of the art in 2016. Reprod. Biomed Online. 2016;32 (5):474-89.
8. Eftekhar M, Tabibnejad N, Tabatabaie AA. (2017). The thin endometrium in assisted reproductive technology: An ongoing challenge. [online]. Available from https://www.sciencedirect.com/science/article/pii/S1110569017302947?via%3Dihub. [Accessed February 2018].
9. Papanikolaou EG, Kyrou D, Zervakakou G, et al. Follicular HCG endometrium priming for IVF patients experiencing resisting thin endometrium. A proof of concept study. J Assist Reprod Genet. 2013;30:1341-5.
10. Ke H, Jiang J, Xia M, et al. The effect of tamoxifen on thin endometrium in patients undergoing frozen-thawed embryo transfer. Reprod Sci. 2017:1933719117698580.
11. Eid ME. Sildenafil improves implantation rate in women with a thin endometrium secondary to improvement of uterine blood flow; "pilot study". Fertil Steril. 2015;104(3):e342.
12. Takasaki A, Tamura H, Miwa I, et al. Endometrial growth and uterine blood flow: a pilot study for improving endometrial thickness in the patients with a thin endometrium. Fertil Steril. 2010;93:1851-8.
13. Gleicher N, Vidali A, Barad DH. Successful treatment of unresponsive thin endometrium. Fertil Steril. 2011;95:13-7.
14. Xu B, Zhang Q, Hao J, et al. Two protocols to treat thin endometrium with granulocyte colony-stimulating factor during frozen embryo transfer cycles. Reprod Biomed Online. 2015;30 (4):349-58.
15. Nagori CB, Panchal SY, Patel H. Endometrial regeneration using autologous adult stem cells followed by conception by in vitro fertilization in a patient of severe Asherman's syndrome. J Hum Reprod Sci. 2011;4(1):43-8.
16. Singh N, Mohanty S, Seth T, et al. Autologous stem cell transplantation in refractory Asherman's syndrome: a novel cell based therapy. J Hum Reprod Sci. 2014;7(2):93-8.
17. Chang Y, Li J, Chen Y, et al. Autologous platelet-rich plasma promotes endometrial growth and improves pregnancy outcome during in vitro fertilization. Int J Clin Exp Med. 2015;8:1286-90.
18. Zadehmodarres S, Salehpour S, Saharkhiz N, et al. Treatment of thin endometrium with autologous platelet-rich plasma: a pilot study. JBRA Assist Reprod. 2017;21(1):54-6.

CHAPTER

# 9

# Personalized Luteal Phase Support in Assisted Reproductive Technology

*Seema Pandey, Sujata Kar*

## ■ INTRODUCTION

Treatments that make assisted reproductive technology (ART) include in vitro fertilization (IVF), intracytoplasmic sperm injection (ICSI), and frozen embryo transfer (FET). These treatments frequently consist of either the transfer of an embryo into a woman who has undergone controlled ovarian hyperstimulation (COH) with oocyte retrieval or a woman receiving an embryo in a nonovulatory cycle (FET or a fresh embryo transfer of embryos from donor eggs into a recipient). In all these situations, there is a luteal phase defect.

Recently lots of focus was given to fragmented IVF cycles in lieu of ovarian hyperstimulation syndrome (OHSS), our main concern, and many clinics worldwide have adopted to freeze all and FET transfers. But still many IVF clinics do not have very good vitrification program and recent research proving increased miscarriage rates in FET cycles than fresh transfers, epigenetic modifications in vitrified embryos, and an increased rates of congenital malformations in a fetus born as a result of ICSI with freeze all and FET.[1,2] This newer concept of individualized luteal phase support, where our aim is to design a protocol which gives an excellent ongoing pregnancies and good live-birth rates irrespective of fresh or frozen transfer and as per the need of the patient.

### What is luteal phase?

From our physiology days, we understand that follicular phase culminates with maturation of Graafian follicle, granulosa cell of this dominant follicle in turn secretes more estradiol and this in return triggers luteinizing hormone (LH) surge from anterior pituitary. This LH surge propagates a series of events:
- Breakdown of the connection of granulosa cells comprising the cumulus oophorus.
- Reentry of the oocyte into the diplotene phase of prophase 1 meiosis.
- Eventual rupture of follicle and extrusion of the oocyte into pelvis.
- Remaining follicular cells are called corpus luteum.
- With luteinization, the basal lamina regresses and the theca cells migrate into the forming corpus luteum.

- There is very prompt neovascularization of this structure (one of the highest blood flow per unit mass in the body).
- This corpus luteum starts secreting progesterone along with other factors and this progesterone converts the proliferative endometrium to a secretary one for implantation of the blast and maintenance of early pregnancy.
- The period of progesterone secretion and implantation collectively called as luteal phase.
- The individual corpus luteum has a programmed life span independent of LH secretion. The normal life span of the corpus luteum is 11–17 days (mean 14.2 days) from the time of ovulation to the menses. If not rescued by human chorionic gonadotropin (hCG) production from a newly implanted pregnancy, the corpus luteum will regress into an avascular structure called corpus albicans.[3,4]

## ■ LUTEAL PHASE DEFECT

It is a condition where there is insufficient progesterone exposure to maintain a normal secretory endometrium, which is required for embryo implantation and growth. Luteal phase defect is sometimes, clinically manifested by a shortened luteal phase lasting less than 9 days, from the day of ovulation to bleeding.[5,6]

### Why assisted reproductive technology pregnancies need luteal phase support?

The need for progesterone supplementation is obvious in cases of donor cycles where women are anovulatory and there is no inherent corpus luteum. In FET cycles (downregulated ones) there is no natural cyclicity in form of follicular and luteal phase, so follicular phase is mimicked with estradiol supplementation to produce a proliferative endometrium.[7] While preparing this endometrium for implantation of an embryo (blast), the luteal phase is mimicked by exposing endometrium to progesterone. The appropriate duration of exposure to progesterone is must for implantation of embryos. But how does hyperstimulated fresh cycles become defective is still not clear. Few proposed mechanisms for dysfunctional luteal phase are following:
- Due to destruction of granulosa cells during oocyte aspiration, which were destined to become corpus luteum later in the cycle.
- The administration of hCG to mimic LH surge by causing inhibition to endogenous LH secretion from the pituitary.
- Due to gonadotropin-releasing hormone (GnRH) agonist downregulation there is suppression of LH secretion during luteal phase.
- The most widely accepted theory of luteal phase defect after ART is secretion of supraphysiological steroid hormone levels from multiple corpus luteum in early luteal phase of an IVF cycle, causing direct inhibition of LH secretion via negative feedback on the hypothalamopituitary axis.

# LUTEAL PHASE SUPPORT IN ASSISTED REPRODUCTIVE TECHNOLOGY

The optimal success of ART depends not only on creating high quality embryos but also on the establishment of a receptive endometrium. To achieve this numerous modality have been tried but progesterone was always a mainstay in the list. Here are few agents which were used as luteal phase support since the infancy of ART:
- Progesterone
- Human chorionic gonadotropin
- Gonadotropin-releasing hormone agonist
- Estradiol.

## Progesterone

Progesterone is available in synthetic as well as natural forms with all the possible routes of administration for the ease of the patient. Commonly used routes are oral, intramuscular (IM), vaginal, sublingual, per rectal, and latest subcutaneous, our new kid on the block.

In a summary of a meta-analysis done in 2014, of 284,600 IVF cycles were taken from 82 separate centers worldwide, 77% of the cycles were performed with vaginal progesterone only, and an additional 17% used either oral or IM in combination. Only 5% cycles were on IM progesterone only while only 0.5% was on oral progesterone exclusively.[8]

Area wise preference was also noted, while north Americans were more pro toward IM preparations, Europeans were more comfortable with vaginal route.

### *Oral Micronized Progesterone*

Oral micronized progesterone was in vogue in 1980s, however, it has since proven to be a poor option due to its inconsistent bioavailability which is only 10% of IM. Serum levels take 2–4 hours to reach its peak and remain so for 6–7 hours only, thus frequent dosing is required.

### *Dydrogesterones*

An oral progestin with improved bioavailability compared to oral micronized progesterone. In a randomized controlled trial (RCT), pregnancy rates were higher in females undergoing IVF using oral dydrogesterones for luteal support versus micronized vaginal progesterone (41.0% vs. 29.4%; $p < 0.1$).[9,10]

Cochrane review analysis also favored the use of synthetic progesterone compared with micronized progesterone for clinical pregnancy [odds ratio (OR), micronized progesterone use; 0.79, 95% confidence interval (CI); 0.65–0.69].[11]

### Intramuscular Progesterone

It was first used as luteal phase support in IVF in 1985. Due to injection site pain, skin rashes, inflammatory reaction, and rare abscess formation, it is not very popular amongst patients. Due to stable serum level of progesterone it is a favorable route by many especially in FET cycles.

### Vaginal Progesterone

Most popular route amongst clinicians and patients both. The main benefit is its first pass uterine effect due to which the drug concentration is maximum in the endometrial tissues. Vaginal progesterone is available in tablet form, suppositories, and gel form. Tablets are to be used at least twice or thrice a day, vaginal gel (8%) is used either once or twice. Suppository use is discouraged because of fluctuating bioavailability.

In a large multicentric randomized trial the live-birth rate was almost same in three studied groups, one taking vaginal micronized progesterone twice a day, second taking it thrice a day while third group was using vaginal progesterone gel (progesterone twice a day 35%, thrice a day 38%, and vaginal gel 38%).[8]

The only complaint is difficulty in administration and occasional vaginal discharge.

### Subcutaneous Water-soluble Progesterone

Though it is too early to comment upon its efficacy but the trials available indicate an equal efficacy without skin site pain and other side effects.[12,13]

### When to start progesterone for luteal phase support in an in vitro fertilization cycle?

There is no consensus about starting time, but it is usually either from the day of pickup or within 2 days of oocyte retrieval with no obvious change in pregnancy rates.[14,15]

Prapas and colleagues concluded that implantation and clinical pregnancy rates were better in narrow window of progesterone exposure. They studied the exposure of 2–6 days in fresh and donor cycles as an optimum period.[16]

Similarly, there is no clear-cut consensus on how long progesterone has to be given. In a recent meta-analysis, it was concluded that there is no additional benefit of progesterone supplementation once the beta-HCG value comes positive, either in live-birth rates [relative risk (RR); 0.95, CI; 0.86–1.05], ongoing pregnancy rates (RR; 0.97, CI; 0.9–1.05), and miscarriage rates (RR; 1.01, CI; 0.78–1.3).[16] Despite these data more than 70% of clinics continue progesterone either up to 8 weeks or beyond and only 15% stop it at positive beta-HCG value.[8]

## Human Chorionic Gonadotropins

In women undergoing ART cycle with pituitary downregulation (lacking significant LH production), early ovarian progesterone production can be stimulated with a supplementation of hCG, an LH analog. Further, the profound and rapid variation in progesterone levels throughout the luteal phase closely mimics LH pulsatility in the human and rhesus.

Detailed protocols of hCG supplementation are described in later part of this chapter. The basic principle is to rescue more corpus luteum and stimulate endogenous progesterone production along with other growth factors.

### Gonadotropin-releasing Hormone Analogs

It is hypothesized that, if we supplement GnRHa as an adjuvant on day 5-6 of luteal phase, it stimulates LH secretion and in turn progesterone production is increased through corpus luteum. GnRHa is also said to have direct positive effect on endometrial receptors and embryo itself.[17]

In a Cochrane meta-analysis 2010, they found that pregnancy rates were higher in the groups who received a single dose of GnRHa on posttransfer day 5 or 6, in both long agonist protocol as well as an antagonist cycle (42.4% vs. 35.7%, OR: 1.33, 95% CI; 1.08–1.64). A subgroup analysis was performed and results were more in favor of antagonist cycle with analog supplementation. These findings were replicated as favorable outcome in later RCTs as well but we need more such studies to highlight the exact mechanism of action.[18]

### Estradiol Supplementation in Luteal Phase

Adjuvants to progesterone as luteal phase supports are given on the basis that corpus luteum does not only secrete progesterone but estrogen and other factors too.

However, a Cochrane meta-analysis in 2008, which was again revised in 2015, concluded that there is no additional benefit of adding estradiol to progesterone in terms of biochemical pregnancies, ongoing pregnancy rates, and live births, but an additional subgroup analysis showed that progesterone alone performed worse than the combination of progesterone with estradiol patches and we could say that more than supplementing the route of estrogen supplementation matters.[18]

## ■ LUTEAL PHASE SUPPORT IN FROZEN EMBRYO TRANSFER AND DONOR AND RECIPIENT CYCLES

These cycles are different from COH cycles as there is no endogenous estrogen, no corpus luteum so no progesterone. These cycles should not be deal with the way we deal fresh transfers in self cycles. Here we give estrogen from exogenous source to mimic proliferative phase and then exogenous progesterone is introduced to make the endometrium receptive for a cleavage stage of embryo or a blastocyst. We do not have dose finding studies for these drugs as well as there is no information regarding how many days of progesterone exposure is needed before the embryo transfer. Arbitrarily, we give 3–4 days of progesterone before a cleavage stage embryo transfer and around 5–6 days before a blast transfer. Regarding the route of supplementation there is no fixed guideline. While Americans prefer IM progesterone, Europeans they give vaginal progesterone before transfer. In earlier studies, there was no difference in ongoing pregnancy rates when both the routes were compared but later studies have claimed a better pregnancy rate with IM progesterone. However, we need larger RCTs to clear all these differences and come forward with a clear-cut guideline. Till then we have to judge it on individual basis.[19]

## What is individualized luteal phase support and how can we individualize the luteal phase protocols?

We are already aware of conventional ART cycles, where women undergo COH, hCG is used as conventional trigger, oocytes are retrieved, and exogenous progesterone given by various routes before embryo transfer, followed by luteal phase support basically in form of progesterone.

The individualization starts from the day a particular patient is registered for an ART treatment. Based on her antral follicle count (AFC) and anti-Müllerian hormone (AMH) the dose of gonadotropin and a protocol (downregulation vs. antagonist) is decided. The aim is to promote fresh cycle transfer as it will reduce the cost of vitrification and prevent the fetus from unwanted and unknown side effects of frozen-thaw transfer along with the stress of prolonged treatment. As the cycle proceeds we come to know the real picture in terms of expected number of oocytes, her risk of OHSS, etc. The key point is selection of trigger as "hCG" is main culprit in precipitating OHSS. Therefore, a hyperresponder woman, based on the numbers of oocytes expected we can either adopt a policy of freeze all after giving an analog trigger or we can use low dose of hCG along with analog trigger to rescue the cycle.

After more than a decade of GnRHa triggering we know that due to its shorter half-life and corpus luteum lytic action, fresh cycle transfer gives poorer pregnancy rates as compared to hCG trigger. So, our aim is to add hCG in these women. Now a million-dollar question is when to do it.

Many American and European working groups are fine tuning the protocols in last few years. While American people are fond of exogenous supplementation of steroid hormones along with adjuvants, the European group believes in endogenous production of steroid hormones through corpus luteum by regular supplementation of either hCG in low dose or LH analog. The aim of both these protocols is to facilitate fresh embryo transfer in an analog cycle with excellent reproductive outcome and no severe OHSS.

Shapiro, who was the first person to introduce dual trigger in ART by using GnRHa along with hCG. Out of all the widely studied was introduction of hCG at either 12 hours' post-GnRHa or 35 hours. It has almost become certain that the addition of hCG just after oocyte pickup gives better result in form of rescuing the corpus luteum. The dose of hCG varies between 1,000 units and 2,000 units. As per the timings there are three possible protocols:

1. *Dual trigger:* Where GnRHa is given along with low dose of hCG
2. *Segmented trigger:* Here hCG is introduced at least 12 hours after GnRHa
3. Supplementation of hCG immediately after oocyte pickup (35 hours).

## ■ LUTEAL PHASE SUPPORT POSTANALOG TRIGGER

Intensive luteal phase support is needed in these patients because of lots of evidences regarding defective luteal phase steroid secretion in these patients. While the trusted exogenous progesterone and estrogen plus progesterone support did not work in these women, after multiple experiments there came a reasonable protocol which gave an ongoing pregnancy rate at par with those women who had received conventional hCG trigger. There are two basic approaches:
1. American way
2. European way.

## American Way

Starting oil-based progesterone 50 mg IM from the day of oocyte retrieval till 10 weeks of gestation along with regular steroid hormone measurement (progesterone and estradiol weekly) and estradiol supplementation in form of transdermal patches. Dosages are to be increased as per the measurement. IM progesterone was increased up to 75 mg with additional vaginal micronized progesterone if serum concentration was found to be less than 20 ng/dL on any given day. Ideal luteal phase support is still to be found for these cycles. But using IM route to supplement progesterone is in the lieu of constant blood level and the measurements. Similarly, estradiol supplementation is given on the assumption of defective corpus luteum function in this group of patients. The preference for transdermal route is based on the avoidance of "first pass metabolism" of estradiol which takes place when it is given orally. Third important thing is that these exogenous steroid supplementations should not be stopped early in the pregnancy as the endogenous hCG produced in these patients may not be sufficient to rescue the pregnancy alone in GnRHa trigger cycles.[20]

### Human Chorionic Gonadotropin Supplementation

As already mentioned Shapiro was the first person to introduce the concept of dual trigger. He has used 4 mg of leuprolide along with 1,000–2,500 IU of hCG according to the body weight, number of follicles, and the expected risk of OHSS in his patients and found encouraging results.[21,22] Unfortunately, it was not a randomized prospective trial and the higher dose of hCG made clinicians skeptical about OHSS, but it gave us a food for thought to rescue these analog cycles. Later various protocols of adding hCG came into vogue, in one study Peter Humaidan used 1 mg of leuprolide along with fixed dose of 1,000 IU hCG in combination with intensive luteal phase support in patients with serum estradiol level more than 4,000 pg/mL and reported very good implantation and ongoing pregnancy rates (41.9% vs. 22.1%; P < 0.1) and minimum risk of OHSS. It was clear by this study that these patients with more than 4,000 pg/mL estradiol could be optimize for good outcome by giving low-dose dual trigger.

However, this is still not clear that these patients do they benefit by dual trigger or by supplementing hCG immediately after oocyte pickup.

### European Way

After devastating results in terms of ongoing pregnancy rates with GnRHa trigger, a newer and innovative concept was needed as hCG and LH share more than 80% of beta-subunit amino acids and bind to and activate the same receptors. The hCG has longer half-life so it is taken as surrogate for LH and rescues the early corpus luteal function for longer time in terms of progesterone production while exogenous progesterone (vaginal) takes care of late luteal phase until the embryo starts secreting its own hCG. In contrast GnRHa per se would induce less LH activity in early and midluteal phase and for shorter duration (75% reduced LH activity than natural cycle). It was thought to add low-dose hCG in a GnRHa cycles, the idea was to supplement high enough dose of hCG to rescue some of the corpus luteal functions but at the same time low enough to prevent OHSS and the purpose is not defeated.

To test all the earlier points various hCG protocols were tested in pilot studies. In one of the studies addition of 1,500 IU hCG at 12 hours' post-GnRHa trigger and 35 hours along with regular luteal phase support was compared and the results were in favor of 35 hours' group (though both the groups were rescued but midluteal phase progesterone and ongoing pregnancy was better in 35 hours' group). One added advantage of 35 hours was a dissociation of trigger from luteal phase.[20]

### Recombinant Luteinizing Hormone Supplementation

Few clinicians have tried recombinant LH supplementation for the same purpose of rescuing corpus luteum and endogenous progesterone secretion but study could not be continued because of the withdrawal of LH from American market.

## ■ PROGESTERONE-FREE LUTEAL PHASE

No more messy progesterone, discharge per vagina, painful injections, days are not far when you just need few hCG shots postembryo transfer and it is done. The principle is same, by providing hCG from outside in an analog cycle one is promoting endogenous progesterone production along with other growth factors. This protocol cannot be compared with traditional hCG trigger cycle as these are selected group of patients who have received analog as trigger and their corpus luteal function is being restored partially by these small fragmented doses of hCG.[23]

## CONCLUSION

- Personalized luteal phase preparation starts the moment patient is registered for an ART treatment.
- There are two ways to support luteal phase, one is exogenous supplementation of progesterone and progesterone plus adjuvants like estradiol and second is to promote corpus luteum to secrete progesterone along with other growth factors.
- Endogenous boost is acquired by supplementing low and continuous dose of hCG, in cases where there is no risk of frank OHSS.
- Frozen cycles and donor cycles get more benefit by IM progesterone.
- The aim of personalized care is to promote optimum success along with least side effects to the woman undergoing ART as fertility treatments are complex, lots of things are at stake, and if anyone step falters, the whole cycle goes into drain.

## REFERENCES

1. Tomás C, Alsbjerg B, Marlikainen H, et al. Pregnancy loss after frozen-embryo transfer—a comparison of three protocols. Fertil Steril. 2012;98:1165-9.
2. Belva F, Henriet S, Vanden Abdeel E, et al. Neonatal outcome of 937 children born after transfer of cryopreserved embryos obtained by ICSI and IVF and comparison with outcome data of fresh ICSI and IVF cycles. Hum Reprod. 2008;23:2227-38.
3. Fritz MA, Speroff L. Clinical Gynecologic Endocrinology and Infertility. Philadelphia: Lippincott Williams and Wilkins; 2012.
4. Barbiery RL. The endocrinology of menstrual cycle. Methods Mol Biol. 2014;1154:145-69.
5. Caspo AL, Pulkkinen MO, Ruttner B, et al. The significance of the human corpus luteum in pregnancy maintenance. Am J Obstet Gynecol. 1972;112:1061-7.
6. Practice Committee of the American Society for Reproductive Medicine. The clinical relevance of luteal phase deficiency: a committee opinion. Fertil Steril. 2012;98:1112-7.
7. Kerin JF, Broom TJ, Ralph MM, et al. Human luteal phase function following oocyte aspiration from the immediately preovular graffian follicle of spontaneous ovular cycle. Br J Obstet Gynecol. 1981;88:1021-8.
8. Vaisbuch E, de Ziegler D, Leong M, et al. Luteal phase support in assisted reproduction treatment: real life practices reported worldwide by an updated website-based survey. Reprod Biomed Online. 2014;28:330-5.
9. Practice Committee of the American Society for Reproductive Medicine. Progesterone supplementation during the luteal phase and in early pregnancy in the treatment of infertility: an educational bulletin. Fertil Steril. 2008;89:789-92.
10. Patki A, Pawar VC. Modulating fertility outcome in assisted reproductive technologies by the use of dydrogesterone. Gynecol Endocrinol. 2007;23:68-71.
11. Van der Linden M, Buckingham K, Farquhar C, et al. Luteal phase support for assisted reproduction cycles. Cochrane Database Syst Rev. 2011;(10):CD009154.

12. Zarutskie PW, Philips JA. A meta-analysis of the route of administration of luteal phase support in assisted reproductive technology: vaginal versus intramuscular progesterone. Fertil Steril. 2009;92:162-9.
13. Sator M, Radisioni M, Cometti B. Pharmacokinetics and safety profile of a novel progesterone aqueous formulation administered by the SC route. Gynecol Endocrinol. 2013;29:205-8.
14. Sonntag B, Ludwig M. An integrated view on luteal phase: diagnosis and treatment in subfertility. Clin Endocrinol (Oxf). 2012;77:500-7.
15. Fatemi HM. The luteal phase after 3 decades of IVF—What do we know? Reprod Biomed Online. 2009;19:1-13.
16. Liu XR, Mu HQ, Shi Q, et al. The optimal duration of progesterone supplementation in pregnant women after IVF/ICSI: a meta-analysis. Reprod Biol Endocrinol. 2012;10:107.
17. Oliviera JB, Baruffi R, Peterson CG, et al. Administration of single-dose GnRH agonist in luteal phase in ICSI cycles: a meta-analysis. 2010;8:107.
18. Kolibianakis EM, Venetis CA, Papanicolaou EG, et al. Estrogen addition to progesterone for luteal phase support in cycles stimulated with GnRH-analogues and gonadotrophins for IVF: a systemic review and meta-analysis. Hum Reprod. 2008;23:1346-54.
19. Casper RF. Luteal phase support for frozen embryo transfer cycles: IM or vaginal progesterone? Fertil Steril. 2014;101:627-8.
20. Humaidan P, Engmann L, Benadiva C. Luteal phase supplementation after gonadotropin releasing hormone agonist trigger in fresh embryo transfer: the American versus European approaches. Fertil Steril. 2015;103:879-85.
21. Iloiodromiti S, Blockeel C, Tremellen KP, et al. Consistent high clinical pregnancy rates and low ovarian hyperstimulation syndrome rates in high risk patients after GnRH agonist triggering and modified luteal support: a retrospective multicenter study. Hum Reprod. 2013;28:2529-36.
22. Shapiro BS, Daneshmand ST, Garner FC, et al. Comparison of "triggers" using leuprolide acetate alone or in combination with low dose HCG. Fertil Steril. 2011;95:2715-7.
23. Humaidan P, Ejdrup Bredkjaer H, Wartergard LG, et al. 1500 IU hCG administered at oocyte retrieval rescues the luteal phase when GnRHa is used for ovulation induction: a prospective, randomized controlled study. Fertil Steril. 2010;93:847-54.

# CHAPTER 10

# Endometrial Preparation for Frozen Embryo Transfer

*Kuldeep Jain, Bharti Jain, Maansi Jain*

## ■ INTRODUCTION

Frozen embryo transfer (FET) is an important arm of assisted reproductive technology (ART). The technology is now increasingly offered to patient undergoing ART procedures for making it more cost effective, to minimize ovarian hyperstimulation syndrome (OHSS), and for optimization of outcome. As per World Report 2014, FET cycles estimated at 27.4% of the total ART cycles.[1] According to a report of Society of Assisted Technique, a clear trend toward increased use of FET is noticed when compared with fresh cycles 82.5% versus 3.1% during 2006-2012 (Fig. 1). Trends in estimated numbers of live births with fresh transfer and FET also showed a positive shift toward FET outcome (Fig. 2).[2]

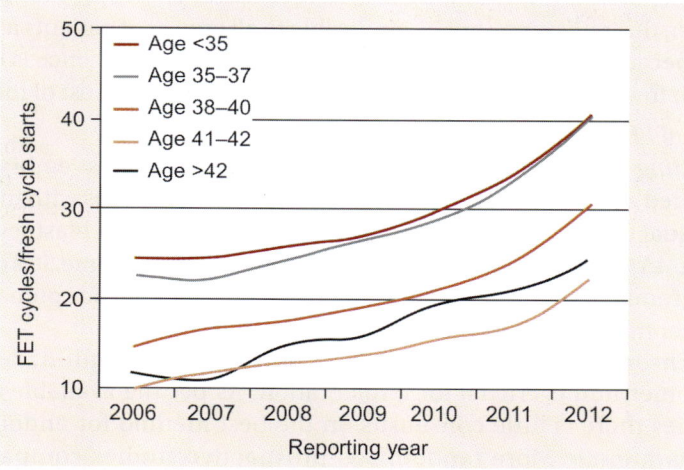

**Fig. 1:** Trends in the ratio of the numbers of reported frozen-thawed embryo transfers to reported fresh cycle in each SART age group. (FET: frozen embryo transfer)

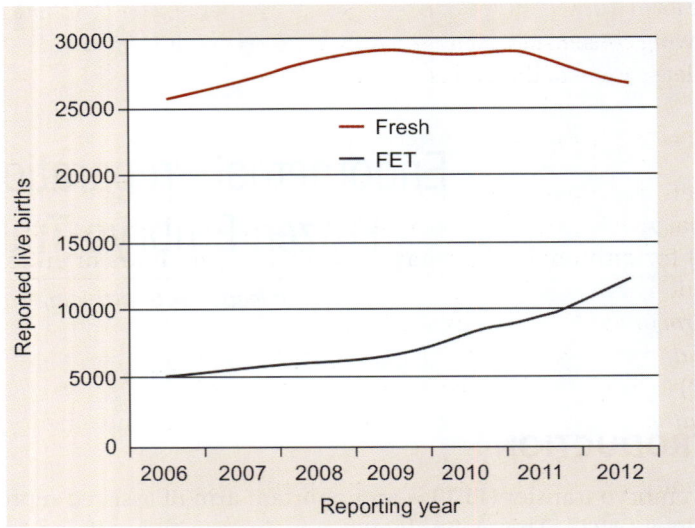

**Fig. 2:** Trends in estimated numbers of live births with fresh transfer and frozen embryo transfer (FET).

The clinical pregnancy rates with frozen cycles varies widely because of different protocols used by different clinics, policies in respect to day of freezing as well as quality of embryos and technique used. Optimization of laboratory conditions, better techniques of vitrification coupled with limitations on the number of embryos [single embryo transfer (ET)] to be transferred have led to an increase in FET cycles. There is a growing evidence that culturing up to blastocyst stage, transferring a single embryo, and freezing of surplus embryo is quite acceptable to patients and can increase the cumulative pregnancy rates.[3,4] However, this policy may not be applicable to all groups of patients and for all clinics because of multiple factors involved. The current practice is deciding between fresh cycles versus FET on a case to case basis in most of the clinics.

*Success of FET depends on:*
- *Selecting proper embryos:* It is a valuable parameter. Best embryos to be selected are cleavage stage embryos (grade 3)/d3 embryos with more than or equal to eight blastomeres or if vitrification is done at blastocyst stage, grade 4AA/3AA/4AB (4 Gartner) is desirable for best outcome. It is observed that if embryos are of lower grades then outcome may not be optimal though conceptions do occur with these embryos.
- *Synchronization of endometrium and embryo:* A good, receptive endometrium is crucial for implantation. As per the available research studies there is little consensus on the best method for endometrium preparation.[5,6] More randomized prospective studies comparing the different protocols are required to reach a consensus.
- *Providing sufficient luteal support:* This area also remains a debatable area as available literature is inconclusive. However, most of the programs use

some form of luteal support to optimize the outcome in FET cycles as there is a growing consensus that luteal support might provide an added advantage in at least some of the cycles.

## METHODS OF ENDOMETRIAL PREPARATION

Endometrial preparation protocols may vary depending on the ovarian hormonal activity. However, there is little consensus till date on the optimal method for endometrial preparation. Various methods of endometrial preparation are:
- *Natural or modified natural cycle:* In ovulatory patients with regular cycles
- *Gonadotropin-releasing hormone agonist:* Hormone replacement therapy (HRT) in irregular or anovulatory ovarian cycles
- *Ovulation induction by ovulatory drugs:* In irregular or anovulatory ovarian cycles
- *Hormone replacement therapy:* In quiescent ovaries.

## Natural Cycle for Frozen Embryo Transfer

Natural cycle for FET is feasible only in females with regular cycles and proven ovulation. The endogenous steroids from a developing follicle prime the endometrium and the time of ET is determined by detecting spontaneous luteinizing hormone (LH) surge. The monitoring is done by ultrasonography (USG) which measures the ET (thickness and type), follicular growth rate, and ovulation in conjunction with LH surge (urine or blood) and/or serum progesterone levels. Based on various studies, it is assumed that ovulation occurs 36–40 hours after LH surge (LH surge implies a rise of 180% from the baseline). Also it is to be kept in mind that urinary LH surge lags 21 hours behind serum LH surge. The day of ovulation corresponds to the day of ovum pickup (OPU) and ET is done 3–5 days after ovulation depending on stage at which the embryo is frozen. Luteal phase support is done with progesterone. A mock cycle before actual cycle is recommended to optimize the outcome while using this method.

The disadvantage of natural cycle for FET is that even with regular cycles, ovulation may not occur always. Also LH surge is transitory so for its detection. Estimation is to be done daily or twice daily. Also the variable LH threshold of LH kits should be kept in mind (there is a risk of 30% false negative). Risk of desynchronization and premature LH surge remain even after mock cycle.

## Modified Natural Cycle for Frozen Embryo Transfer

It overcomes the disadvantage of LH monitoring. In this approach human chorionic gonadotropin (hCG) (5,000–10,000 IU) is administered to initiate luteinization once the follicle reaches the size of at least 18 mm. Ovulation is expected to occur 36–38 hours later. Monitoring of these cycles can be with USG alone or USG combined with serum E2 levels (450–550 pmol/L). However, there is a risk of unexpected ovulation leading to cycle cancelation. Evidence supporting luteal phase support is scant, some argue that as corpus luteal formation is not hampered and luteal phase support is not required. Literature review shows no significant difference in outcome in natural cycle FET versus modified FET cycles.

## Hormone Replacement Cycle

Indicated for females with irregular cycles but remaining ovarian function. It has an advantage as it allows a greater flexibility in planning and control in timing of transfer. Endometrium is prepared with estradiol valerate, either in incremental/step up low-dose regime or fixed dose regimen without suppressing pituitary by gonadotropin-releasing hormone agonist (GnRHa). Early administration (D2–D3) of estrogen causes proliferation of the endometrium and added suppression of the growth of follicles.

Most common route to administer estrogen is by oral route, however, it can also be given by subcutaneous patches or gel or as vaginal rings.

In step up regimen, estrogen is given as 2 mg OD, followed by 2 mg BID for 4 days and then 2 mg TDS for 4–5 days depending on endometrial response. Usually a 10–12 days exposure is enough for optimal response, i.e. 8–12 mm thickness with trilaminar morphology. Transdermal estradiol patch 100 μg, increased to 200 μg, and then 300 μg/day can be applied to nonhairy part of body like inner aspect of thigh, arms. In the fixed dose regime, 2 mg thrice a day estradiol valerate is given for 10 days continuously. No difference has been found till date between two protocols in terms of success rate or cancelation rates. Estrogen can also be given in subcutaneous gel form or as vaginal ring.

Endometrium is evaluated (thickness and type) and the dose titrated to achieve an optimal response. In cases of suboptimal response one can increase the duration and/or the dose (12–14 mg/day). Even though the endometrium receptivity is optimal when follicular phase or duration of estrogen exposure is 12–19 days, studies have shown that endometrium development is unaffected by length of follicular phase. No adverse effect in terms of implantation rates, pregnancy rates, or cancelation rates have been noted by varying the exposure time from as minimum as 7 days or as long as 35 days.

The desired effect is an endometrial thickness more than 7 mm with type b morphology without follicular activity. The administration of estrogen and progesterone does not guarantee complete pituitary suppression. There can be a dominant follicle or premature exposure to progesterone causing luteinization in which case the ET is canceled. Primed by estrogen with an endometrial thickness of at least 7 mm, progesterone is added to initiate secretory changes to mimic the physiologic midcycle estrogen–progesterone transition.

It is the endometrial thickness and not the duration of estrogen exposure which should be the deciding factor to start progesterone.[7,8] Embryo thawing and subsequently ET is timed according to the day of progesterone supplementation. The day of starting progesterone is considered to be the ovulation/OPU day to decide the time of transfer. Progesterone can be given by oral, intramuscular (IM), or vaginal route. Glujovsky et al.[9] could not detect any difference between vaginal and IM administration when comparing the pregnancy rates. Progesterone given by IM (natural progesterone dose 50–100 mg/day) or intravaginal (micronized progesterone dose 300 mg or 600 mg/day) is the most frequently used progesterone preparations. Orally administered micronized progesterone was shown not to be suitable for preparing the endometrium for implantation.

For ET, blastocyst transfer is done after 6–7 days of progesterone and in D3 cleavage stage, transfer is done after 4 days of progesterone exposure. It is followed by luteal phase support by estrogen and progesterone. The length of the follicular phase can be varied without detrimental effects to implantation rate or pregnancy rate or cancelation rate. Literature review has shown a higher implantation and pregnancy rate when compared to natural cycle with less cycle cancelation rates.[10]

## Downregulation with Gonadotropin-releasing Hormone Agonist and Hormone Replacement

This is the most popular protocol used for endometrial preparation. GnRH agonist is used to downregulate pituitary to avoid follicular growth, avoiding spontaneous LH surge, and ovulation thus providing increased flexibility of scheduling as per the requirement of the ART clinic. Estradiol valerate is started from D2 to D3 of cycle and continued after titration to achieve desired response before addition of progesterone. The cancelation rates are low and this protocol is best suited for polycystic ovary syndrome (PCOS), adenomyosis, endometriosis, and patients with history of FET cancelation because of premature luteinization and premature ovulation.[11,12] No endocrine monitoring is required and cycle can be managed with help of ultrasound only.

Limitation and disadvantage of this regime are the higher cost, prolonged injection schedule, and risk of hypoestrogenic side effects. As per Cochrane database 2010 which reviewed 22 randomized controlled trials (RCTs), no significant benefit was seen when compared with natural cycle FET.[9] However, a significant higher live-birth rate, clinical pregnancy rate, and better endometrial thickness were demonstrated with downregulated protocol when compared with HRT alone.[5]

## Stimulated Frozen Embryo Transfer Cycle

This protocol is best suited for ovaries with functional activity but with anovulatory, irregular cycles, and especially in those cases which are refractory to exogenous estrogen. Stimulation can be done with clomiphene, aromatase inhibitors, or gonadotropins depending on previous response. However, clomiphene is not the ideal drug because of antiestrogenic effect on endometrium. Gonadotropins use increase the cost, the compliance is poor, and there is a risk of premature luteinization requiring antagonist administration to prevent cancelation.

## ■ COMPARATIVE EFFICACY OF VARIOUS PROTOCOLS

Literature review showed five studies comparing NC versus modified NC representing 1,965 cycles. Analysis of pooled result of all studies showed no significant difference with regard to clinical pregnancy [odds ratio (OR) 0.91, 95% confidence interval (CI) 0.74–1.1], ongoing pregnancy (OR 1.0, 95% CI 0.66–1.6), and live birth (OR 1.0, 95% CI 0.63–1.6).[6,13-15]

In two of the five studies effect of luteal support on clinical pregnancy rate and ongoing pregnancy rate was analyzed.[15] (Tomax et al. 2012) Clinical pregnancy rates were comparable between the studies using luteal phase support and those without luteal phase support (OR 0.80, 95% CI 0.61–1.0 vs. OR 1.1, 95% CI 0.79–1.5, respectively). Test for subgroup differences showed no significant difference between both subgroups ($P = 0.16$). Moreover, comparable results were observed in ongoing pregnancy rates with and without luteal phase support, respectively (OR 0.82, 95% CI 0.62–1.1 vs. OR 1.5, 95% CI 0.58–4.0) and there was no significant difference between subgroups ($P = 0.23$).

## ■ NATURAL CYCLE VERSUS ARTIFICIAL CYCLES

Eight retrospective studies representing 8,152 cycles and one RCT representing 111 cycles were included. In seven studies luteal phase support was used.[16,17] (Kawamura, 2007; Givens et al. 2009; Xiao et al. 2011; Hancke et al. 2012; Tomax et al. 2012) No significant difference in clinical pregnancy rates was obtained (OR 1.2, 95% CI 0.86–1.6). The pooled result of the retrospective studies is consistent with the only included prospective study. No significant difference in either ongoing pregnancy rates (OR 1.2, 95% CI 0.95–1.5) or live-birth rates (OR 1.2, 95% CI 0.93–1.6) were observed. Tests for heterogeneity showed evidence for a high level of heterogeneity for all endpoints.[16,17]

The primary reasons why the natural cycle appears to yield better reproductive results are as follows:
- Except for estrogen and progesterone, the implantation and maintenance of pregnancy depends on the complicated interaction of multiple hormones of which secretion may be suppressed in HRT cycle
- Many cytokines participate in the process of implantation which, depending of their level may reduce in HRT cycle, for example, glycodelin.[18,19]
- Small follicle development in HRT cycle adversely influences the endometrial receptivity.

## ENDOMETRIAL PARAMETERS AND OUTCOME IN FROZEN EMBRYO TRANSFER CYCLES

Ultrasound is the mainstay to evaluate endometrial thickness and pattern in both fresh and frozen cycles. It helps the clinicians to prognosticate and counsel the patients about the expected outcome. The addition of Doppler has been proposed by few workers to increase the sensitivity of evaluation. Most of the studies have failed to demonstrate a difference between conception and nonconception cycle based on the endometrial thickness.[20,21] However, a recent large retrospective study has concluded that a thickness between 7 mm and 14 mm was associated with significantly better implantation and clinical pregnancy rates in nondownregulated but supported FET cycles.[22] Other studies have evaluated the effect of pattern of endometrium and conception in FET cycles but did not find any association with pregnancy rate and presence of trilaminar pattern as seen in fresh cycles.[21,23] Studies on Doppler parameters and its effect on conception in FET cycles remain inconclusive.[21,23]

## ADVANTAGES OF FROZEN EMBRYO TRANSFER OVER FRESH EMBRYO TRANSFER

- Permits transfer of reduced the number of embryos.
- Lowers the risk of multiple pregnancies.
- Increases the cumulative pregnancy rate.
- Additional clinical safety in the presence of ovarian hyperstimulation with prevention of late-onset OHSS.
- Higher live-birth rate as the freezing the embryos and performing a subsequent FET cycle prevents the premature rise of progesterone. In contrast the fresh cycles have frequently been seem to be associated with an elevated progesterone levels on the day of trigger which is negatively associated with live-birth rate.
- The defective luteal phase associated with the GnRH agonist trigger given in fresh cycles is not seen.
- Frozen embryo transfer cycles have been shown to be associated with reduced risks of low-birth weight and prematurity.
- It also permits genetic screening because embryos can be frozen while awaiting the test results.
- Transfer of confirmed euploid embryos and better endometrial receptivity in the absence of ovarian stimulation may contribute to increasing FET success rates.[24]

However, some studies have shown FET has the following disadvantages:
- Pregnancy rates, live-birth rates in FET cycles are usually lower than that of fresh transferred embryos.[25]
- Frozen embryo transfer is associated with increased risks of macrosomia and large for gestational age.

- Salumets et al. report a higher rate of biochemical pregnancy and clinical abortion was reported 15–20% and 20–25% after FET, respectively likely caused by the damage to embryos occurring during the freezing and thawing procedures.

Freeze all policy is it the future of ART. Currently the proposed freeze all policy is in the research stage, limited by the fact that most of the retrospective trials have been small in scale with limited power. So, it may be best to follow an individualized approach, balancing fresh transfer, and embryo cohort cryopreservation options while considering patient characteristics, cycle parameters, and clinic success rates. Also, the current data does not support any method of endometrial preparation. We require larger, variable controlled RCT considering the effect of implantation potential of the cryopreserved embryo (number, grade, storage duration, and developmental stage of embryo at freezing), cause of infertility, the endometrial thickness at the transfer time, and the technique of the operator. Additionally number of canceled cycles, visits, costs, and other logistics of the laboratory and hospital, patient and doctor preference should be taken into account.

## CONCLUSION

Recently worldwide use of FET is an integral part of art, with an increasing potential for increasing trend due to increase in success rates coupled with reduced risks.

## REFERENCES

1. Mansour R, Ishihara O, Adamson GD, et al. International Committee for Monitoring Assisted Reproductive Technologies World Report: Assisted Reproductive Technology 2006. Hum Reprod. 2014;29:1536-51.
2. Society for Assisted Reproductive Technology. IVF Success Rate Reports: 2006-2012; 2014.
3. Csokmay JM, Hill MJ, Chason RJ, et al. Experience with a patient-friendly, mandatory, single-blastocyst transfer policy: the power of one. Fertil Steril. 2011;96:580-4.
4. Martini S, Van Voorhis BJ, Stegmann BJ, et al. In vitro fertilization patients support a single blastocyst transfer policy. Fertil Steril. 2011;96:993-7.
5. Ghobara T, Vandekerckhove P. Cycle regimens for frozen-thawed embryo transfer. Cochrane Database Syst Rev. 2008;(1):CD003414.
6. Weissman A, Levin D, Ravhon A, et al. What is the preferred method for timing natural cycle frozen-thawed embryo transfer? Reprod Biomed Online. 2009;19: 66-71.
7. Nawroth F, Ludwig M. What is the 'ideal' duration of progesterone supplementation before the transfer of cryopreserved–thawed embryos in estrogen/progesterone replacement protocols? Hum Reprod. 2005;20:1127-34.
8. El-Toukhy T, Coomarasamy A, Khairy M, et al. The relationship between endometrial thickness and outcome of medicated frozen embryo replacement cycles. Fertil Steril. 2008;89:832-9.

9. Glujovsky D, Pesce R, Fiszbajn G, et al. Endometrial preparation for women undergoing embryo transfer with frozen embryos or embryos derived from donor oocytes. Cochrane Database Syst Rev. 2010;(1):CD006359.
10. Pados G, Camus M, Van Waesberghe L, et al. Oocyte and embryo donation: evaluation of 412 consecutive trials. Hum Reprod. 1992;7:1111-7.
11. Devroey P, Palermo G, Bourgain C, et al. Progesterone administration in patients with absent ovaries. Int J Fertil. 1988;34:188-93.
12. Kalem Z, Kalem MN, Gürgan T. Methods for endometrial preparation in frozen-thawed embryo transfer cycles. J Turk Ger Gynecol Assoc. 2016;17:168-72.
13. Fatemi HM, Kyrou D, Bourgain C, et al. Cryopreserved-thawed human embryo transfer: spontaneous natural cycle is superior to human chorionic gonadotropin-induced natural cycle. Fertil Steril. 2010;94:2054-8.
14. Chang EM, Han JE, Kim YS, et al. Use of the natural cycle and vitrification thawed blastocyst transfer results in better in-vitro fertilization outcomes: cycle regimens of vitrification thawed blastocyst transfer. J Assist Reprod Genet. 2011;28:369-74.
15. Weissman A, Horowitz E, Ravhon A, et al. Spontaneous ovulation vs hCG triggering for timing natural cycle frozen thawed embryo transfer—a randomized study. Reprod Biomed Online. 2011;23:484-9.
16. Loh SK, Leong NK. Factors affecting success in an embryo cryopreservation program. Ann Acad Med Singapore. 1999;28:260-5.
17. Morzov V, Ruman J, Kenigsberg D, et al. Natural cycle cryo-thaw transfer may improve pregnancy outcome. J Assist Reprod Genet. 2007;24:119-23.
18. Lindhard A, Bentin-Ley U, Ravn V, et al. Biochemical evaluation of endometrial function at the time of implantation. Fertil Steril. 2002;78:221-33.
19. Dalton C, Bolton AE, Ling E, et al. An analysis of the variation of plasma concentrations of placental protein 14 in artificial cycles. Fertil Steril. 1992;57:776-82.
20. Check JH, Dietterich C, Graziano V. Effect of maximal endometrial thickness on outcome of frozen embryo transfer. Fertil Steril. 2004;81:1399-400.
21. Coulam CB, Bustillo M, Soenksen DM, et al. Ultrasound predictors of implantation after assisted reproduction. Fertil Steril. 1994;62:1004-10.
22. El-Toukhy T, Coomarasamy A, Khairy M, et al. The relationship between endometrial thickness and outcome of medicated frozen embryo replacement cycles. Fertil Steril. 2008;89:832-9.
23. Ng EH, Chan CC, Tang OS, et al. The role of endometrial and subendometrial vascularity measured by three-dimensional power Doppler ultrasound in the prediction of pregnancy during frozen-thawed embryo transfer cycles. Hum Reprod. 2006;21:1612-7.
24. Salumets A, Suikkari AM, Makinen S, et al. Frozen embryo transfers: implications of clinical and embryological factors on the pregnancy outcome. Hum Reprod. 2006;21:2368-74.
25. Song T, Liu L, Zhou F, et al. Frozen-thawed embryo transfer (FET) versus fresh embryo transfer in clinical pregnancy rate during in vitro fertilization-embryo transfer. Zhonghua Yi Xue Za Zhi. 2009;89:2928-30.

CHAPTER
11

# Role of Hormone Analysis in ART

*SK Goswami, Radhika L Kundul, Manjusree Chakrabarty*

## INTRODUCTION

Assisted reproduction is the jewel in the crown of reproductive medicine. Assisted reproduction is a vast field encompassing both the sublime secrets of how two haploid cells combine to create a diploid zygote that contains all the information necessary to grow and develop into a complex mammal and the pragmatically empirical application of the technology to treat infertility.

Successful capacitation of sperm in vitro and fertilization of human oocytes matured in vitro were followed by the insight that preovulatory oocytes were optimal for in vitro fertilization (IVF). These exploratory steps culminated in 1978 with a term birth resulting from the IVF of a single preovulatory oocyte obtained from a natural menstrual cycle, transferred to the uterus at an eight-cell stage. Since then assisted reproductive technology (ART) has evolved into a scientific field applying knowledge of laboratory scientists to the standardization of infertility treatment. This chapter reviews the role of hormonal analysis in the practice of ART.[1]

There is considerable debate and substantial individual variation in clinical practice regarding what hormones should be assessed in all patients prior to commencing and while monitoring IVF treatment.[2] While it would appear logical to measure multiple hormones such as gonadotropins [follicle-stimulating hormone (FSH), luteinizing hormone (LH)], steroids (estradiol, testosterone, 17 hydroxy-progesterone), prolactin, and thyroid function tests in all women, the utility of such an extensive hormone analysis in the average ovular patient less certain. In today's environment of escalating medical expenses it is imperative that we only order tests that have potential clinical value.

Success of the cycle is critically dependent on generating an adequate number of mature follicles that contain developmentally competent oocytes [controlled ovarian stimulation (COS)] not conceding on the complication rate like multiple gestation and ovarian hyperstimulation (OHSS). Prediction of poor response to stimulation is also a very important concern for the infertility specialists.

Hormone analysis in ART[1] is essential for assessment at various levels:
1. Baseline hormonal evaluation—to predict the ovarian response to gonadotropins
2. Evaluate pituitary downregulation
3. To monitor the response to ovarian stimulation
4. For prevention of OHSS
5. To assess the precise timing for administration hCG injection.

## ■ BASAL HORMONAL EVALUATION AND PITUITARY DESENSITIZATION

Response to COS during IVF treatment is highly variable, even among women of similar age. This undoubtedly reflects the wide variation in ovarian reserve between different women. Performing hormone assessments of ovarian reserve before commencing a first cycle of IVF treatment may allow a more accurate prediction of a woman's anticipated response to COS, allowing for deciding on the type of stimulation, optimal dose of gonadotropins required and anticipate complications like OHSS and poor ovarian response.

The traditional hormones used for assessment of ovarian reserve include early follicular phase FSH/estradiol, serum inhibin B, and anti-Müllerian hormone (AMH).

## Gonadotropins

Follicle-stimulating hormone plays a crucial role in the recruitment, selection and dominance processes during the whole follicular phase. LH acts directly on the theca cells where LH receptors are present and ensure a tonic production of androgens during the follicular phase. LH induces a dose dependent protein synthesis (aromatase activity). FSH is the main therapeutic agent for folliculogenesis except in hypogonadotropic hypogonadism. A minimal amount of LH (LH threshold) is essential for dose-dependent increase in estradiol production and hence the required endometrial preparation for embryo implantation. During the follicular phase, serum levels of LH and FSH by radioimmunoassay range from 4 mIU/mL to 15 mIU/mL, although individual laboratory ranges may vary.

Traditionally a day 3 FSH exceeding 15 IU/L has been seen as a very poor prognostic sign and has been used by many clinics to exclude patients from IVF treatment.

High levels of LH, with increased LH/FSH ratios are found in about 50% of women with PCOS and are at a higher risk of OHSS. High endogenous LH levels are often associated with an increased incidence of infertility or miscarriages.

High levels of serum FSH and LH are typical of diminished ovarian reserve and may require a higher dose of gonadotropins for stimulation.

Measurements of plasma LH are routinely performed at the time of pituitary desensitization to ensure downregulation of endogenous hormones with GnRH agonist.

Apart from alterations in FSH and LH associated with various disorders and physiologic states, FSH levels are increased by Levodopa and ketoconazole and decreased by the administration of estrogens and phenothiazines. LH is increased by ketoconazole and decreased by administration of sex steroids, phenothiazines, digoxin and propranolol.

## Estradiol

Serum estradiol levels range from 20 pg/mL to 80 pg/mL during the early to mid-follicular phase of the menstrual cycle in most of the laboratories. It is commonly stated that plasma E2 level must be lower than 50 pg/mL to make sure that hypophyseal desensitization is effective at the ovarian level in a long-term GnRH agonist protocol cycle. In every situation, it is recommended to start ovarian stimulation with FSH only when ovarian activity is suppressed.

## Anti-Müllerian Hormone

Anti-Müllerian Hormone (Müllerian-inhibiting substance), a member of the transforming growth factor-β family and predominantly a product of preantral and small antral follicles[3] and thereby a close correlate of AFC, is not only predictive of the ovarian responses to ovarian stimulation,[4-6,9] but it is also able to predict clinical pregnancy and live birth.[9]

Furthermore, AMH levels in most studies are stable across the menstrual cycle,[7,8,10] removing the constraint of early follicular blood samples or ultrasound scans.

A review of over 2,000 cycles of IVF from 20 individual studies has concluded that AMH is abetter marker for predicting ovarian response to COS than patient age, day 3 FSH, estradiol and inhibin B. All of the available data show a strong positive correlation between basal serum AMH levels and the number of retrieved oocytes in women undergoing ovarian stimulation. Several authors have investigated the utility of AMH in the prediction of poor response to FSH. The reported sensitivity and specificity for predicting poor response are in the range 44–97% and 41–100% respectively, depending on the "cut off" serum AMH value used in the individual study.

While serum AMH appears to be an excellent marker of quantitative ovarian reserve, it appears to have very limited usefulness as a marker of oocyte quality. Serum AMH levels do not predict embryo morphology or the rate of embryo aneuploidy.

AMH levels in women with polycystic ovarian syndrome (PCOS) are on average 2–3 higher than their age matched ovulatory peers, with serum AMH having a relatively high sensitivity and specificity (92% and 67% respectively) for diagnosing the presence of polycystic ovaries on scan and predict the occurrence of OHSS during IVF treatment. AMH can facilitate individualization of treatment and improve outcomes.

## Inhibin-B

Inhibins A and B are secreted from granulosa cells following FSH stimulation and regulate FSH secretion by negative feedback. Small antral follicles have the potential to secrete inhibin-B whereas preovulatory follicles may secrete inhibin-A. Serum inhibin-B value in the early follicular phase of the menstrual cycle is a valuable tool to evaluate the size of follicular cohort that is destined to form mature oocytes. During the early stage of ovarian stimulation, inhibin-B measurement helps the clinicians decide on cycle cancellation or modulation of the gonadotropin dose.

## ■ OTHER TESTS

Clomiphene citrate challenge test is done to assess the ovarian reserve and was considered more valuable than a single measurement of FSH and estradiol on day 3. Clomiphene 100 mg is administered on days 5 through day 9 of the cycle. An abnormal FSH level in this setting is a value of more than 10–12 mIU/mL. However recent data suggest that this test may not be more valuable than baseline FSH assessments.

Serum progesterone levels are low in the follicular phase, less than 1.5 ng/mL. Elevated values during pituitary desensitization are deleterious for the subsequent ART cycle. It requires continuation of GnRH analogs and postponement of ovarian stimulation.

Serum estradiol level more than 50 pg/mL or serum progesterone level more than 1 ng/mL or an LH level more than 2 mIU/mL following pituitary desensitization suggests the presence of a persistent corpus luteum or an ovarian cyst which needs to be addressed prior to ovarian stimulation.

## ■ ASSESSMENT OF THYROID DYSFUNCTION

Hypothyroidism is relatively common in the infertile population, affecting 5–6% of women with idiopathic or anovulatory infertility and 2% of women with tubal or male factor infertility. Hyperthyroidism is significantly less common, affecting between 0.1% and 1% of women in the reproductive age group. The treatment of women with previously undiagnosed hypothyroidism with thyroxin replacement can itself result in natural conception, removing the need for IVF treatment. Furthermore, undiagnosed hypothyroidism may adversely affect the IVF cycle as it has been linked with failed oocyte fertilization despite the use of good quality sperm. Untreated hypothyroidism may lead to pregnancy complications such as miscarriage, growth restriction, and preterm delivery and a possible reduction in the neuropsychomotor development of the child conceived by fertility treatment. It has been suggested that thyroid function is best assessed in infertile women with both a TSH and FT4 test, since isolated hypo-FT4 (normal TSH) has been reported in up to 2% of pregnancies and may still interfere with the child's neurological development. Compared to natural conception, IVF treatment itself may exacerbate hypothyroidism since the supraphysiological levels of estradiol seen during COS results in an increase in production of thyroxin-binding globulin, thereby reducing the concentration of biologically active free thyroxin hormone. It would therefore appear prudent to order a screening TSH and FT4 test on all women before commencing IVF treatment.

## ■ ANDROGENS

Plasma androgen levels namely testosterone and androstenedione are not routinely determined in clinical practice. Assessment of ovarian morphology by transvaginal ultrasound (TVUS) allows a more accurate evaluation of polycystic ovaries than measurement of plasma androgens. Androgens exert a stimulatory effect on granulosa cell proliferation and may be involved in follicular recruitment. Hence plasma androgen evaluation may be useful in research scenarios.

## ■ BASAL HORMONE LEVELS FOR STIMULATION

| Hormone | Normal range |
| --- | --- |
| FSH | < 15 mIU/ml |
| LH | |
| E2 | < 80 pg/ml |
| Progesterone | < 1.5 pg/ml |

## ■ AFTER PITUITARY DESENSITIZATION

| Hormone | Normal range |
| --- | --- |
| LH | <1.8 mIU/ml |
| E2 | <50 pg/ml |
| Progesterone | < 1.5 pg/ml |

## ■ MONITORING THE ART CYCLE

There is an extensive literature regarding the use of serum estradiol and TVUS for monitoring of ART cycles, but none has been proven to be superior over the other. There are data that ultrasound alone is sufficient for monitoring of follicular and endometrial growth.

It has been suggested that combined monitoring is time consuming, expensive and inconvenient for women and that simplification of IVF and ICSI therapy by using TVUS only should be considered.[11]

Monitoring of ART cycles is mainly done by ultrasound in the present clinical scenario. Addition of hormonal analysis to sonographic monitoring can be valuable when ultrasound shows adequate follicular growth but inadequate endometrial growth indicating a low estrogen production per follicle due to low endogenous LH level. This may require addition of LH component to ovarian stimulation. Monitoring with ultrasound is used for timing and estradiol to avoid complications during the ART cycle.

Plasma estradiol measurement is a good indicator of granulosa cell differentiation and is helpful to evaluate follicular maturity before triggering ovulation. In clinical practice, determination of E2 response to the flare-up effect of the agonist is relevant for an early detection of potential poor responders and for tailoring gonadotropin administration accordingly. It was suggested that an increase in the plasma E2 concentrations for 6 consecutive days would be optimal for the success of an IVF cycle. But a plateau of E2 level for more than 3 days is usually associated with a poor outcome.

In case of poor responders, analysis of estradiol on day 5 of stimulation is useful in manipulation of dosage at an earlier stage. Arbitrarily, if serum E2 less than 700 pmol/L, FSH dose can be safely increased by 75–150 IU followed by ultrasound monitoring.

Before the introduction of GnRH analogs in ART cycles, detection of premature endogenous LH surges was a constant concern. Despite an effective suppression of endogenous gonadotropins by the analogs, a small increment in the plasma progesterone has been reported in upto 20% of stimulated cycles. It hampers the oocyte quality and the implantation rate. Plasma progesterone determination has been performed to seek for any premature luteinization. It is hypothesized that increase in circulating progesterone concentration from nonluteinized tissues may lead to advances in the development of endometrium and effectively reduce the window of implantation. Elevated serum progesterone more than 1.35 ng/mL on the day of hCG is detrimental to both positive beta hCG test and clinical pregnancy rate.[12] The duration of preovulatory serum progesterone elevation before hCG administration is detrimental to the outcome of IVF/ICSI cycles by causing an early closure of the implantation window.[13]

On the day of hCG trigger, estradiol level of more than 5,000 and more than 18 follicles above 10 mm in size have a 83% sensitivity and 84% specificity for prediction of OHSS. Coasting is initiated when follicles are 15–16 mm in diameter and serum E2 levels more than 3,000 pg/mL.

With the wide usage of antagonist cycles and development of good cryo/vitrification programs coasting are becoming redundant. Patients at risk of OHSS are taken for an antagonist cycle, GnRH agonist trigger, freeze all and transfer in natural or HRT cycle.

## KEY POINTS

- Monitoring of ART cycles are center specific. Commonly used modalities are transvaginal ultrasonography and serum estradiol levels. But combined monitoring for all cycles is time consuming, expensive and inconvenient.
- Two-dimensional ultrasound scanning of follicular growth is the method of choice for monitoring IVF cycles. Serum estradiol estimation is useful in monitoring poor responders and those at risk for OHSS.
- Fine tuning of COS on the basis of hormonal measurements has given us new treatment strategies to ensure optimal outcomes.

## REFERENCES

1. Carmina E, Lobo RA. Evaluation of hormonal status. In: Strauss J, Barbieri R (Eds). Yen and Jaffe`s Reproductive Endocrinology, 6th edition. Philadelphia: Saunders; 2009. pp. 801-23.
2. Wikland M, Hillensjo T. Monitoring IVF cycles. In: Gardner Dk, Weissman A, Howles CM, Shoham Z (Eds). Textbook of Assisted Reproductive Technologies. Florida: CRC Press; 2004. pp. 553-64.
3. Weenen C, Laven JS, Von Bergh AR, et al. Anti-Müllerian hormone expression pattern in the human ovary: potential implications for initial and cyclic follicle recruitment. Mole Hum Reprod. 2004;10:77-83.
4. van Rooij IA, Broekmans FJ, te Velde ER, et al. Serum anti-Müllerian hormone levels: a novel measure of ovarian reserve. Hum Reprod. 2002;17 3065-71.
5. Penarrubia J, Fabregues F, Manau D, et al. Basal and stimulation day 5 anti-Müllerian hormone serum concentrations as predictors of ovarian response and pregnancy in assisted reproductive technology cycles stimulated with gonadotropin-releasing hormone agonist gonadotropin treatment. Hum Reprod. 2005;20 915-22.
6. Fleming R, Harborne L, MacLaughlin DT, et al. Metformin reduces serum müllerian-inhibiting substance levels in women with polycystic ovary syndrome after protracted treatment. Fertil Steril. 2005;83:130-6.
7. Cook CL, Siow Y, Taylor S, et al. Serum müllerian-inhibiting substance levels during normal menstrual cycles. Fertil Steril 2007;3:859-61.
8. La Marca A, Giulini S, Orvieto R, De Leo V & Volpe A 2005 Anti-Müllerian hormone concentrations in maternal serum during pregnancy. Human Reproduction 20 1569–1572.
9. Nelson SM, Yates RW, Fleming R. Serum anti-Müllerian hormone and FSH: prediction of live birth and extremes of response in stimulated cycles–implications for individualization of therapy. Hum Reprod. 2007;22:2414-21.
10. Streuli I, Fraisse T, Pillet C, et al. Serum antimüllerian hormone levels remain stable throughout the menstrual cycle and after oral or vaginal administration of synthetic sex steroids. Fertil Steril. 2008:90:395-400.

11. Kwan I, Bhattacharya S, Kang A, et al. Monitoring of stimulated cycles in assisted reproduction (IVF and ICSI). Cochrane Database Syst Rev. 2008;8:CD005289.
12. Papaleo E, Corti L, Vanni VS, et al. 2014. Basal progesterone level as the main determinant of progesterone elevation on the day of hCG triggering in controlled ovarian stimulation cycles. Arch Gynecol Obstet. 2014;290:169-76.
13. Huang CC, Lien YR, Chen HF, et al. The duration of pre-ovulatory serum progesterone elevation before hCG administration affects the outcome of IVF/ICSI cycles. Hum Reprod. 2012:27:2036-45.

CHAPTER
12

# Role of Transvaginal Sonography in Assisted Reproductive Technology

*Sanghamitra Ghosh, Nitin Gupta, Monica Chetani, Mumtaz Sanghamita*

## ■ INTRODUCTION

Transvaginal ultrasonography has provided new anatomic and pathophysiologic information about the female pelvis. It offers a significantly accurate, quick, and reproducible assessment of female pelvic anatomy and other important female factors of infertility. Resolution is dramatically improved in transvaginal sonography (TVS) because of probe proximity to the organ of interest and higher insonating frequency.

Transvaginal sonography has an important role from baseline workup till ovum pickup in management of infertility patients, especially those needing assisted reproductive technology (ART). Physiologic information concerning the endometrium and ovarian follicles has vastly improved diagnosis and treatment.

Introduction of three-dimensional (3D)-TVS and color Doppler has opened a new dimension in diagnosis of factors responsible for female infertility. TVS is not only useful for prediction of ovulation timing, endometrial preparation but also is a useful adjunct for ovum pickup. 3D-TVS is the modality of choice in evaluation of female infertility.

Pelvic assessment by TVS can be done in the following manner:
- *Basic infertility workup:* It includes anatomic assessment of uterus, endometrial cavity, myometrium, ovaries, and fallopian tubes.
- *Assessment of index in vitro fertilization cycle:* It includes baseline scan for antral follicle count (AFC) and endometrial study. Thereafter, TVS is used for follicular monitoring to assess response to stimulation, endometrial preparation (endometrial thickness, blood flow, and volume assessment), culminating in oocyte retrieval (OCR).

## ■ BASIC INFERTILITY WORKUP

- *Uterus:* Uterine dimensions, cervical corporeal ratio, myometrium, endomyometrial junction, and endometrial cavity are assessed. Normal uterine dimensions for reproductive age group female are: length 6–9 cm, height 3–5 cm, and width 3–5 cm.

Normal cervical corporeal ratio is 1:2. It is helpful to rule out infantile type of uterus.
- *Myometrial assessment:* Myometrial assessment for fibroids, focal adenomyoma, and adenomyosis. Adenomyotic uterus appears bulky and shows Swiss cheese pattern and loss of differentiation of endomyometrial junction. It can be assessed both by two-dimensional (2D) and 3D-TVS (Figs. 1 and 2).
- *Endometrial cavity:* Three-dimensional TVS is an essential modality to assess endometrial cavity, as it not only delineate the endometrial cavity but also informs about myometrium and fundal contour of uterus (Figs. 3A to E). Saline infusion 3D-TVS increase the accuracy for assessment of endometrial polyp, submucous fibroid, and adhesions in the cavity (Figs. 4A to C). Müllerian anomalies are also better depicted by 3D-TVS.

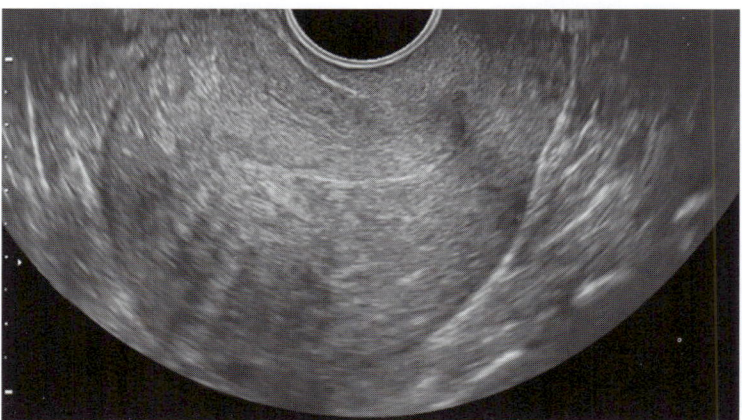

**Fig. 1:** Adenomyosis Swiss cheese appearance (TVS-2D). (2D: two-dimensional; TVS: transvaginal sonography)

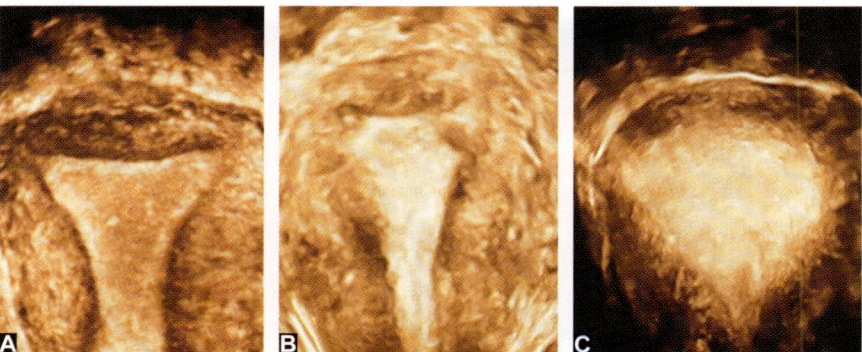

**Figs. 2A to C:** Normal versus adenomyotic uterus (TVS-3D). (3D: three-dimensional; TVS: transvaginal sonography)

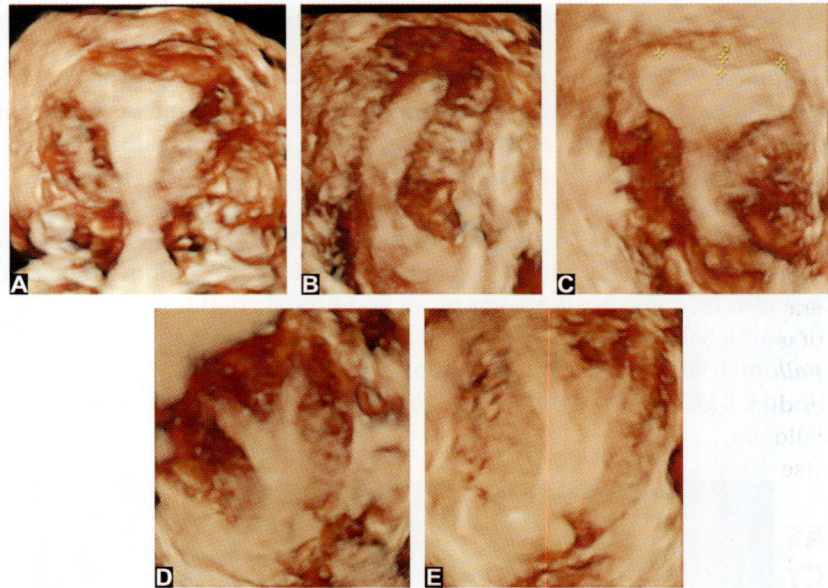

**Figs. 3A to E:** (A) Normal cavity; (B) Unicornuate; (C) Bicornuate; (D) Septate; and (E) Arcuate.

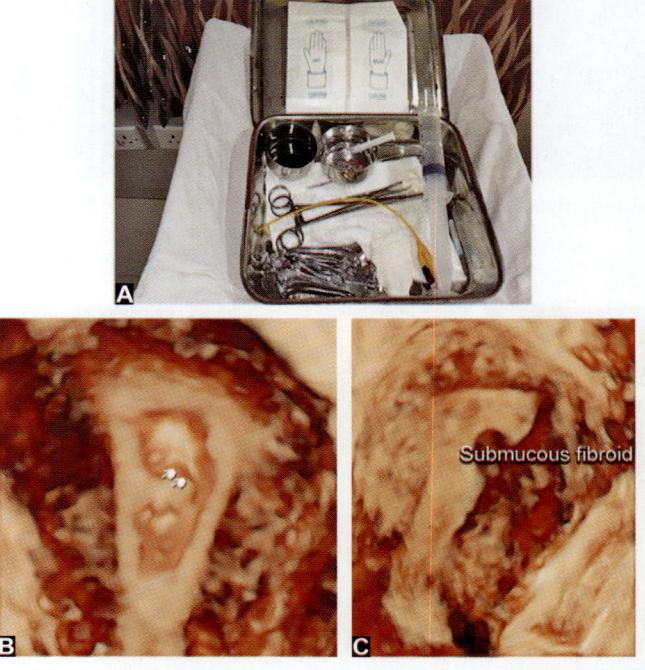

**Figs. 4A to C:** (A) Saline infusion sonography (SIS) tray; (B) Endometrial polyp; and (C) Submucous fibroid.

– *Saline infusion sonography:* This helps in better assessment of uterine cavity and tubes. In this procedure, total pain score is significantly lower than for hysterosalpingography (HSG). It also reduces the number of laparoscopies and allows patients to proceed for corrective surgeries if needed. The contraindications are—bilateral hydrosalpinx, pelvic infection.
- *Ovaries:* Ovarian morphology for size, shape, volume is assessed. Endometriotic, hemorrhagic, dermoid, and other cystic lesions of ovary can also be nicely depicted by TVS (Figs. 5A to D). TVS is also very useful tool for assessment of severity of endometriosis. Intestinal involvement in endometriosis can be assessed by adherence of intestine with posterior wall of uterus (restriction of free mobility of intestine).
- *Fallopian tubes:* Tubal disease (hydrosalpinx, hematosalpinx, and tubal endometriosis) can be assessed by routine TVS, however, patency of fallopian tubes can only be assessed by saline infusion sonography (SIS). Use of ultrasound contrast can also depict the anatomy of fallopian tube.

# ASSESSMENT OF INDEX IN VITRO FERTILIZATION CYCLE

## Baseline Scan

Transvaginal sonography is performed on D2/D3 of cycle for assessment of ovarian reserve. It includes AFC and endometrial assessment. It gives absolute

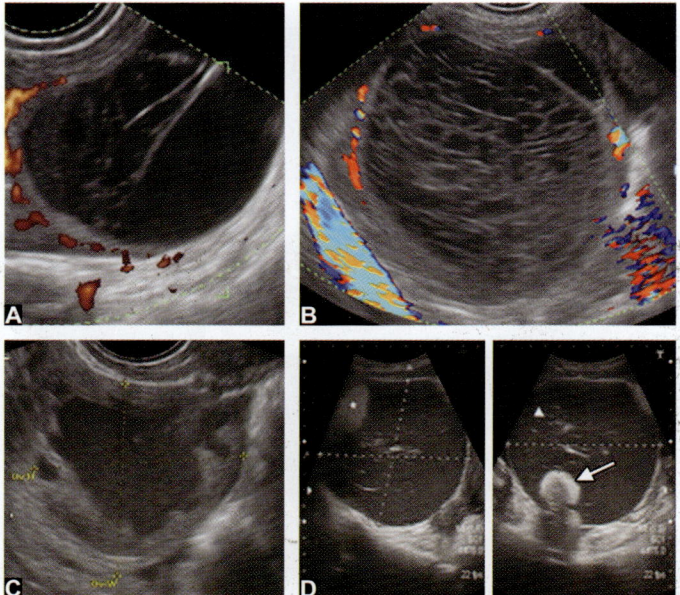

**Figs. 5A to D:** (A) Corpus luteum cyst; (B) Hemorrhagic cyst; (C) Endometrioma; and (D) Dermoid cyst.

baseline status of ovaries. AFC count along with follicle-stimulating hormone (FSH) and anti-Müllerian hormone (AMH) are the most important parameters to decide the stimulation protocol.

## Antral Follicle Count

Transvaginal sonography is used for assessment of ovarian reserve. Ultrasonography is a significant part of the tests now being used to investigate follicular dynamics in women, as are endocrine-based tests.[1-4] Follicles measuring between 2 mm and 9 mm are defined as antral follicle. AFC includes all these follicles in both ovaries. The number of antral follicles (2-9 mm) in both ovaries is clearly related to reproductive age and could well reflect the size of the remaining primordial follicle pool. AFC less than 5 is considered as poor responder.[5,6] AFC 5-15 are considered as normal responder. AFC more than 15 are considered as hyperresponder and have high chances of developing ovarian hyperstimulation syndrome (OHSS) (Figs. 6A and B).

Sono automated volume calculation (AVC) is a 3D tool and can be used for reliable AFC in polycystic ovary syndrome (PCO) patients. In PCO patients, as number of follicles are significantly higher, it avoids recounting of the same follicle. Predominant hyperechoic stroma is most reliable factor for diagnosis of PCO (Figs. 7A to C).

## Ovarian Volume

Another 3D tool named as virtual organ computer-aided analysis (VOCAL) can be used for assessment of ovarian and stromal volume. Ovarian volume may predict ART outcomes better than FSH concentration on day 3.[7,8] Measurement of ovarian volume by TVS before ovulation induction can predict poor response.[6]

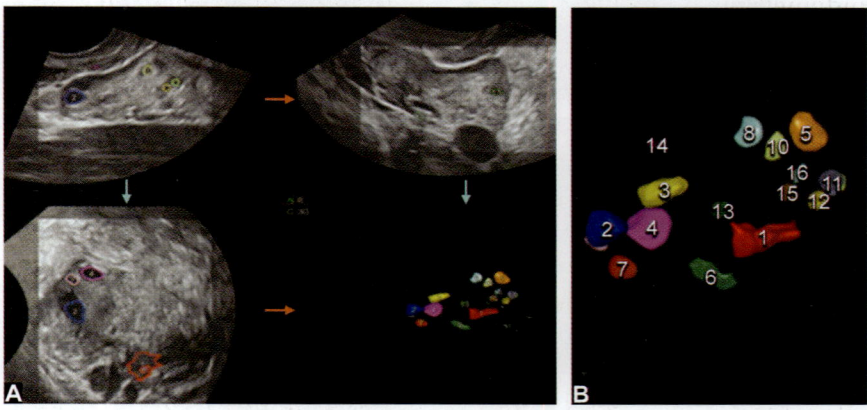

**Figs. 6A and B:** Antral follicle count (AFC).

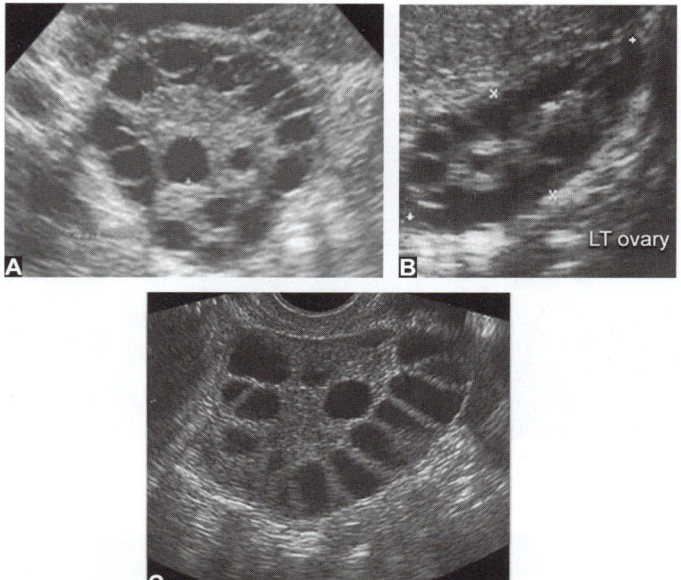

**Figs. 7A to C:** Polycystic ovaries.

## Ovarian Vascularity

Ovarian stromal blood flow can also be assessed with power Doppler. Normal RI values are 0.6–0.7 and peak systolic values are 5–10 cm/sec for stromal vessels. Ovaries having peak systolic velocity (PSV) more than 10 cm/sec at baseline scan are highly prone for hyperstimulation and ovarian stimulation in the index cycle should be planned accordingly.

## Endometrium

Endometrium on baseline scan by TVS is thin, as it has shed off during menstruation (Fig. 8).

Endometrial volume and endometrial vascularity (vascularity index, flow index, and vascularity flow index) can also be assessed by 3D-TVS and color Doppler (Fig. 9).

Endometrial volume of 3–5 cc has shown favorable outcome in in vitro fertilization (IVF)-embryo transfer (ET) cycle in many studies (Figs. 10A and B).[9-11]

## Follicular Tracking (Monitoring)

Follicle monitoring is started on D5/D6 of ovarian stimulation. Follicle size is assessed till it becomes dominant and mature follicle. When a follicle reaches a size of 10 mm, it is considered as dominant follicle. It grows at a rate of 2–3

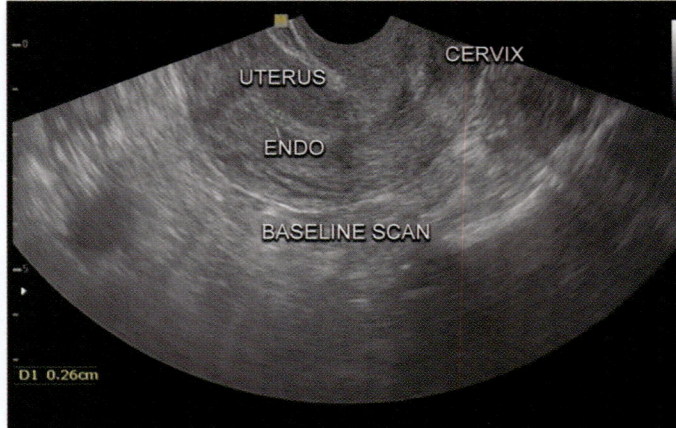

**Fig. 8:** Endometrium at baseline scan.

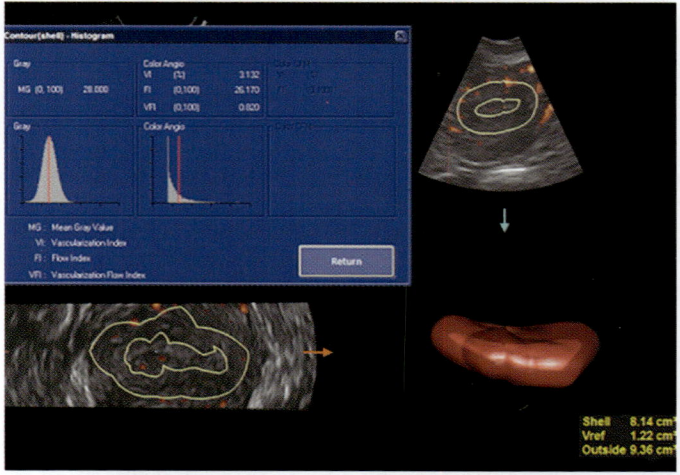

**Fig. 9:** Endometrial vascularity—VI, FI, and VFI. (FI: flow index; VI: vascularity index; VFI: vascularity flow index)

mm/day. When leading follicle reaches 18 mm, human chorionic gonadotropin (hCG) trigger is given. Subsequently ovum pickup is scheduled 34–35 hours later.

## Color Doppler Evaluation of Ovarian Follicles

Along with cyclical changes in ovarian follicles there is change in Doppler wave pattern in ovarian and follicular vascularity. Color Doppler can identify dominant follicles easily. Due to neovascularization of growing follicle, dominant follicle develops a low impedance shunt. Some changes also happen

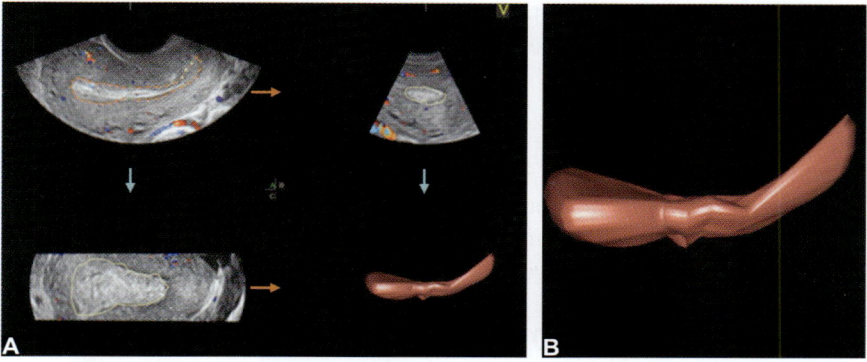

**Figs. 10A and B:** Endometrial volume.

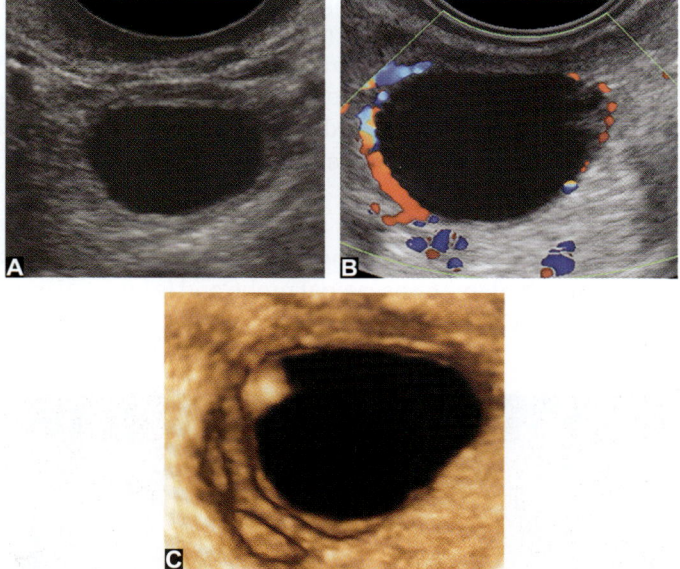

**Figs. 11A to C:** Follicle more than or equal to 16 mm; (B) More than or equal to third-fourths of vascularity; and (C) Cumulus oophorus.

in the corpus luteum. The changes in Doppler wave patterns in growing dominant follicle and developing corpus luteum are high diastolic flow, low impedance, and increased intraovarian vascularity (Figs. 11A to C).

There is a significant relationship between PSV of perifollicular blood flow and quality of oocytes, and preimplantation embryos. When PSV is greater than 10 cm/sec there is a 70% chance of formation of a grade I embryo.[12]

## Endometrial Assessment

Endometrium is assessed for thickness, volume, vascularity, and pattern. A triple-layered 8–10 mm thick, slightly hyperechoic endometrium is most receptive for embryo implantation. Endometrial vascularity can be assessed by color Doppler. Vascularity in zone 3 and 4 are highly favorable for successful embryo implantation. Endometrial vascularity has been classified by "Applebaum" as follows:

- *Zone 1:* A 2 mm thick area surrounding the hyperechoic outer layer of endometrium
- *Zone 2:* The hyperechoic outer layer of endometrium
- *Zone 3:* The hypoechoic inner layer of endometrium
- *Zone 4:* The inner most layer of endometrial cavity (Figs. 12A to D).

## TRANSVAGINAL SONOGRAPHY IN OOCYTE RETRIEVAL (OVUM PICKUP)

The most visible use of TVS imaging in IVF has been the tremendous advancement facilitated by transvaginal retrieval of oocyte. The first description of oocyte collection with transvaginal transducer was done by Matts Wikland in 1985.[13,14] OCR has become easier and safer with TVS. It has also simplified the OCR technique enabling the procedure to be performed under sedation. Transvaginal OCR has completely replaced laparoscopic OCR under general anesthesia (Figs. 13A and B).[15]

Retrieval of oocytes in IVF cycles is now routinely performed under transvaginal ultrasound (TVUS) guidance. An aspirating needle is introduced through a guide attached to a transvaginal probe and is inserted into first one ovary, then the other, via the vaginal fornices. Almost all aspiration needles

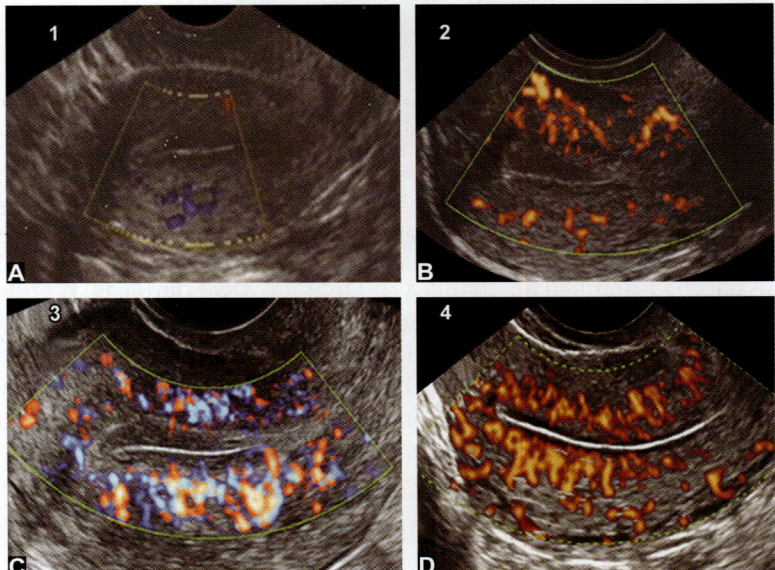

**Figs. 12A to D:** Endometrial vascularity.

# Role of Transvaginal Sonography in Assisted Reproductive Technology

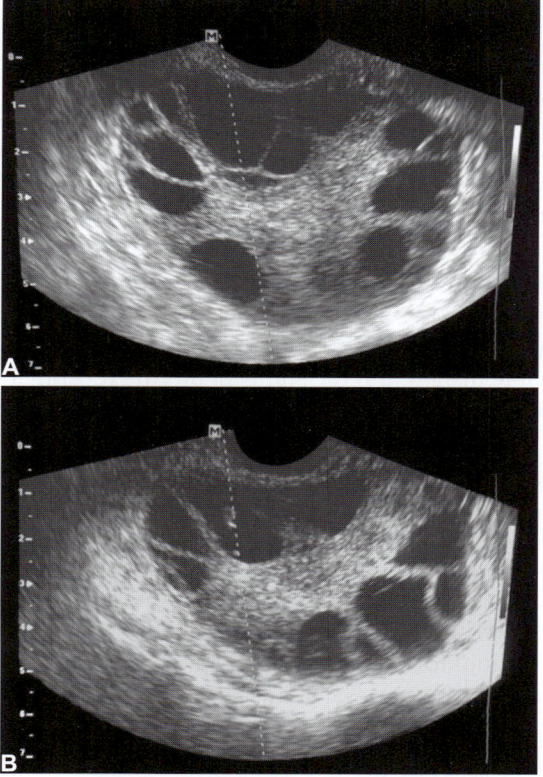

**Figs. 13A and B:** Oocyte retrieval.

now in common use have a small band of highly reflective surface near the tip of the needle to facilitate visualization as the needle enters the ovary and once it is in the follicles. The path of the OCR needle may be accurately visualized within biopsy guidelines imposed on the ultrasound screen as it is guided into each ovarian follicle. The highly reflective echoic tip of the needles makes identifying their path quite easy in most cases. The needle tip can be observed directly as it is maneuvered within the ovaries and into each follicle. The follicular fluid containing the oocyte-cumulus complex is then aspirated by application of gentle suction. The walls of the follicle collapse as the fluid is aspirated and the needle moved within the follicle to ensure that all of the follicular fluid is withdrawn.[16-18]

## ■ TRANSVAGINAL ULTRASOUND-GUIDED EMBRYO TRANSFER IN IN VITRO FERTILIZATION

The percentage of pregnancies per transfer is significantly increased when the transfer is performed under TVUS guidance.[19] Ultrasound-guided embryo transfer (UGET) was associated with an increase in the chance of a clinical pregnancy or live birth.[20]

## Uterine Receptivity

It is one among several factors contributing to implantation. Use of high-resolution TV ultrasonography is a noninvasive method of assessment of uterine receptivity. A trilaminar endometrial pattern and a thickness between 7 mm and 12 mm are indirect evidence of a receptive endometrium.[21-23] Recently a 3D approach of monitoring the endometrial volume,[10,11] uterine artery blood flow, and endometrial tissue vascular flow has been proposed to give a better understanding of endometrial receptivity.[9] Color Doppler along with TVS also provides valuable insight into the status of uterine receptivity. Vascularity in zone 3 and zone 4 are highly favorable for successful embryo implantation.

## Transvaginal Sonography in Complications of Assisted Reproductive Technology

Ovarian hyperstimulation syndrome is the most significant complication of ART (Fig. 14). TVS helps in prediction of the syndrome and it is also needed for aspiration of ascitic fluid when patient needs symptomatic relief. TVS is also an efficient tool for diagnosing ectopic pregnancies or pregnancies of unknown location.

## ■ TRANSVAGINAL SONOGRAPHY IN INTRAUTERINE INSEMINATION

Transvaginal sonography is routinely used in intrauterine insemination (IUI) for assessment of endometrium and folliculometry. TVS provides detailed information of follicle number and size in each ovary. Under best situation

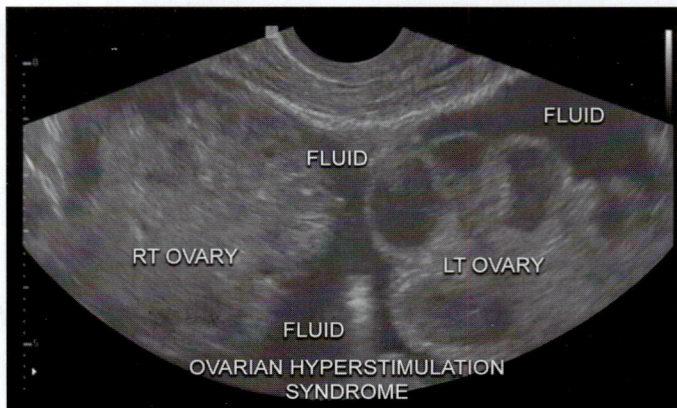

**Fig. 14:** Ovarian hyperstimulation syndrome.

a follicle in the ovary can be seen from a diameter of 2–3 mm. Follicles usually grow by 2–3 mm daily. In an ART cycle, the frequency of ultrasound examination depends on the type of ovarian stimulation and patient's response to it. Endometrium is also monitored simultaneously. It usually grows 0.5–2 mm per day.

Prediction of ovulation by TVS can be done when dominant follicle is 18–24 mm in size. hCG is administered at this stage. The dominant follicle has sonolucent halo 24 hours prior to ovulation, vascularity around third-fourths of the follicle, and cumulus-like echoes in certain cases. Ovulation is confirmed when follicle disappears or collapses. There may be small amount of fluid in the pouch of Douglas (POD) as seen by TVS. IUI is done after ovulation.

## CONCLUSION

Transvaginal sonography is one of the most clinically important diagnostic instruments in assisted conception. Advanced TVS, including 3D, color Doppler, power Doppler, hysterosalpingo-contrast-sonography (HyCoSy), and SIS, is accurate for diagnosis and differentiation of uterine anomalies and provide valuable information about endometrial receptivity. It is an indispensable tool for ovarian assessment. It is comprehensive, cost effective, and minimally invasive. It saves highly valuable time of the childless couple as well as the ART professional. Addition of color Doppler along with TVS helps in prediction of success and avoids complications. 3D-TVS has given us a new dimension of volume and provides us with sculpture like images.

Transvaginal ultrasound has revolutionized the practice of ART. It is unthinkable to practice infertility and/or ART without TVS in this modern era of technology.

## REFERENCES

1. Bukulmez O, Arici A. Assessment of ovarian reserve. Curr Opin Obstet Gynecol. 2004;16(3):231-7.
2. Hansen KR, Hodnett GM, Knowlton N, et al. Correlation of ovarian reserve tests with histologically determined primordial follicle number. Fertil Steril. 2011;95(1):170-5.
3. Wallace WH, Kelsey TW. Ovarian reserve and reproductive age may be determined from measurement of ovarian volume by transvaginal sonography. Hum Reprod. 2004;19(7):1612-7.
4. Wallace WH, Kelsey TW. Human ovarian reserve from conception to the menopause. PLoS One. 2010;5(1):e8772.
5. Hendriks DJ, Mol BW, Bancsi LF, et al. Antral follicle count in the prediction of poor ovarian response and pregnancy after in vitro fertilization: a meta-analysis and comparison with basal follicle-stimulating hormone level. Fertil Steril. 2005;83(2):291-301.

6. Lass A, Skull J, McVeigh E, et al. Measurement of ovarian volume by transvaginal sonography before ovulation induction with human menopausal gonadotrophin for in-vitro fertilization can predict poor response. Hum Reprod. 1997;12(2):294-7.
7. Syrop CH, Dawson JD, Husman KJ, et al. Ovarian volume may predict assisted reproductive outcomes better than follicle stimulating hormone concentration on day 3. Hum Reprod. 1999;14(7):1752-6.
8. Erdem A, Erdem M, Biberoglu K, et al. Age-related changes in ovarian volume, antral follicle counts and basal FSH in women with normal reproductive health. J Reprod Med. 2002;47(10):835-9.
9. Ledee N. Uterine receptivity and the two and three dimensions of ultrasound. Ultrasound Obstet Gynecol. 2005;26(7):695-8.
10. Raga F, Bonilla-Musoles F, Casañ EM, et al. Assessment of endometrial volume by three-dimensional ultrasound prior to embryo transfer: clues to endometrial receptivity. Hum Reprod. 1999;14(11):2851-4.
11. Schild RL, Indefrei D, Eschweiler S, et al. Three-dimensional endometrial volume calculation and pregnancy rate in an in-vitro fertilization programme. Hum Reprod. 1999;14(5):1255-8.
12. Nargund G, Bourne T, Doyle P, et al. Associations between ultrasound indices of follicular blood flow, oocyte recovery and preimplantation embryo quality. Hum Reprod. 1996;11(1):109-13.
13. Wikland M, Enk L, Hammarberg K, et al. Use of a vaginal transducer for oocyte retrieval in an IVF/ET program. J Clin Ultrasound. 1987;15(4):245-51.
14. Wikland M, Enk L, Hammarberg K, et al. Oocyte retrieval under the guidance of a vaginal transducer. Ann N Y Acad Sci. 1988;541(3):103-10.
15. Schulman JD, Dorfmann AD, Jones SL, et al. Outpatient in vitro fertilization using transvaginal ultrasound-guided oocyte retrieval. Obstet Gynecol. 1987;69(4):665-8.
16. Feichtinger W. Current technology of oocyte retrieval. Curr Opin Obstet Gynecol. 1992;4(5):697-701.
17. Gembruch U, Diedrich K, Welker B, et al. Transvaginal sonographically guided oocyte retrieval for in-vitro fertilization. Hum Reprod. 1988;3(Suppl 2):59-63.
18. Feldberg D, Goldman JA, Ashkenazi J, et al. Transvaginal oocyte retrieval controlled by vaginal probe for in vitro fertilization: a comparative study. J Ultrasound Med. 1988;7(6):339-43.
19. Larue L, Keromnes G, Massari A, et al. Transvaginal ultrasound-guided embryo tranfer in IVF. J Gynecol Obstet and Hum Reprod. 2017;46(5):411-16.
20. Cochrane Review (March 2016).
21. Oliveira JB, Baruffi RL, Mauri AL, et al. Endometrial ultrasonography as a predictor of pregnancy in an in-vitro fertilization programme after ovarian stimulation and gonadotrophin-releasing hormone and gonadotrophins. Hum Reprod. 1997;12(11):2515-8.
22. Zhang X, Chen CH, Confino E, et al. Increased endometrial thickness is associated with improved treatment outcome for selected patients undergoing in vitro fertilization—embryo transfer. Fertil Steril. 2007;88(1):74-81.
23. McWilliams GD, Frattarelli JL. Changes in measured endometrial thickness predict in vitro fertilization success. Fertil Steril. 2007;88(1):74-81.

CHAPTER
13

# Tests for Endometrial Receptivity

*Moumita Naha, Gautam Khastgir*

## ■ INTRODUCTION

Endometrial receptivity is defined as a temporary unique sequence of factors that make the endometrium receptive to the embryonic implantation.[1] The endometrium acquires the capacity to welcome the embryo during a restrictive time period in the mid-luteal phase called "window of implantation (WOI)". Thus it is critical to recognize the time of maximum endometrial receptivity for embryo transfer, which should best correspond with the window of implantation. With the increasing popularity of single embryo transfer, the knowledge of endometrial receptivity has now become even more relevant and major focus in the leading assisted reproductive technology (ART) centers of the world.

## ■ CLINICAL APPLICATION OF ENDOMETRIAL RECEPTIVITY ASSAY

- The most important group of patients that would get benefit from this assay and possible interventions suggested by this assay is patients with recurrent implantation failure with good quality embryo.
- It is known that ovarian hyperstimulation during in vitro fertilization (IVF) has detrimental effect on endometrial receptivity. If a reliable, noninvasive and quick test is available which can be applied during treatment cycle, clinician can decide whether to go ahead with embryo transfer or to freeze all embryos.
- A reliable and affordable test would allow its application as a screening test for endometrial receptivity disorders in all infertile patients in future.

## ■ ASSESSMENT FOR ENDOMETRIAL RECEPTIVITY

### Histology

Back in 1950, Noyes et al. first described endometrial dating by histology.[2] With slight modification of their original work [luteinizing hormone (LH) surge or ultrasound (USG) to predict ovulation instead of basal body temperature], histological dating of endometrium is still being considered as a routine workup of infertile couple in many centers. If menstrual cycle date based on histological features as per Noyes criteria lags behind the actual cycle date for more than 2 days, endometrium is considered "out of phase".

Later studies, however, pointed out a number of flaws of histological dating:

Dating appears to be more accurate in early and late luteal phase but not in the implantation window.[3]

There are significant intra- and interobserver variability. Intraobserver variability was more prevalent among infertile women during implantation window.[3,4]

It was also shown that the prevalence of "out of phase" endometrium was quite high in fertile women and even more than that of infertile couple (49% vs 43%).[5]

Hence, it can be concluded that histological dating provides very little information pertaining to the evaluation of endometrial receptivity.

## Ultrastructural Assessment of Endometrium

Ultrastructural changes in the surface epithelium seem to be another promising marker for receptivity. Scanning electron microscopy (SEM) shows that microvilli of apical membranes convert into smooth projection called pinopodes during window of implantation. Pinopodes expression is progesterone dependent, limited to a brief period of 2 days in menstrual cycle and embryo transfer done on the day of mature pinopodes formation has shown to increase pregnancy rate.[6]

Later studies, however, showed poor intrapatient consistency in consecutive cycles and presence of pinopodes till the end of luteal phase thus making it a poor predictor of window of implantation. Furthermore, presence of equivalent number of pinopodes in infertile females as fertile controls at the time of implantation window makes it an unsatisfactory test for endometrial receptivity.[6]

## Functional Assessment of Endometrium

### *Molecular Markers*

A large number of molecular markers have been investigated to be involved in early fetomaternal cross-talks. They are expressed in window of implantation under influence of ovarian hormones and include cytokines, growth factors, adhesion molecules, prostaglandin, etc. Test for $\alpha V \beta 3$ integrin and endometrial function test (EFT) which is immune-histochemical staining of endometrium with markers for cyclin E and P27 are only commercially available tests for biomarkers.[7]

The use of biomarkers has not been adopted in routine infertility practice as it seems unlikely that a single or two biomarkers would represent the entire genetic pool alteration during window of implantation. Recent researches thus have focused on microassay or global gene analysis to assess endometrial receptivity.

## Endometrial Receptivity Array

It is a molecular diagnostic tool based on transcriptomics signature (characterization of gene expression at mRNA level) that can identify the time of maximum endometrial receptivity.

An endometrial biopsy is taken on Day 21 (LH +7 or 6 days after follicular rupture) in a natural cycle or 7 days after hCG administration or after 5 days of progesterone in a HRT cycle. The sequencing expression of the 238 genes that are involved in endometrial receptivity is then analyzed by using a customized DNA microarray and the endometrial receptivity status is assessed by the ERA computational predictor.[8] The endometrial receptivity array (ERA) test diagnoses the endometrial samples as receptive (R) or nonreceptive (NR) with an associated diagnostic probability. The initial result is validated by performing a second endometrial biopsy and ERA analysis on the day recommended by first ERA result. Once the personalized WOI is identified, a personalized embryo transfer (pET) plan is developed to transfer the embryo according to the day in which the endometrium is receptive (Flow chart 1).

Initial studies of ERA have shown promising result in patients with recurrent implantation failure (RIF). However, further studies are required before its implementation in routine practice.[9-11]

The major disadvantage of endometrial tissue based approach is that being an invasive procedure, it cannot be applied in the treatment cycle. Noninvasive tests like study of proteins or lipids in endometrial fluid derived from aspiration or lavage (secretomics, lipidomics), study of circulating micro RNA (miRNA) derived from endometrium in the peripheral blood are now an active area of research.[12]

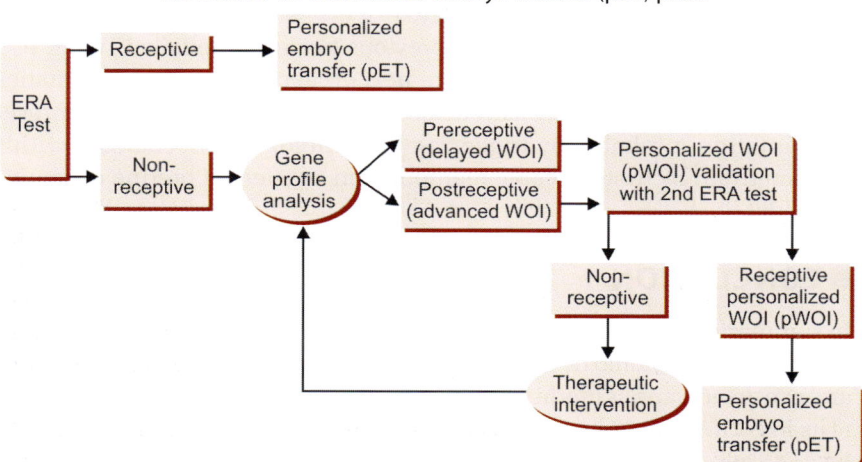

**Flowchart 1:** Personalized embryo transfer (pET) plan.

## ■ MORPHOLOGICAL ASSESSMENT OF ENDOMETRIAL RECEPTIVITY

Functional markers of endometrial receptivity, although promising, are invasive, expensive and circumstantial.

Transvaginal ultrasonography (TVS) has been proposed as an alternative, noninvasive tool to assess receptivity of endometrium. It has been reported that endometrial thickness between 7 mm and 14 mm, a triple layer pattern, endometrial volume of more than 2 mm in 3D scan and good subendometrial blood flow on the day before oocyte retrieval may indicate a receptive endometrium.[13-17]

Recent studies have shown that individually these USG parameters have poor specificity and positive predictive value, but reasonably good negative predictive value for successful implantation.[18,19]

### Uterine Biophysical Profile

A scoring system combining various USG parameters has been proposed to predict receptive endometrium in IVF cycles. Initial results are promising, however, more studies are required before its routine application.[20]

Another major advantage of USG is that it can detect some intrauterine pathologies that can be detrimental to implantation process, e.g. uterine polyp, submucous or intramural fibroid distorting uterine cavity, intrauterine septa etc. Use of 3D scan or saline infusion sonography can improve detection of these potential anatomic causes of reduced fertility.

### Hysteroscopy

Hysteroscopy is considered gold standard to detect intrauterine pathology. In 18.50% patients undergoing IVF with normal USG report, hysteroscopy detected subtle intrauterine pathology.[21]

It is shown that in patients with previous two or more failed IVF or ICSI cycle, hysteroscopy performed before next cycle can improve implantation rate.[22,23] Even when no abnormality detected, diagnostic hysteroscopy improved implantation, probably by triggering immunological mechanism within endometrium by hysteroscopic manipulation or effect of uterine distention by media.[24]

## ■ CONCLUSION

In summary, till date there is no perfect diagnostic tool to assess endometrial receptivity. USG should be the frontline test as it is noninvasive, easy to perform and can detect various uterine pathologies. More sophisticated transcriptomics tests like ERA should be reserved for patients with RIF. More research must be done in search of noninvasive proteomics or secretomics tests that can be applied during treatment cycle. However, even with transfer of euploid embryo within personalized WOI, it appears impossible to achieve an implantation rate of 100% in IVF as embryo-endometrial cross talk that takes place during implantation process can reduce the practical value of any preimplantation endometrial assessment.

## REFERENCES

1. Bergh PA, Navot D. The impact of embryonic development and endometrial maturity on the timing of implantation. Fertil Steril. 1992;58:537-42.
2. Noyes RW, Hertig AT, Rock J. Dating the endometrial biopsy. Am J Obstet Gynecol. 1975;122:262-3.
3. Myers ER, Silva S, Barnhart K. Interobserver and intraobserver variability in the histological dating of the endometrium in fertile and infertile women. Fertil Steril. 2004;82:1278-82.
4. Murry MJ, Meyer WR, Zaino RJ. A critical analysis of the accuracy, reproducibility, and clinical utility of histologic endometrial dating in fertile women. Fertil Steril. 2004;81:1333-43.
5. Coutifaris C, Myers ER, Diamond MP, et al. Histological dating of timed endometrial biopsy tissue is not related to fertility status. Fertil Steril. 2004;82:1264-72.
6. Nikas G. Pinopodes as markers of endometrial receptivity in clinical practice. Hum Reprod. 1999;14(Suppl 2):99-106.
7. Cakmak H, Taylor HS. Assessment of uterine receptivity. In: Nagy Z, Varghese A, Agarwal A (Eds). Practical manual of in vitro fertilization. New York: Springer; 2012. pp. 559-66.
8. Diaz-Gimeno P, Horcajadar JA, Martinez-Conejero JA, et al. A genomic diagnostic tool for human endometrial receptivity based on transcriptomic signature. Fertil Steril. 2011;95 (1):50-60.
9. Diaz-Gimeno P, Ruiz-Alonso M, Blesa D, et al. Transcriptomics of human endometrium. Int J Dev Biol. 2014;58:127-37.
10. Ruiz-Alonso M, Blesa D, Diaz-Gimeno P, et al. The endometrial receptivity assay for diagnosis and personalized embryo transfer as a treatment for patients with repeated implantation failure. Fertil Steril. 2013;100(3):818-24.
11. Mahajan N. Endometrial receptivity array: clinical application. J Hum Reprod Sci. 2015;8(3):121-9.
12. Edgell TA, Rombauts LJ, Salaonsen LA. Assessing receptivity in the endometrium: the need for a rapid, non-invasive test. Reprod Biomed Online. 2013;27:486-96.
13. Elnashar A, Afifi A, Donia O. Endometrial thickness and pregnancy rates in infertile couples undergoing AIH. Benha M J. 1998;12:1-9.
14. Weissman A, Gotilieb L, Casper R. The detrimental effect of increased endometrial thickness on implantation and pregnancy rates and outcome in an in vitro fertilization program. Fetil Steril. 1999;71:147-9.
15. Leibovitz Z, Grinin V, Rabia R, et al. Assessment of endometrial receptivity for gestation in patients undergoing in vitro fertilization, using endometrial thickness

and the endometrium-myometrium relative echogenicity co-efficient. Ultrasound Obstet Gynecol. 1999;143:194-9.
16. Raga F, Bonilla-Musoles F, Casan EM, et al. Assessment of endometrial volume by three dimensional ultrasound prior to embryo transfer; clues to endometrial receptivity. Hum Reprod. 1999:14: 2851-4.
17. Kupesic S, Bekavac I, Bjelos D, et al. Assessment of endometrial receptivity by transvaginal color Doppler and three dimensional power Doppler ultrasonography in patients undergoing in vitro fertilization procedures. J Ultrasound Med. 2001;20:125-34.
18. Ernest Hung Yu NG, Pak Chung HO. Ultrasound Assessment of Endometrial. Receptivity in in vitro Fertilization Treatment. DSJUOG. 2010;4 (2):179-88.
19. Abdallah Y, Naji O, Saso S, et al. Ultrasound assessment of the peri-implantation uterus: a review. Ultrasound Obstet Gynecol. 2012;39:612-9.
20. Malhotra N, Malhotra J, Malhotra N, et al. Endometrial receptivity and scoring for prediction of implantation and newer markers. DSJUOG. 2010;4(4):439-46.
21. Doldi N, Persico P, Di Sebastiano F, et al. Pathologic findings in hysteroscopy before in vitro fertilization-embryo transfer (IVF-ET). Gynecol Endocrinol. 2005;21:235-7.
22. Demirol A, Gurgan T. Effect of treatment of intrauterine pathologies with office hysteroscopy in patients with recurrent IVF failure. Reprod biomed Online. 2004:8:590-4.
23. Rama Raju GA, Shashi Kumari G, Krishna KM, et al. Assessment of uterine cavity by hysteroscopy in assisted reproduction program and its influence on pregnancy outcome. Arch Gynecol Obstet. 2006;274:160-4.
24. Mansour RT, Aboulghar MA. Optimizing the embryo transfer technique. Hum Reprod. 2002;17:1149-53.

# CHAPTER 14

# Endometrial Markers of Receptivity

*Simi Mohandas, Shaweez, Sankalp Singh*

*"A nourishing soil is the holy grail for the birth of a seed."*

## ■ INTRODUCTION

The human endometrium, under the influence of hormones, goes through precisely regulated cyclical changes of proliferation and differentiation followed by regression. The initial proliferation, superseded by secretory changes occurs in anticipation of the implantation of a healthy embryo, failing which the endometrium dutifully undergoes regression and shedding. The astounding phenomenon of implantation of a healthy embryo into a receptive endometrium is an evidence of the well-orchestrated role of each factor involved in the maternal-embryo crosstalk interface.

The window of implantation (WOI) lasts only 4 days in the mid secretory phase which is between days 20 and day 24 of the menstrual cycle. WOI in simple word means, the time period during which the maternal endometrium will permit a blastocyst to implant.

Apposition, adhesion and invasion are the three steps involved in implantation of the embryo to the luminal epithelium of the endometrium. The dialogue between the implanting blastocyst and receptive endometrium is played by several genes, molecular markers, growth factors, cytokines—the contribution of each being accurately defined.

Advances in the field of ART research has brought us a long way from the historical endometrial biopsy and dating by Noyes' criteria.[1] The lack of consensus among the studies for the assessment of these markers limits the application of any single test to define endometrial receptivity (ER). The current emphasis is on the diagnostic method to be noninvasive with reliable, reproducible results with fairly accurate prediction of ER status, ideally in the index cycle planned for embryo transfer (ET).

## REGULATION OF ENDOMETRIAL RECEPTIVITY

The quintessential step of implantation of a healthy embryo is undoubtedly a result of the intricate interplay of several factors. Specifically during the window of implantation, the epithelial estrogen receptor alpha (ESR1) is downregulated and progesterone along with progesterone receptor (PR) is shifted from glandular to the stromal compartment. The presence of pinopodes-endometrial protrusions with the expression of αVβ3 integrin and osteopontin at implantation site, has been evaluated as a biomarker of endometrial receptivity. However, few studies have refuted the association of pinopodes due to inconsistent scoring methods and their questionable timing of expression. Several molecular markers, to name a few adhesion molecules, cytokines, growth factors and lipids, have been noted to play a role in implantation. αVβ3, a cellular adhesion molecule (CAM), is proven to predict success in IVF cycles. Other CAM such as troponin, CD 44 and cadherin have also been studied. Glycoprotein molecules, Mucin 1 (MUC1) and glycodelin, have been proposed as markers of endometrial receptivity although with conflicting consensus.

Mucin 1 (MUC1), is present on the luminal surface epithelium. Its role as an antiadhesion molecule has been proven as it is absent on pinopodes and it has a putative role in protecting the implanting blastocyst against other antiadhesion molecules during the peri-implantation period. Glycodelin, primarily an immunomodulator prevents the rejection of the embryo as an allograft. Cytokines and growth factor such as leukemia inhibitory factor (LIF), HOXA-10 transcription, factor, heparin binding growth factor (HB-GF), insulin like growth factor II, L-selectin and its ligand and calcitonin are few of many factors which play an important role in implantation.[2]

## ASSESSMENT OF ENDOMETRIAL RECEPTIVITY

Constant research in the field of assisted reproductive technology (ART) has led to advancement in gamete and embryo factors. However, conclusive assessment of the receptivity of endometrium is still far behind.

The tool for determining the receptivity is unavailable in the armamentarium of fertility specialists as the endometrium is a dynamic tissue that poses certain limitations such as lack of global representation, high cycle to cycle variability, varying factors of infertility and induction of receptivity by a good embryo. The availability of an affordable, reproducible and a reliable test will help us in treating women with recurrent implantation failure (RIF) and in determining the advancement of endometrium at the end of a COS. If the ideal endometrial receptivity test is cost effective and noninvasive, it can be offered to all patients undergoing ET.

This chapter will shed light on the pros and cons of the currently available tools of assessment of ER.

## ULTRASOUND MARKERS OF RECEPTIVITY

Ultrasound is the most widely used and the only noninvasive technique to assess ER.

### Endometrial Thickness

Numerous studies have supported as well as refuted a significant correlation between endometrial thickness and pregnancy rate. Thin endometrium has been associated with a lower implantation rate, but no cutoff exists. Pregnancies have been reported in cycles with endometrium less than 6 mm and even 4 mm. Noyes et al.[3] found that clinical pregnancy rate and live birth rate were significantly lower when endometrial thickness was less than 7 mm than when endometrial thickness was more than or equal to 9 mm. In a recent meta-analysis Kasius et al. showed that more than the positive predictive value, the endometrial thickness less than 7 mm definitely has a negative role in implantation.[4]

Why does a thinner endometrium result in failure of implantation? Casper RF[5] hypothesized that when the thickness measured by ultrasound is less than 7 mm, the functional layer is thin or absent. This brings the embryo to extreme proximity to the underlying spiral arteries which have increased blood flow. This compromises the physiological hypoxic niche essential for the implanting embryo.

Weissman et al.[6] showed that pregnancy rate was significantly lower above a maximum thickness of 14 mm, and they also suggested a possible increase in spontaneous abortion rates.

### Endometrial Pattern

The synchronized maturation of the endometrium and the embryo is one of the preliminary steps to a successful implantation. The estrogen primed endometrium undergoes decidualization under the influence of progesterone. These steroid hormones bring about histological changes which are reflected in the ultrasound as the loss of the trilaminar pattern. Broadly these patterns can be categorized as trilaminar, homogenous hyperechoic and an intermediate pattern. The presence of trilaminar pattern is suggested to be most favorable for implantation.[7] Few studies have implicated that the trilaminar pattern in the presence of a comparatively thin endometrium suffices the prerequisite for a positive result[8] whereas others have refuted this. While few studies noted the endometrial pattern on the day of ovulation trigger, others based their results on the pattern on embryo transfer (ET) day, hence leading to diverse conclusions. There is no consensus on the predictive value of endometrial morphology on implantation.

### Endometrial and Subendometrial Blood Flow

The uterine artery pulsatility index (PI) has been applied as a predictor of implantation in the past. However, there was no significant association between this marker and ER. It has been proposed that as the endometrium is the recipient of the implanting embryo, measurement of blood flow to the endometrium and subendometrial regions would be more meaningful. Sardana D et al.[9] using 2D power Doppler, noted that the clinical pregnancy rate and implantation rate were significantly higher in patients undergoing frozen embryo transfer (FET) with endometrial-subendometrial blood flow when compared to absence of blood flow. A Nandi et al.[10] have evaluated the role of 3D power Doppler (3DPD) in assessing the uterine vascularity but did not find any significant correlation for endometrial receptivity.

The ultrasound, due to its obvious advantages in addition to operational ease and familiarity among the clinicians seems to be a popular option. This has been proven by the attempts to explore and correlate every measurable feature to ER. However it may be too simple a tool to assess the multidimensional, complex process of implantation. This has urged researchers to explore other domains involved in receptivity of the endometrium.

At this point of time, the only ultrasound parameter to have a certain correlation to pregnancy rate seems to be the endometrial thickness.

## ■ HISTOLOGICAL MARKERS

Noyes et al.[1] morphological criteria to evaluate endometrial development and receptivity. Inspite of having poor reproducibility this remained the main stay for assessing ER for many years. The accuracy of Noyes criteria to predict the WOI has been questioned and invalidated by randomized studies,[11] suggesting a 60% interobserver and intercycle variability. Endometrial pinopods identified on electron microscopy also was suggested as a marker of ER. Pinopods are cytoplasmic projections of the luminal epithelial cells, abundant during the WOI, thought to promote blastocyst adhesion. The pinopods was also demonstrated in postreceptive endometrium, and this prevented their use as a useful marker of ER.[12]

## ■ TRANSCRIPTOMICS FOR ENDOMETRIAL RECEPTIVITY

The simultaneous evaluation of several thousands of genes is now possible following the advent of microarray technology. The genes which are actively being expressed by a cell population are portrayed by the transcriptome. Transcriptomics thus represents gene expression at the mRNA level, thereby defining the "transcriptomic signature." of tissue function or disease phenotype.

Ongoing research in the field of transcriptomics focusing on endometrial receptivity and its alterations has led to discovery of a "genomic signature" of various phases of the endometrium and its alterations in gynecological pathology such as cancers, endometriosis, infertility, RIF and during COS.[13]

The secretory phase, divided into the early (pre-receptive), mid (receptive/WOI) and late (postreceptive) expresses a wide variety of genes which modulate implantation. The early secretory phase shows elevated levels of molecular markers for transport, germ cell migration and cellular metabolism such as eicosanoids, fatty acids and amino alcohols. This occurs as a result of increased metabolic activity in preparation for the process of implantation. The downregulation of growth factors leads to a transient decline in the mitotic division of cells during this phase.

This is followed by the receptive phase, associated with upregulation of several genes responsible for a wide range of secretory and metabolic functions as well as immune modulation, thereby allowing a healthy blastocyst to implant into a "receptive"' endometrium. The late secretory phase coinciding with the closure of WOI, is characterized by alterations in gene expression of humoral and cellular immune factors, steroidogenesis, prostaglandin metabolism and coagulation.[14,15]

The simultaneous evaluation of thousands of genes by microarray technology was utilised by researchers analyzing more than 12,000 genes. The studies varied significantly in the number of genes which were upregulated and downregulated during the WOI due to methodological differences. The consensus genes were—osteopontin (structural protein), apolipoprotein D (transporter), and Dickkopf/DKK1 (signaling). This posed the difficulty in bringing forth a standardized gene-based marker.[15]

## ■ ENDOMETRIAL RECEPTIVITY ARRAY AND PERSONALIZED EMBRYO TRANSFER

Endometrial receptivity assay (ERA) is a commercially available diagnostic tool. ERA uses microarray to characterize the transcriptomic profile of 238 genes, thereby classifying the biopsied endometrium as receptive, pre-receptive, or postreceptive is gaining popularity in this era of advanced diagnostics. RNA is obtained from endometrial tissue biopsied in a natural cycle on day 7 after the luteinizing hormone peak (LH+7), or day 5 of progesterone administration (P+5) following estrogen priming in a hormonal replacement therapy cycle. A computational predictor aided by cluster analysis against sample training models then recognizes the profile according to its receptivity status. The inter rater variability was better for ERA when compared to the histological sample.[16,17] The reproducibility of this method to 40 months is an added advantage to the improved accuracy when compared to histological dating methods

Katzorke et al.[18] analyzed over 6000 ERA results and concluded that 30 % biopsied samples may demonstrate a nonreceptive profile, further classifying this group as pre-receptive (85%) or postreceptive (12.6%). The salient feature of this predictive model is its clinical application to a personalized embryo transfer (pET). Treatment with progesterone can be commenced based on individualized WOI status, thence improving the success rates of the "personalized" ET. It has been observed in several elegant studies that a pET based on ERA, one out of four patients had a displaced WOI and pET helped in improving implantation and pregnancy rates.[15,19]

The value of ERA in routine embryo transfer is presently being investigated in an international, multicenter, prospective RCT "The ERA as a diagnostic guide for personalized embryo transfer"—comparing fresh embryo transfer versus elective delayed embryo transfer or pET (Clinical trails.gov, Identifier: NCT01954758).

## ■ MICRORNA: THE NOVEL GENE-BASED MARKER

Unlike mRNAs, which code for proteins, MiRNAs are noncoding RNA sequences comprising of 18–25 nucleotides regulating post-transcriptional gene expression thereby functioning as gene silencers.[20]

Studies have shown that different miRNAs are upregulated and downregulated during the menstrual cycle. MiRNAs are noted to be secreted by the endometrium as well as the embryo as a mediator of their communication during the WOI. The upregulation of hsa-miR-30b and hsa-miR-30-d has been documented in acquisition of endometrial receptivity.[21] The preimplantation embryo can internalize miRNA hsa-miR-30d secreted into the endometrial fluid by the endometrium and modify its transcriptome. MiRNAs are thus potential molecules which can be utilized in the uterine fluid for prediction of the ER.

## ■ THE UTERINE SECRETOME

A noninvasive means of analyzing the molecules involved in implantation is being evaluated. Several factors such as growth factors, cytokines, proteins, electrolytes, urea, glucose, enzymes like metalloproteinases, immunoglobulins, transferrin and haptoglobulins play an indispensible role in this crucial step of implantation.[22]

The analysis of these factors was earlier studied by biopsy of the endometrium. Since this method represented a focal area of 2–4% of the endometrium, analysis of a more global representation of the uterine secretome was suggested. Cheong et al. has elaborated on this method where endometrial fluid is aspirated with a 2 mL syringe attached to an embryo transfer catheter.[23]

Attempts of elaborating the protein repertoire of the uterine fluid had been done in many studies. Casado-Vela et al. using three different proteomic strategies identified 803 proteins of the uterine fluid but cycle dependent shift of proteins was not addressed in this study.[24] Scotchie et al. used two-dimensional differential in gel electrophoresis (2D DiGE) technique to identify 468 proteins out of which 82 showed differential abundance in receptive phase.[25] Alpha-2-macroglobulin, serum albumin, activin receptor type-2B, AAT, interalpha-trypsin inhibitor family heavy chain-related protein) were identified by studies as the proteins which had abundance during receptive compared to pre receptive phase.[26]

Uterine fluid acts as mirror for endometrial regulation and dysregulation. Hence analyzing the secretome along with advances in metabolomics and proteomics can lead to an era in ART where the ET can be done after confirming that the endometrium is receptive.

## CONCLUSION

The key factors in implantation still remain an enigma. This is one of the bottle necks in improving the ART pregnancy rates. The search for the ideal test continues and the omics technology—the genomics and secretomics; decoding the functional regulation of implantation can be the light house to the lost sailor.

## KEY POINTS

- Endometrial thickness of less than 7 mm have a high but not absolute negative predictive value.
- ERA has a better accuracy than the histological dating and is reproducible up to 60 months.
- The uterine secretome once fully deciphered would be a major player in determining the day of embryo transfer.

## REFERENCES

1. Noyes RW, Hertig AI, Rock J. Dating the endometrial biopsy. Fertil Steril. 1950;1:3-25.
2. Fox C, Morin S, Jeong JW, et al. Local and Systemic Factors and Implantation: what is the Evidence? Fertil Steril. 2016;105(4):873-84.
3. Noyes N, Hampton BS, Berkeley A, et al. Factors useful in predicting the success of oocyte donation: a 3-year retrospective analysis. Fertil Steril. 2001;76:92-7.
4. Kasius A, Smit JG, Torrance HL, et al. Endometrial thickness and pregnancy rates after IVF: a systematic review and meta-analysis. Human Reprod Update. 2014;20(4):530-41.
5. Casper RF. It's time to pay attention to the endometrium. Fertil Steril. 2011;96:519-21.
6. Weissman A, Gotlieb L, Casper RF. The detrimental effect of increased endometrial thickness on implantation and pregnancy rates and outcome in an in vitro fertilization program. Fertil Steril. 1999;71:147-9.
7. Zhao J, Zhang Q, Li Y. The effect of endometrial thickness and pattern measured by ultrasonography on pregnancy outcomes during IVF-ET cycles. Reprod Biol Endocrinol. 2012;10:100.
8. Chen SL, Wu FR, Luo C, et al. Combined analysis of endometrial thickness and pattern in predicting outcome of in vitro fertilization and embryo transfer: a retrospective cohort study. Reprod Biol Endocrinol. 2010; 8:30.
9. Sardana D, Upadhyay AJ, Deepika K, et al. Correlation of subendometrial-endometrial blood flow assessment by two-dimensional power Doppler with

pregnancy outcome in frozen-thawed embryo transfer cycles. J Hum Reprod Sci. 2014;7(2):130-5.
10. Nandi A, Martins WP, Jayaprakasan K, et al. Assessment of endometrial and subendometrial blood flow in women undergoing frozen embryo transfer cycles. Reprod Biomed Online. 2014;28:343-51.
11. American Society for Reproductive Medicine. A Practice Committee report: Optimal evaluation of the infertile female. ASRM. Fertil Steril. 2012;98:302-7.
12. Quinn CE, Casper RF. Pinopodes: a questionable role in endometrial receptivity. Hum Reprod Update. 2009;15(2):229-36.
13. Altmäe S, Martínez-Conejero JA, Salumets A, et al. Endometrial gene expression analysis at the time of embryo implantation in women with unexplained infertility. Basic Sci Reprod Med. 2010;16(3):178-87.
14. Critchley HO, Kelly RW, Brenner RM, et al. The endocrinology of menstruation—A role for the immune system. Clin Endocrinol (Oxf). 2001;55:701-10.
15. Ruiz-Alonso M, Blesa D, Simon C. The genomics of the human endometrium. Biochim Biophys Acta. 2012;1822:1931-42.
16. Diaz-Gimeno P, Horcajadas JA, Martínez-Conejero JA, et al. A genomic diagnostic tool for human endometrial receptivity based on the transcriptomic signature. Fertil Steril. 2011;95:50-60.
17. Diaz-Gimeno P, Ruiz-Alonso M, Blesa D, et al. The accuracy and reproducibility of the endometrial receptivity array is superior to histology as a diagnostic method for endometrial receptivity. Fertil Steril. 2013;99:508-17.
18. Katzorke N, Vilella F, Ruiz M, et al. Diagnosis of endometrial-factor infertility: current approaches and new avenues for research. Geburtshilfe und Frauenheilkunde. 2016;76(6):699-703.
19. Ruiz-Alonso M, Galindo N, Pellicer A, et al. What a difference two days make: "personalized" embryo transfer (pET) paradigm: a case report and pilot study. Hum Reprod. 2014;29:1244–1247.
20. Vilella F, Moreno-Moya JM, Balaguer N, et al. Hsa-miR-30d, secreted by the human endometrium, is taken up by the pre-implantation embryo and might modify its transcriptome. Development. 2015;142:3210-21.
21. Sha AG, Liu JL, Jiang XM, et al. Genome-wide identification of micro-ribonucleic acids associated with human endometrial receptivity in natural and stimulated cycles by deep sequencing. Fertil Steril. 2011;96:150-5.
22. Parmar T, Gadkar-Sable S, Savardekar L, et al. Protein profiling of human endometrial tissues in the midsecretory and proliferative phases of the menstrual cycle. Fertil Steril. 2009;92(3):1091-103.
23. Cheong Y, Boomsma C, Heijnen C, et al. Uterine secretomics: a window on the maternal-embryo interface. Fertil Steril. (2013);99(4):1093-9.
24. Casado-Vela J, Rodriguez-Suarez E, Iloro I, et al. Comprehensive proteomic analysis of human endometrial fluid aspirate. J Proteome Res. 2009;8:4622-32.
25. Scotchie JG, Fritz MA, Mocanu M, et al. Proteomic analysis of the luteal endometrial secretome. Reprod Sci. 2009;16:883-93.
26. Bhusane K, Bhutada S, Chaudhari U, et al. Secrets of endometrial receptivity: some are hidden in uterine secretome. Am J Reprod Immunol. 2016;75:226-36.

CHAPTER
# 15

# Challenges during Assisted Reproductive Technology in Polycystic Ovary Syndrome

*Duru Shah*

## ■ HIGHLIGHTS

- Characteristics that affect ovarian stimulation in polycystic ovary syndrome (PCOS) patients
- Accepted treatment protocols to minimize risks and maximize outcomes
- Clinical ovarian stimulation protocols used during assisted reproductive technology (ART) in PCOS patients.

## ■ INTRODUCTION

Polycystic ovary syndrome (PCOS) is a common gynecological endocrine disorder affecting 4–12% of women in the reproductive age group.[1] Some of the cardinal manifestations of PCOS include hyperandrogenism, ovulatory dysfunction, and polycystic ovaries in its complete phenotype.[2] PCOS is the primary cause of hyperandrogenism and oligo-anovulation at the reproductive age and is often associated with infertility, with a prevalence between 70% and 80% in this particular cohort.[3]

Oligo-ovulation or anovulation in women with PCOS is a major cause of infertility, and such women might require ovulation induction or assisted reproductive technology (ART) to achieve successful conception.[4]

This chapter focuses on the barriers to successful pregnancy outcomes and the challenges during ART in women with PCOS.

## ■ APPROACHES FOR MANAGING INFERTILITY IN POLYCYSTIC OVARY SYNDROME

The evaluation of infertility in women with PCOS or other causes of subfertility should start after 6 months of attempting pregnancy without success if the couple has regular sexual intercourse without the use of contraceptives as per the recommendations from the American Society for Reproductive Medicine (ASRM). The primary approaches for managing infertility in PCOS can broadly be classified as follows:[5]

- Preconception counseling along with lifestyle changes
- Drugs to induce mono- or bifollicular ovulation
- Use of exogenous gonadotropins
- Laparoscopic ovarian drilling
- Assisted reproductive technology/in vitro fertilization (IVF).

Essentially the choice of treatment depends on the age of the patient, presence of any other compounding factor leading to infertility, previous experience with any treatment modality, and the anxiety of the couple to conceive. Finally, it must be emphasized that treatment should be individualized after careful evaluation of the clinical presentation, desire to conceive, and the risk of developing long-term complications.

## ■ CHALLENGES IN POLYCYSTIC OVARY SYNDROME PATIENTS DURING ASSISTED REPRODUCTIVE TECHNOLOGY

Generally, lifestyle changes, ovulation induction, and pharmacological measures such as use of insulin sensitizing agents, gonadotropins, and gonadotropin-releasing hormone (GnRH) analogs, and laparoscopic ovarian surgery are tried before initiating ART like IVF. However, in presence of complicating factors like tubal damage, severe endometriosis, preimplantation genetic diagnosis, and male factor infertility, ART may become the first treatment of choice in PCOS patients.[5]

The principal challenges faced in implementing ART protocols in PCOS patients are:[6]
- Lack of any tool/method to predict response to ovarian stimulation
- Suppression of luteinizing hormone (LH) levels
- Choosing the right dose and protocol
- Preventing ovarian hyperstimulation syndrome (OHSS).

Influence of patient characteristics must also be taken into account when evaluating PCOS patients for ART. Some of the major considerations include:
- Obesity
- Baseline luteinizing hormone:follicle-stimulating hormone (LH/FSH) ratio
- Gonadotropin requirements.

### Obesity: More than Just a Weighty Problem in Polycystic Ovary Syndrome

The cause of obesity in PCOS remains unknown but may be the result of hyperinsulinemia. Weight gain usually precedes the onset of clinical features of PCOS in majority of patients. 50% of PCOS patients are obese, and obesity tends to be abdominal/visceral. Visceral obesity is associated with hyperandrogenemia, insulin resistance (IR), and dyslipidemia, and worsens the metabolic and reproductive parameters of PCOS.[7]

Obesity, particularly the abdominal type, has a major impact on reproductive function in women with PCOS. Obesity is related to more severe hirsutism, more frequent anovulatory cycles, and increased frequency of infertility in women with PCOS.[8,9]

There is also evidence of a higher incidence of blunted responsiveness to pharmacological treatments that induce ovulation and a reduced pregnancy rate in obese PCOS patients.[10] To compound these issues, obesity is also associated with lower embryo quality and a decreased rate of implantation by IVF treatment.[11]

A study by Tarlatzis et al. demonstrated that ovulation rates in obese women with PCOS following gonadotropin induction were half of those seen in nonobese women with PCOS. This clearly highlights the fact that obesity is a major challenge during ART in PCOS patients.

## Baseline (Luteinizing Hormone/Follicle-stimulating Hormone) Ratio

This is another characteristic that is thought to be important in determining the success of ART in PCOS. The prognostic value of the LH-FSH ratio continues to be debated, but a study demonstrated that a high basal LH:FSH ratio appears to have an adverse effect on the number of follicles and oocytes, as well as on oocyte maturity and may also predict a greater possibility for miscarriage.[11]

The study also highlighted that administration of GnRHa in the long protocol seems to reverse the adverse effect on follicle and oocyte development, but did not influence the risk of miscarriage in any way.[11]

## Gonadotropin Requirements: Less is More

Gonadotropin therapy plays an integral role in ovarian stimulation for infertility treatments such as ART. Studies have demonstrated a negative correlation between total gonadotropin dosage and live-birth rate for fresh autologous cycles of IVF regardless of age of patient or number of oocytes retrieved.[12]

However, a study by Ryan et al. suggests that prolonged duration of stimulation is associated with decreased ART success for all couples, except for women with PCOS where a "low and slow" approach might be beneficial.[13]

The take home message as far as the gonadotropin requirement in PCOS is concerned is that the clinician must customize approaches based on individual needs and prevalent patient characteristics.

## ■ POLYCYSTIC OVARY SYNDROME AND ASSISTED REPRODUCTIVE TECHNOLOGY: OVARIAN STIMULATION

Ovarian stimulation and the outcomes associated with it are a critical part of any ART undertaken in PCOS. A meta-analysis of outcomes of conventional

IVF in women with PCOS demonstrated increased cancellation rates, more oocytes retrieved per retrieval, and lower fertilization rate in PCOS during ART. The duration of stimulation was significantly longer in the PCOS group as compared to the non-PCOS group, underlining the "low and slow" approach undertaken in many studies.

However, this meta-analysis also surprisingly found no difference in pregnancy and live-birth rates between PCOS and non-PCOS patients.[14]

## ■ POLYCYSTIC OVARY SYNDROME AND ASSISTED REPRODUCTIVE TECHNOLOGY: MANAGING INSULIN RESISTANCE

The presence of hyperinsulinemia due to increased IR, and hyperandrogenemia lead to the appearance of multiple antral follicles and frequently a multifollicular response to gonadotropin stimulation for ART in PCOS patients. Research has highlighted a positive correlation of homeostatic model assessment of insulin resistance (HOMA-IR) levels above a threshold level of 2.5 and a continuous positive correlation of free androgen index (FAI) to total ovarian follicle count following controlled ovarian hyperstimulation (COH) in the non-PCOS patient.[15]

Prudent use of insulin sensitizers such as metformin may help in such cases.

## ■ POLYCYSTIC OVARY SYNDROME AND ASSISTED REPRODUCTIVE TECHNOLOGY: PREVENTING OVARIAN HYPERSTIMULATION SYNDROME

Ovarian hyperstimulation syndrome complicates a small percentage of IVF treatments, but its incidence is increasing in lean, young women with PCOS. Vasoactive substances, secreted by the ovaries under human chorionic gonadotropin (hCG) stimulation play a key role in triggering this syndrome. It is important to prevent OHSS in this patient cohort. Some of the accepted strategies are outlined in Box 1.[16,17]

## ■ POLYCYSTIC OVARY SYNDROME AND ASSISTED REPRODUCTIVE TECHNOLOGY: CLINICAL IMPLICATIONS OF USE OF GONADOTROPIN-RELEASING HORMONE AGONISTS VERSUS ANTAGONISTS[18]

A recent Cochrane review evaluated the efficacy and safety of GnRH antagonists compared to the more widely used GnRH agonists in subfertile couples undergoing ART. The review summarized that the evidence suggested that if the chance of live birth following GnRH agonist is assumed to be 29%, the

## Box 1  Prevention of OHSS.[16,17]

- Use of the long protocol with recombinant FSH especially in patients with PCOS
- Withholding the hCG or reducing the dose of hCG trigger
- Continuation of GnRH analog
- Use of GnRH analog to trigger ovulation (adequate luteal support is required, particularly ideal for donor cycles)
- Coasting: Complete discontinuation of exogenous gonadotropins while administration of GnRH agonist is continued, with administration of hCG after E2 levels reach below 3,000 pg/mL
- Aspiration of all the follicles
- Use of progesterone for luteal support
- Cryopreservation (oocyte/embryo-freeze all) and replacement of frozen–thawed embryos in a subsequent cycle
- Use of dopamine agonist cabergoline
- Use of GnRH antagonist protocol
- Coasting with GnRH antagonist
- Limiting the starting dose of FSH in high responders or tapering the FSH dose once the mature follicles are recruited
- Use of metformin
- Low-dose aspirin during IVF cycle.

(FSH: follicle-stimulating hormone; GnRH: gonadotropin-releasing hormone; hCG: human chorionic gonadotropin; IVF: in vitro fertilization; OHSS: ovarian hyperstimulation syndrome; PCOS: polycystic ovary syndrome)

chance following GnRH antagonist would be between 25% and 33%. However, the OHSS rates were much higher after GnRH agonist. The evidence suggested that if the risk of OHSS following GnRH agonist is assumed to be 11%, the risk following GnRH antagonist would be between 6% and 9%.

The authors concluded that there is moderate quality evidence that the use of GnRH antagonist compared with long-course GnRH agonist protocols is associated with a substantial reduction in OHSS without reducing the likelihood of achieving live birth.

## GONADOTROPIN-RELEASING HORMONE AGONIST AND ANTAGONIST PROTOCOLS IN POLYCYSTIC OVARY SYNDROME

With regard to the protocols themselves, there are multiple options. When it comes to GnRH agonist protocols, the following choices are available for clinicians:
- Ultrashort protocol
- Short protocol
- Long protocol
- Variable long protocol.

There has been a lot of debate as well as research into the question of which protocols are appropriate for women with subfertility such as those with PCOS. GnRH agonist protocols have long been viewed as a "gold standard" in ovarian stimulation, in fact, GnRH antagonists are preferred as second-line agents in patients who are poor responders, in the elderly, and in the ones with previous IVF failures.[19]

In recent years, this tide seems to be shifting in favor of GnRH antagonist protocols. Some of the advantages cited by researchers and clinicians alike advocating the use of GnRH antagonist protocols over GnRH agonist protocols include:
- Shorter treatment duration.[20]
- Lack of hypoestrogenism.[20]
- Lower gonadotropin requirement.[20]
- Lower incidence of OHSS.[20]
- No risk of withdrawal symptoms.[19]
- No risk of cyst formation and accidental administration of GnRH analogs during early pregnancy.[19]
- More patient friendly than agonist protocols.[19]

In fact a recent Cochrane review by Al-Inany et al. in 2016 seemed to settle the debate in favor of the GnRH antagonist protocols given the near-equivalent numbers as far as live births were concerned. This review demonstrated that although more number of embryos were available and the cryopreservation rate was higher in the agonist group, there was no significant difference in cumulative clinical pregnancy rate and live-birth rate. The review also stressed that significant reduction in the incidence of severe OHSS in the antagonist group could have a direct impact on the reduction of cost of cycle, thereby making the GnRH antagonist protocols an attractive choice.[18]

On the flip side, researchers contend that there is still no sound evidence as far as pregnancy rates with either protocol is concerned. When collating the clinical experiences on IVF outcomes, it was found that the day of hCG trigger is crucial for IVF success in patients who were given the GnRH antagonist protocol and not the long GnRH agonist one. Furthermore, for patients undergoing GnRH antagonist ovarian stimulation protocols should be triggered whenever the ratio of estradiol concentration to number of follicles of more than 14 mm on the day of hCG administration is lower than 100 pg/mL/follicle.[20]

In such a scenario, where the choice of appropriate protocols is heavily debated, it is worthwhile to look at what the clinical practice guidelines have to say. Various recommendations from the ASRM practice guidelines, the European Society of Human Reproduction and Embryology (ESHRE) guidelines, and the National Institute for Health and Care Excellence (NICE) recommendations probably give a clearer picture on which protocol is appropriate for patients with PCOS.

The NICE recommendations from the UK clearly specify procedures to follow pretreatment and during treatment in subfertile women.[21]

## Pretreatment[21]

Advise women that using pretreatment (with either the oral contraceptive pill or a progestogen) as part of IVF does not affect the chances of having a live birth.

Consider pretreatment in order to schedule IVF treatment for women who are not undergoing long downregulation protocols.

## Downregulation and Other Regimens to Avoid Premature Luteinizing Hormone Surges in In Vitro Fertilization[21]

- Use regimens to avoid premature luteinizing hormone surges in gonadotropin-stimulated IVF treatment cycles
- Use either GnRH agonist downregulation or GnRH antagonists as part of gonadotropin-stimulated IVF treatment cycles
- Only offer GnRH agonists to women who have a low risk of OHSS
- When using GnRH agonists as part of IVF treatment, use a long downregulation protocol.

## Controlled Ovarian Stimulation in In Vitro Fertilization[21]

- Use ovarian stimulation as part of IVF treatment
- Use either urinary or recombinant gonadotropins for ovarian stimulation as part of IVF treatment
- When using gonadotropins for ovarian stimulation in IVF treatment it is recommended to use an individualized starting dose of FSH, based on factors that predict success, such as: age, body mass index (BMI), presence of polycystic ovaries, ovarian reserve, and not use a dosage of FSH of more than 450 IU/day.
- Offer women for ultrasound monitoring (with or without estradiol levels) for efficacy and safety throughout ovarian stimulation (new 2013).
- Inform women that clomiphene citrate-stimulated and gonadotropin-stimulated IVF cycles have higher pregnancy rates per cycle than natural cycle of IVF
- Do not offer women for natural cycle of IVF treatment
- Do not use growth hormone or dehydroepiandrosterone (DHEA) as adjuvant treatment in IVF protocols.

## ■ POLYCYSTIC OVARY SYNDROME AND ASSISTED REPRODUCTIVE TECHNOLOGY: LUTEAL PHASE SUPPORT[22]

Luteal phase insufficiency is one of the reasons for implantation failure and is responsible for miscarriages and unsuccessful ART. Luteal phase defect is seen in women with PCOS, thyroid, and prolactin disorders.

Progesterone is known to induce secretory changes in the lining of the uterus essential for successful implantation of a fertilized egg. It has been suggested that a causative factor in many cases of miscarriage may be inadequate secretion of progesterone. Therefore, progestogens have been used, beginning in the 1st trimester of pregnancy, in an attempt to prevent spontaneous miscarriage.

Polycystic ovary syndrome women are thought to have the higher possibility in early pregnancy loss than non-PCOS patients. A study done to clarify the relation between corpus luteum function and early pregnancy loss in PCOS women showed no significant difference in progesterone and estrogen concentration in the midsecretory phase. The progesterone production in 5-week pregnancy, on the other hand, demonstrated a remarkable change; $27.5 \pm 10.8$ ng/mL (mean $\pm$ SD) in PCOS group and $32.4 \pm 14.3$ ng/mL in control, respectively ($P < 0.05$). In addition, PCOS women with early pregnancy loss demonstrated lower progesterone production at 5-week gestational stage than those without miscarriage. Serum testosterone level did not affect corpus luteum function in both midsecretory and early pregnancy stage.

Thus, for the PCOS patients with episodes of early pregnancy loss, progesterone supplementation, if low at 5 weeks gestation, might restore the fetal growth and then avoid recurrent miscarriages. In ART cycles involving use of a GnRH agonists or antagonists, progesterone supplementation yields higher pregnancy rates.

## ■ POLYCYSTIC OVARY SYNDROME AND ASSISTED REPRODUCTIVE TECHNOLOGY: OPTIMIZING OUTCOMES

Lifestyle modifications continue to be the mainstay of optimizing outcomes. Guidelines from the ESHRE and the ASRM state:[6]

- Experience from other areas of medicine suggests lifestyle modifications as the first-line treatment of obesity in PCOS
- Weight loss prior to infertility treatment improves ovulation rates in women with PCOS
- The best diet and exercise regimens are unknown, but caloric restriction and increased physical activity are recommended
- Treatment of adverse lifestyles, including obesity and physical inactivity, should precede ovulation induction
- The ideal amount of weight loss is unknown, but a 5% decrease of body weight might be clinically meaningful.

## KEY POINTS

- Lifestyle modifications continue to be important in determining overall success of ART in PCOS patients.
- Choosing the right dose and protocol is of critical importance during ART in PCOS patients.
- Gonadotropin-releasing hormone antagonist protocols seem to be gaining popularity for ovarian stimulation in PCOS patients.
- The NICE recommendations advocate use of GnRH agonist downregulation or GnRH antagonists as part of gonadotropin-stimulated IVF treatment cycles.
- Contemporary approach to ovarian stimulation with low-dose FSH, GnRH antagonist, triggering with an agonist, and small doses of hCG may be helpful in the luteal phase.

## REFERENCES

1. Melo AS, Vieira CS, Barbieri MA, et al. High prevalence of polycystic ovary syndrome in women born small for gestational age. Hum Reprod. 2010;25(8):2124-31.
2. Iftikhar S, Collazo-Clavell ML, Roger V, et al. Risk of cardiovascular events in patients with polycystic ovary syndrome. Neth J Med. 2012;70(2):74-80.
3. Azziz R, Woods KS, Reyna R, et al. The prevalence and features of the polycystic ovary syndrome in an unselected population. J Clin Endocrinol Metab. 2004;89(6):2745-9.
4. Rajashekar L, Krishna D, Patil M. Polycystic ovaries and infertility: our experience. J Hum Reprod Sci. 2008;1(2):65-72.
5. Thessaloniki ESHRE/ASRM-Sponsored PCOS Consensus Workshop Group. Consensus on infertility treatment related to polycystic ovary syndrome. Hum Reprod. 2008;23(3):462-77.
6. Shrestha D, La X, Feng HL. Comparison of different stimulation protocols used in in vitro fertilization: a review. Ann Transl Med. 2015;3(10):137.
7. Shah D, Rasool S. Polycystic ovary syndrome and metabolic syndrome: the worrisome twosome? Climacteric. 2016;19(1):7-16.
8. Ozgun MT, Uludag S, Oner G. The influence of obesity on ICSI outcomes in women with polycystic ovary syndrome. J Obstet Gynaecol. 2011;31(3):245-9.
9. Pasquali R, Gambineri A, Pagotto U. The impact of obesity on reproduction in women with polycystic ovary syndrome. BJOG. 2006;113(10):1148-59.
10. Galtier-Dereure F, Pujol P, Dewailly D, et al. Choice of stimulation in polycystic ovarian syndrome: the influence of obesity. Hum Reprod. 1997;12 Suppl 1:88-96.
11. Tarlatzis BC, Grimbizis G, Pournaropoulos F, et al. The prognostic value of basal luteinizing hormone:follicle-stimulating hormone ratio in the treatment of patients with polycystic ovarian syndrome by assisted reproduction techniques. Hum Reprod. 1995;10(10):2545-9.
12. Baker VL, Brown MB, Luke B, et al. Gonadotropin dose is negatively correlated with live birth rate: analysis of over 650,000 ART cycles. Fertil Steril. 2015;104(5):1145-52.e1-5.
13. Ryan A, Wang S, Alvero R, et al. Prolonged gonadotropin stimulation for assisted reproductive technology cycles is associated with decreased pregnancy rates for all women except for women with polycystic ovary syndrome. J Assist Reprod Genet. 2014;31(7): 837-42.

14. Heijnen EM, Eijkemans MJ, Hughes EG, et al. A meta-analysis of outcomes of conventional IVF in women with polycystic ovary syndrome. Hum Reprod Update. 2006;12(1):13-21.
15. Dickerson EH, Cho LW, Maguiness SD, et al. Insulin resistance and free androgen index correlate with the outcome of controlled ovarian hyperstimulation in non-PCOS women undergoing IVF. Hum Reprod. 2010;25(2):504-9.
16. Humaidan P, Quartarolo J, Papanikolaou EG. Preventing ovarian hyperstimulation syndrome: guidance for the clinician. Fertil Steril. 2010;94(2):389-400.
17. Alper MM, Smith LP, Sills ES. Ovarian hyperstimulation syndrome: current views on pathophysiology, risk factors, prevention, and management. J Exp Clin Assist Reprod. 2009;6:3.
18. Al-Inany HG, Youssef MA, Ayeleke R, et al. Gonadotrophin-releasing hormone antagonists for assisted reproductive technology. Cochrane Database Syst Rev. 2016;4:CD001750.
19. Kaur H, Krishna D, Shetty N, et al. A prospective study of GnRH long agonist versus flexible GnRH antagonist protocol in PCOS: Indian experience. J Hum Reprod Sci. 2012;5(2):181-6.
20. Orvieto R, Patrizio P. GnRH agonist versus GnRH antagonist in ovarian stimulation: an ongoing debate. Reprod Biomed Online. 2013;26(1):4-8.
21. National Institute for Health and Care Excellence (NICE) (2013). Fertility problems: assessment and treatment. [online] Available from www.nice.org.uk/guidance/cg156/chapter/Recommendations#procedures-used-during-ivf-treatment. [Accessed February, 2018].
22. Shah D, Nagrajan N. Luteal insufficiency in first trimester. Indian J Endocrinol Metab. 2013;17(1):44-9.

# CHAPTER 16

# The Assisted Reproductive Technology in Endometriosis: Is it Different?

*Kamini A Rao*

## ■ INTRODUCTION

- Endometriosis is a chronic inflammatory condition characterized by lesions of endometrial-like tissue outside the uterus[1] and is associated with pelvic pain and infertility.
- The prevalence in the general population is still unknown since the definitive diagnosis of endometriosis can be established only at time of laparoscopy.
- Endometriosis occurs in 25–50% of infertile women and 30–50% of women with endometriosis are found to be infertile.[2]
- Prevalence in infertile women undergoing laparoscopic evaluation is about 9–50%.[2,3]
- Endometriosis is 6–7 times more prevalent among infertile women compared to the fertile population.[3]
- The cause of endometriosis is still an enigma. Many theories have been proposed as the cause of endometriosis.
- Due to variation in clinical practice in the management of endometriosis in these women, we often experience difficulties in diagnosing endometriosis. This might result in either delayed care or suboptimal care in these women.[1]

## ■ ENDOMETRIOSIS AND INFERTILITY

The concept that endometriosis might cause infertility or reduce the fecundity is still controversial. Endometriosis can lead to adhesions or pelvic anatomy that might be distorted leading to infertility (Fig. 1).[4]

The monthly fecundity rate in a normal couple is around 15–20% but in untreated women with endometriosis it was reported to be 2–10%.

### Effects of Endometriosis

- On ovarian function (Flowchart 1)
- *On endometrial receptivity:*
  - Defective $\alpha v \beta 3$ integrin expression (a cell adhesion molecule) during the time of implantation.[5]

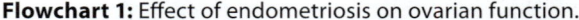

Fig. 1: Mechanisms that link endometriosis and infertility.[4]

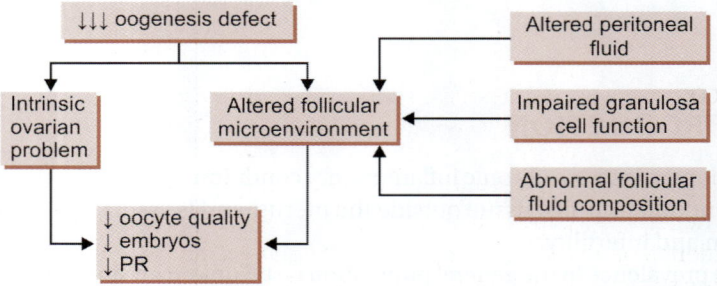

Flowchart 1: Effect of endometriosis on ovarian function.

- Lower levels of an enzyme which is involved as an endometrial ligand for L-selectin synthesis (a protein that coats the trophoblast on the surface of the blastocyst).
- Eutopic endometrium produces more estradiol because of higher aromatase activity hence causing negative impact on implantation.
- Increased levels of immunoglobulin G (IgG), IgA antibodies, and lymphocytes in the endometrium might alter the receptivity of the endometrium and affects the embryo implantation.
- Absence of midluteal rise of HOXA10.[6]
- Increased oxidative stress also affects the endometrium and embryo.

## ■ ASSISTED REPRODUCTIVE TECHNOLOGY IN ENDOMETRIOSIS

American Society for Reproductive Medicine guidelines regarding management of endometriosis in infertile women is described in Flowchart 2.

### Medical Therapy in Infertile Women: Is It Worth?

Endometriosis is an estrogen-dependent condition. Therefore, suppression with hormones might be an attractive approach medically to treat the women and also to alleviate the symptoms.

Hormonal treatment in endometriosis has been found to induce a state that mimics either like pregnancy or menopause. Gonadotropin-releasing hormone

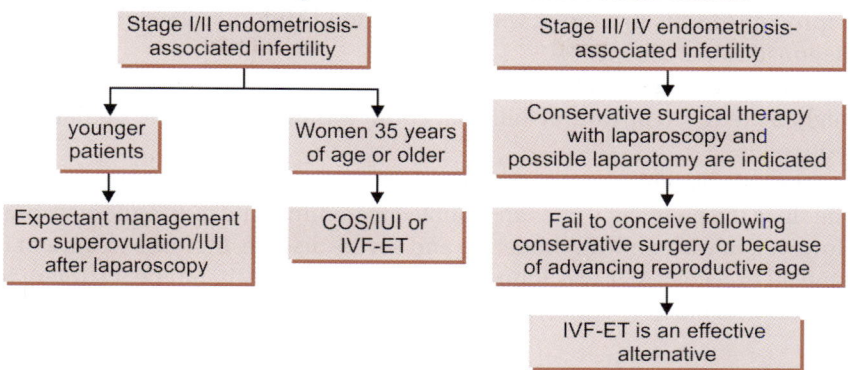

**Flowchart 2:** Management of endometriosis in infertile women.

(COS: controlled ovarian stimulation; ET: embryo transfer; IUI: intrauterine insemination; IVF: in vitro fertilization)

(GnRH) agonist causes a pseudomenopausal state that is an estrogen deficient state where the endogenous hormonal levels are suppressed.

Incidence of disease recurrence at 5-year follow-up was found to be 20% following surgery and 50% following medical treatment.

Hence, in infertile women presenting with endometriosis hormonal treatment should not be prescribed to improve fertility by causing suppression of ovarian function.[4,7]

## Surgery Before Infertility Treatment: What Evidence Suggest?

Whether to operate or to pursue assisted reproductive technology (ART) directly in an infertile women with endometriosis will depend on factors such as symptoms of the patient, ovarian reserve, any ultrasound feature of complex mass, risk of surgery, and finally the cost of the procedure.

## American Society for Reproductive Medicine Stage 1 and 2 Endometriosis

Cochrane review has suggested to perform operative laparoscopy (either ablation or excision of the endometriosis lesions) including adhesiolysis instead of diagnostic laparoscopy only in order to improve on-going pregnancy rates.[8]

Carbon dioxide ($CO_2$) laser vaporization was found to be better than monopolar electrocoagulation in terms of cumulative spontaneous pregnancy rate.[9]

The combined data from ENDOCAN study and GISE study has concluded that surgery was beneficial in terms of ongoing pregnancy rate and live-birth rate.[10,11]

Adhesiolysis with ablation of the endometriotic lesion is effective in improving fertility in women with minimal-mild endometriosis compared to diagnostic laparoscopy.[11]

Following surgery anti-Müllerian hormone, a marker of ovarian reserve might be reduced but antral follicular count was not found to be significantly reduced.[12]

Surgical ablation or excision of endometrioisis can be recommended as first line since the pregnancy rates are doubled in minimal and mild endometriosis. However, in women with moderate and severe disease, first-line treatment is surgical excision. ART was found to be more effective than repeat surgery in women who failed to conceive after surgery.[12]

## American Society for Reproductive Medicine Stage 3 and 4 Endometriosis

In women with stage 3 and 4 endometriosis instead of expectant management, consider operative laparoscopy in order to improve the spontaneous pregnancy rate.[13,14]

## Combined Medical and Surgical Therapy: Is It Recommended?

Combined therapy for endometriosis consists of medical therapy either preoperatively or postoperatively.

Although advantageous theoretically, there is no evidence to suggest that combination of medical-surgical treatment might enhances fertility.

Postoperative therapy might help to eradicate residual implants in women with severe endometriosis where resection of all endometriotic implants is inadvisable or impossible, however, it should not be prescribed to improve the pregnancy rates.[15]

## ■ MANAGEMENT FOR ENDOMETRIOMA IN INFERTILE WOMEN (TABLE 1 AND FLOWCHART 3)[16,17]

Prior to surgery counsel the women regarding the risk of decreased ovarian function after ovary and there might be a possibility of loss of ovary.[4]

No evidence to suggest that cystectomy prior to ART treatment might improve the pregnancy rate if endometrioma size is more than 3 cm.[4,18]

However, if the endometrioma size is more than 3 cm we can consider cystectomy prior to ART, only to improve associated pain or for easy accessibility of the follicles.[4]

Cochrane review has suggested to perform excision of the endometrioma instead of drainage and electrocoagulation of the endometrioma wall in order to increase the pregnancy rates.[19]

**Table 1:** Clinical parameters to be considered to decide on the management of endometrioma in women undergoing in vitro fertilization (IVF).[16]

| Characteristics | Favors surgery | Favors expectant management |
|---|---|---|
| 1. Previous interventions for endometriosis | None | ≥ 1 |
| 2. Ovarian reserve | Intact | Damaged |
| 3. Pain symptoms | Present | Absent |
| 4. Bilaterality | Monolateral disease | Bilateral disease |
| 5. Sonographic feature of malignancy | Present | Absent |
| 6. Growth | Rapid growth | Stable |

**Flowchart 3:** Flowchart for the management of endometrioma prior to IVF.[17]

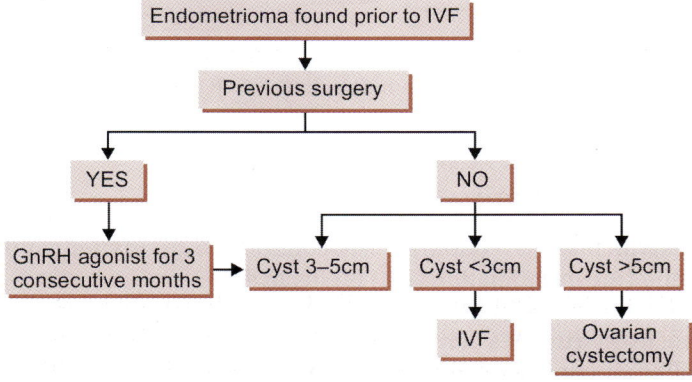

(GnRH: gonadotropin-releasing hormone; IVF: in vitro fertilization)

Still optimal surgery is controversial since each approach has its own pros and cons like in cyst drainage and ablation approach, cyst wall containing normal ovarian tissue might be removed which could potentially compromise the ovarian reserve.

And in ultrasound-guided aspiration method there is a high risk of recurrence, adhesions, and infections. It can be an alternative treatment in case of recurrence or can be done at time of oocyte retrieval. But care should be taken to avoid mixing with the other follicular fluid and should be sent in separate tube.

Laparoscopic cystectomy by using vasopressin injection technique (VIT) was found to be an ideal procedure to reduce damage to the ovaries and also to protect the ovarian reserve as compared to the usual laparoscopic cystectomy.[20] In this technique less coagulation is used, hence it might protect ovarian reserve because of less damage to the ovaries.[5]

## PROS AND CONS IN SURGICAL TREATMENT OF ENDOMETRIOMAS BEFORE IN VITRO FERTILIZATION-INTRACYTOPLASMIC SPERM INJECTION CYCLES (FIG. 2)[21]

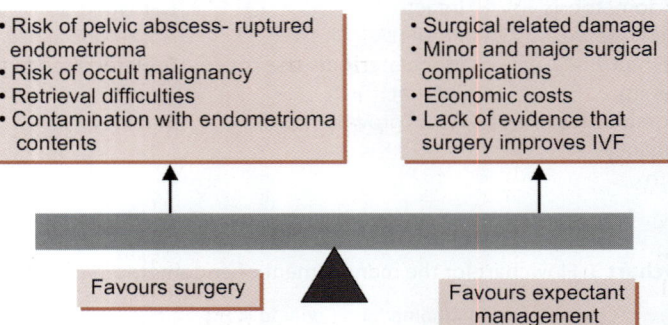

**Fig. 2:** Pros and cons in surgical treatment of endometriomas before IVF-ICSI cycles. (ICSI: intracytoplasmic sperm injection; IVF: in vitro fertilization)

## Controlled Ovarian Stimulation and Intrauterine Insemination

In patients with minimal endometriosis, controlled ovarian stimulation (COS) with intrauterine insemination (IUI) is effective.[22]

Controlled ovarian stimulation and IUI were associated with good outcome in terms of live-birth rates in women with minimal and mild endometriosis.[23]

A small study concluded that COS/IUI may be considered an option instead of in vitro fertilization (IVF) or further surgical therapy, in those women who had a surgical treatment for stage 1 or 2 endometriosis.[24]

In infertile women with ASRM stage 1/2 endometriosis, consider COS with IUI postoperatively within 6 months.[24]

In women with moderate to severe endometriosis, the pregnancy rate was more and had shorter time to pregnancy in IUI with ovarian stimulation group compared with IUI in natural cycle group. So, IUI might be a good option for achieving a pregnancy in this group of women.[25]

There is not much evidence to suggest if COS and IUI is more beneficial after diagnosis and treatment of endometriosis compared to undiagnosed or untreated women with minimal or mild endometriosis.

## Controlled Ovarian Stimulation and In Vitro Fertilization/Intracytoplasmic Sperm Injection

Assisted reproductive technology is recommended if endometriosis is present along with male factor infertility or if tubal function is compromised and/or if other treatments have failed.[4]

# The Assisted Reproductive Technology in Endometriosis: Is it Different?

After surgery, ART should be offered to infertile women with endometriosis as cumulative recurrence rate of endometriosis are not increased after COS and IVF/intracytoplasmic sperm injection (ICSI).[4,26]

The approach to be followed in COS should be that not "one size fits all" and it should be patient-centered individualized approach that takes the recent evidence into consideration.

Worldwide the most commonly used protocol is GnRH antagonist protocol. However, in women with endometriosis the more preferred one is the use of long-term pituitary downregulation by GnRH agonist named as ultra-long protocol. As this might reduce the endogenous hormonal levels as they are elevated in these women.

Both GnRH antagonist and GnRH agonist protocols were found to have similar IVF outcomes in women with mild-to-moderate endometriosis.[27]

However, GnRH agonist protocol had more number of mature oocytes and available embryos significantly compared to women with the antagonist protocol. In the subsequent frozen embryo transfer (ET) cycles, GnRH agonist protocol showed higher cumulative fecundity rate.[27]

A Cochrane review regarding the use of long-term pituitary downregulation in women with endometriosis has concluded that GnRH agonists given for 3–6 months before IVF or ICSI increased the odds of clinical pregnancy by fourfold.[28]

In vitro fertilization/ICSI is a safe procedure in women with severe endometriosis. In women in whom long-term pituitary downregulation were given had a diminished ongoing pregnancy rates after fresh ET. However, in frozen ET cycles it is beneficial in terms of pregnancy rates.[29]

In a study comparing GnRH antagonist protocol and long GnRH agonist protocol had shown similar IVF outcomes in women who underwent IVF postsurgery-laparoscopic endometrioma resection. So, they concluded that higher number of embryos might be obtained by long GnRH agonist protocol which can be cryopreserved and later used for additional ET so no need to undergo COS again.[30]

In a systematic review regarding impact of ovarian endometrioma on IVF outcome and ovarian response to COS have showed that number of retrieved oocytes, mature oocytes, and total embryos were not different between the ovaries affected and contralateral normal ovaries. And also clinical pregnancy rates, live-birth rates were not found to be affected.[31]

Antibiotic prophylaxis may be given at the time of oocyte retrieval to the women with endometrioma, even though risk of forming ovarian abscess is low.[4,32]

## Infertile Women with Recurrent Endometriosis

Surgery should be considered carefully if there is history of previous ovarian surgery.[4]

However, in moderate or severe case of endometriosis if initial surgery fails and fertility is not restored, the effective alternative should be IVF-ET since reoperation is not very beneficial to improve the fertility in these women.[33]

A systematic review regarding the effect of repeat surgery on the reproductive performance in women with recurrent endometriosis showed that the chance of conception after repeat surgery is less compared to primary surgery and in reoperated women IVF results were not inferior.[34]

Hence, second-line surgery is not recommended and IVF-ET is considered as an effective option.

### Pregnancy Outcomes

Adverse obstetrics outcomes are more common in women with endometriosis compared to women without endometriosis.

There is an increased risk of preterm birth, preeclampsia, antepartum bleeding/placental complications, and cesarean section in these women. No increased risk of stillbirth or low-birth weight in them.[35]

## CONCLUSION

- Consider the following parameters like age of the women, infertility duration, pelvic pain, and endometriosis stage before formulating management plan.
- There is insufficient evidence to suggest laparoscopic treatment mainly to improve the likelihood of pregnancy in women with mild-to-moderate endometriosis.
- Expectant management or COS with IUI is the first-line therapy in younger women (<35 years) with stage 1 and 2 endometriosis.
- More aggressive treatment like COS with IUI or IVF should be considered in women more than 35 years of age.
- Conservative surgery with laparoscopy or laparotomy might be beneficial in infertile women with stage 3 and 4 endometriosis.
- Insufficient evidence regarding endometrioma resection for improving IVF outcome.
- In women with stage 3 and 4 endometriosis, IVF-ET is an effective option in women who fail to conceive following surgery or due to advanced age.
- Compared to tubal factor infertility IVF success rates are diminished in women with endometriosis, however, IVF maximizes the cycle of fecundity in these women.
- Compared to women without endometriosis undergoing ART treatment, the incidence of preeclampsia, preterm delivery, cesarean section, and antepartum bleeding/placental complications was found to be higher in women with endometriosis.

## REFERENCES

1. Kennedy S, Bergqvist A, Chapron C, et al. ESHRE guideline for the diagnosis and treatment of endometriosis. Hum Reprod. 2005;20:2698-704.
2. Missmer SA, Hankinson SE, Spiegelman D, et al. Incidence of laparoscopically confirmed endometriosis by demographic, anthropometric, and lifestyle factors. Am J Epidemiol. 2004;160:784-96.

3. Verkauf BS. Incidence, symptoms, and signs of endometriosis in fertile and infertile women. J Fla Med Assoc. 1987;74:671-5.
4. Lessey BA, Castelbaum AJ, Sawin SW, et al. Aberrant integrin expression in the endometrium of women with endometriosis. J Clin Endocrinol Metab. 1994;79:643-9.
5. Saeki A, Matsumoto T, Ikuma K, et al. The vasopressin injection technique for laparoscopic excision of ovarian endometrioma: a technique to reduce the use of coagulation. J Minim Invasive Gynecol. 2010;17:176-9.
6. Dunselman GA, Vermeulen N, Becker C, et al. ESHRE guideline: management of women with endometriosis. Hum Reprod. 2014;29:400-12.
7. Hughes E, Brown J, Collins JJ, et al. Ovulation suppression for endometriosis. Cochrane Database Syst Rev. 2007;(3):CD000155.
8. Jacobson TZ, Duffy JM, Barlow DH, et al. Laparoscopic surgery for subfertility associated with endometriosis. Cochrane Database Syst Rev. 2010;(1):CD001398.
9. Chang FH, Chou HH, Soong YK, et al. Efficacy of isotopic 13CO2 laser laparoscopic evaporation in the treatment of infertile patients with minimal and mild endometriosis: a life table cumulative pregnancy rates study. J Am Assoc Gynecol Laparosc. 1997;4:219-23.
10. Marcoux S, Maheux R, Bérubé S. Laparoscopic surgery in infertile women with minimal or mild endometriosis. Canadian Collaborative Group on Endometriosis. N Engl J Med. 1997;337:217-22.
11. Parazzini F. Ablation of lesions or no treatment in minimal-mild endometriosis in infertile women: a randomized trial. Gruppo Italiano per lo Studio dell'Endometriosi. Hum Reprod. 1999;14:1332-4.
12. Rizk B, Turki R, Lotfy H, et al. Surgery for endometriosis-associated infertility: do we exaggerate the magnitude of effect? Facts Views Vis Obgyn. 2015;7:109-18.
13. Revised American Society for Reproductive Medicine classification of endometriosis: 1996. Fertil Steril. 1997;67:817-21.
14. Vercellini P, Fedele L, Aimi G, et al. Reproductive performance, pain recurrence and disease relapse after conservative surgical treatment for endometriosis: the predictive value of the current classification system. Hum Reprod. 2006;21:2679-85.
15. Yap C, Furness S, Farquhar C. Pre and post operative medical therapy for endometriosis surgery. Cochrane Database Syst Rev. 2004;(3):CD003678.
16. Garcia-Velasco JA, Somigliana E. Management of endometriomas in women requiring IVF: to touch or not to touch. Hum Reprod. 2009;24:496-501.
17. Tsoumpou I, Kyrgiou M, Gelbaya TA, et al. The effect of surgical treatment for endometrioma on in vitro fertilization outcomes: a systematic review and meta-analysis. Fertil Steril. 2009;92:75-87.
18. Benschop L, Farquhar C, van der Poel N, et al. Interventions for women with endometrioma prior to assisted reproductive technology. Cochrane Database Syst Rev. 2010;(11):CD008571.
19. Hart RJ, Hickey M, Maouris P, et al. Excisional surgery versus ablative surgery for ovarian endometriomata. Cochrane Database Syst Rev. 2008;(2):CD004992.
20. Qiong-Zhen R, Ge Y, Deng Y, et al. Effect of vasopressin injection technique in laparoscopic excision of bilateral ovarian endometriomas on ovarian reserve: prospective randomized study. J Minim Invasive Gynecol. 2014;21:266-71.
21. Somigliana E, Vercellini P, Viganó P, et al. Should endometriomas be treated before IVF-ICSI cycles? Hum Reprod Update. 2006;12:57-64.
22. Isaksson R, Tiitinen A. Superovulation combined with insemination or timed intercourse in the treatment of couples with unexplained infertility and minimal endometriosis. Acta Obstet Gynecol Scand. 1997;76:550-4.

23. Tummon IS, Asher LJ, Martin JS, et al. Randomized controlled trial of superovulation and insemination for infertility associated with minimal or mild endometriosis. Fertil Steril. 1997;68:8-12.
24. Werbrouck E, Spiessens C, Meuleman C, et al. No difference in cycle pregnancy rate and in cumulative live-birth rate between women with surgically treated minimal to mild endometriosis and women with unexplained infertility after controlled ovarian hyperstimulation and intrauterine insemination. Fertil Steril. 2006;86:566-71.
25. van der Houwen LE, Schreurs AM, Schats R, et al. Efficacy and safety of intrauterine insemination in patients with moderate-to-severe endometriosis. Reprod Biomed Online. 2014;28:590-8.
26. Benaglia L, Somigliana E, Santi G, et al. IVF and endometriosis-related symptom progression: insights from a prospective study. Hum Reprod. 2011;26:2368-72.
27. Pabuccu R, Onalan G, Kaya C. GnRH agonist and antagonist protocols for stage I-II endometriosis and endometrioma in in vitro fertilization/intracytoplasmic sperm injection cycles. Fertil Steril. 2007;88:832-9.
28. Sallam HN, Garcia-Velasco JA, Dias S, et al. Long-term pituitary down-regulation before in vitro fertilization (IVF) for women with endometriosis. Cochrane Database Syst Rev. 2006;(1):CD004635.
29. Van der Houwen LE, Mijatovic V, Leemhuis E, et al. Efficacy and safety of IVF/ICSI in patients with severe endometriosis after long-term pituitary down-regulation. Reprod Biomed Online. 2014;28:39-46.
30. Bastu E, Yasa C, Dural O, et al. Comparison of ovulation induction protocols after endometrioma resection. JSLS. 2014;18:e2014.
31. Yang C, Geng Y, Li Y, et al. Impact of ovarian endometrioma on ovarian responsiveness and IVF: a systematic review and meta-analysis. Reprod Biomed Online. 2015;31:9-19.
32. Benaglia L, Somigliana E, Iemmello R, et al. Endometrioma and oocyte retrieval-induced pelvic abscess: a clinical concern or an exceptional complication? Fertil Steril. 2008;89:1263-6.
33. Pagidas K, Falcone T, Hemmings R, et al. Comparison of reoperation for moderate (stage III) and severe (stage IV) endometriosis-related infertility with in vitro fertilization-embryo transfer. Fertil Steril. 1996;65:791-5.
34. Vercellini P, Somigliana E, Viganò P, et al. The effect of second-line surgery on reproductive performance of women with recurrent endometriosis: a systematic review. Acta Obstet Gynecol Scand. 2009;88:1074-82.
35. Stephansson O, Kieler H, Granath F, et al. Endometriosis, assisted reproduction technology, and risk of adverse pregnancy outcome. Hum Reprod. 2009;24:2341-7

# CHAPTER 17

# Adenomyosis: A Biggest Challenge in Assisted Reproductive Technology

*Sadhana K Desai, Ritika Rajan*

## ■ INTRODUCTION

Adenomyosis is a benign disorder where basal endometrial glands and stroma are found in the myometrium with reactive hyperplasia of the surrounding smooth muscle myometrial cells.[1] Until recently, adenomyosis had been associated with multiparity, not with impaired fertility. In the last few years, there has been an increasing number of infertile patients getting diagnosed with adenomyosis since women delay their first pregnancy until their late 30s or early 40s.

It is found that approximately 20% of cases of adenomyosis involve women younger than 40 years, and 80% are 40–50 years old. The most severe symptoms are associated with the older group. Adenomyosis is completely asymptomatic in approximately one-third of cases. The most frequent symptoms in the remaining two-thirds are menorrhagia (50%), dysmenorrhea (30%) and metrorrhagia (20%). Dyspareunia may also be a complaint when adenomyosis coexists with endometriosis.

## ■ DIAGNOSIS OF ADENOMYOSIS

Traditionally, the diagnosis was made by means of histopathological examination. With the evolution of magnetic resonance imaging (MRI) and three-dimensional transvaginal sonography (3D TVS) today the diagnosis can be made with a level of accuracy of 80–90% without the need for excisional surgery.

### Imaging Modalities (Table 1)

Various imaging modalities which are used today for the diagnosis of adenomyosis are transabdominal ultrasonography, transvaginal ultrasonography, 3D TVS with color Doppler and MRI. According to Dueholm et al. (2017), MRI and 3D TVS are good at identifying patients with adenomyosis but MRI is superior to TVS to exclude the diagnosis of adenomyosis with equal sensitivity but a higher specificity.

**Table 1:** Imaging modalities.

| Transabdominal ultrasonography | Transvaginal ultrasonography | 3D TVS with color Doppler/ MRI |
|---|---|---|
| • Uterine enlargement without any features of fibroid<br>• Asymmetrical thickening of anterior and posterior walls<br>• Cannot differentiate focal adenomyosis from leiomyoma<br>• Uterine enlargement without any features of fibroid<br>• Asymmetrical thickening of anterior and posterior walls<br>• Cannot differentiate focal adenomyosis from leiomyoma | • To be considered as primary diagnostic tool in suspected case of adenomyosis<br>• Hetrogenous/hypoechoic poorly described areas in the myometrium<br>• Myometrial cysts of various size<br>• Linear striations radiating out from the endometrium into the myometrium<br>• Poor definition of junctional zone<br>• Psuedo widening of the endometrium<br>• Adenomyosis is most often diagnosed in the presence of three or more sonographic criteria | • Junctional zone maximum thickness 8 mm or more, myometrial asymmetry and hypoechoic striations. On color Doppler, there is increased blood flow to the areas affected by adenomyosis.<br>• Gordts et al. (2014) suggested the following adenomyosis classification on MRI<br>• Simple junctional zone hyperplasia – JZ thickness >8 mm but <12 mm in women up to 35 years<br>• Partial or diffuse adenomyosis- JZ thickness >12 mm, involvement of the myometrium, high signal intensity myometrium foci<br>• Adenomyoma- myometrial mass with indistinct margins with primarily low signal intensity |

(TVS: transvaginal sonography; MRI: magnetic resonance imaging)

## ADENOMYOSIS AND SUBFERTILITY

Today increasing numbers of studies have suggested that adenomyosis has a negative impact on female fertility. Success of IVF and embryo transfer and live birth are also affected. The prevalence of adenomyosis in infertile women varies from 7% to 27% as reported by various workers. Several uncontrolled studies with limited data also suggested that treatment of adenomyosis may improve fertility.

Adenomyosis negatively affect implantation by impaired endometrium-myometrium interface, altered uterine peristaltic activity,[2] altered endometrial-myometrial vascular growth, increased levels of prostaglandins in the ectopic endometrial epithelium,[3] higher expression of aromatase cytochrome P450 in the eutopic endometrium,[4] decreased integrin b3, osteopontin, leukemia inhibiting factor, and impaired *HOXA-10 gene* function during the implantation window.[5]

## ■ IMPACT OF ADENOMYOSIS ON ART

Initially, there were not many studies suggesting the impact of adenomyosis on assisted reproductive technology (ART). Now, as increasing number of patients who come for ART are getting diagnosed with adenomyosis, a large number of studies have been carried out to ascertain the role of adenomyosis on female fertility and ART.

On review of literature majority of the published articles were case reports or case series. However, there are 11 good observational studies on the clinical outcome of in vitro fertilization (IVF) in women with adenomyosis compared to IVF in women without adenomyosis. Out of 11, 5 studies are prospective and 6 are retrospective cohort studies. Grace Younes and Togas Tulandi[6] did a meta-analysis of 11 studies for the effect of adenomyosis on fertility and on IVF clinical outcomes. The parameters studied were clinical pregnancy rate, rate of implantation, miscarriage, ongoing pregnancy rate, live birth rate and ectopic pregnancy.

The rates of implantation, clinical pregnancy per cycle, clinical pregnancy per embryo transfer, ongoing pregnancy and live birth among women with adenomyosis were significantly lower than among those without adenomyosis. The miscarriage rate in women with adenomyosis was higher than in those without adenomyosis. The presence of adenomyosis was associated with a 41% decrease in live birth rate.

Another study by Paolo Vercellini et al. (2014) conducted a systemic literature review and meta-analysis of comparative studies published on IVF/intracytoplasmic sperm injection (ICSI) outcome in women with and without adenomyosis.[7] Pooling of results from eight included studies yielded a common relative risk (RR) of 0.72 demonstrating that adenomyosis is associated with a 28% reduction in the likelihood of clinical pregnancy in infertile women undergoing IVF/ICSI.

Martinez Conejero et al. (2011), reported a live birth rate per cycle of 26.8% in the adenomyosis group and 37.1% in the non-adenomyotic group. The difference is statistically significant.[8] The study appears particularly interesting as the use of donated oocytes allow the selective assessment of uterine factor. These authors detected a two-fold risk of miscarriage in women with adenomyosis. This suggests that the adenomyotic uterine environment increases the risk of miscarriage independently of oocyte and embryo quality.

The presence of endometriosis might be a confounding factor. However, even in the studies in which the proportion of patients with endometriosis was low, the presence of adenomyosis led to reduced clinical pregnancy rate and increased miscarriage rate. Dimitrios Mavrelos et al. (2017) in University

College London Hospitals examined the impact of the degree of adenomyosis on the chance of clinical pregnancy after IVF and embryo transfer (IVF–ET) in 375 women out of which 72 had features of adenomyosis. Authors showed that women with any feature of adenomyosis had a lower clinical pregnancy rate 21/72 (29.2%) than those without adenomyosis (42.7%).[9]

In order to stratify women with adenomyosis an "adenomyosis score" was calculated. To calculate the score, each ultrasonic feature of adenomyosis was assigned a value of 1 when present and 0 when absent, giving a minimum score of 0 when no feature of adenomyosis, 1 when a single feature was seen, up to 7 when all seven features were present.

## ■ FEATURES OF ADENOMYOSIS (TABLE 2)

Logistic regression selected an adenomyosis score of 4 or higher as an independent predictor of clinical pregnancy. Estimated probability of clinical pregnancy decreased from 42.7% for women with no adenomyosis features to 22.9% for those with four and 13.0% for those with all seven as shown in Table 2. Women with adenomyosis have lower clinical pregnancy rate after IVF–ET. Condition severity expressed as a number of morphological features on ultrasound scan increases the magnitude of the effect. It was speculated that higher numbers of visible adenomyosis features translate into worse clinical impact through deeper and more extensive myometrial invasion. It is interesting to note that a single feature of adenomyosis associated with dysmenorrhea was a disrupted endometrial-myometrial junction (EMJ), which is also the single feature associated with poor reproductive performance. Women with any feature of adenomyosis were significantly less likely to have a clinical pregnancy following ET.

## ■ MODALITIES OF TREATMENT (TABLE 3)

Usually, treatment of adenomyosis depends on whether it is diffuse or focal. Medical management is for diffuse adenomyosis. It is shown that diffuse adenomyosis fares worse than focal or localized adenomyosis. Furthermore, focal adenomyosis can be easily excised, leading to increased pregnancy

| Table 2: Features of adenomyosis. | | |
|---|---|---|
| 1. | Endometrial striae | |
| 2. | Asymmetric thickening | |
| 3. | Myometrial cyst | |
| 4. | Parallel shadowing | |
| 5. | Adenomyoma | |
| 6. | Irregular endomyometrial junction | |
| 7. | Endometrial islands | |

**Table 3:** Modalities of treatment.

| Medical management | Surgical management | Minimally invasive |
|---|---|---|
| GnRH agonist therapy | Adenomyomectomy | Recent treatment modality |
| Can be combined with conservative surgery both pre- and postoperatively | Two techniques: Old classical incision and transverse H-incision | • Uterine artery embolization<br>• High intensity focused USG |

(USG: ultrasonography; GnRH: gonadotropin-releasing hormone)

rates.[10,11] A few authors have also reported surgical treatment of diffuse adenomyosis, i.e. debulking surgeries.[11] Instead of surgical excision, pre-IVF treatment with the use of gonadotropin-releasing hormone agonists (GnRHa) is certainly less invasive and more practical. GnRH receptors are present in the adenomyotic tissue, and GnRHa induces apoptosis and reduces the inflammatory reaction and angiogenesis.[12] The results show that long-term GnRHa before IVF treatments improved the pregnancy rate.[13,14] The disadvantages of using long-term GnRHa are longer ovarian stimulation and higher gonadotropin doses, especially in the fresh cycle. Its use before frozen cycles could be more cost-effective. Also minimally invasive procedures like uterine arterial embolization or high intensity focused USG can be used although the time period for ART in these procedures are as long as 2–3 years and not many studies have been carried out supporting the positive effect of these new techniques on the pregnancy rate following IVF/ICSI.

## When to Start Treatment

Park CW et al. compared combined GnRHa with add-back or add-back treatment alone before frozen embryo transfer[14] and another compared GnRHa versus no treatment before fresh-embryo transfer. The result showed that pretreatment with GnRHa appears to be beneficial to the pregnancy rate. Also, pre-ART surgery is associated with increased pregnancy rate especially in cases of adenomyosis associated with endometriosis.

Management of adenomyosis in ART patients depends on various factors such as age, AMH, coexisting diseases. The treatment of adenomyosis can start before pick up or after pick up, i.e. segmental transfer.
- Before pick up: Mild disease, young female, good ovarian reserve, postsurgical resection.
- Before embryo transfer: Severely affected, elderly patients, poor ovarian reserve, minimally invasive procedure or medical management.

## IMPACT OF TREATMENT OF ADENOMYOSIS ON FERTILITY

There are four retrospective studies evaluating the effects of surgical and medical treatment of adenomyosis on fertility. Two of four retrospective studies compared fertility outcomes of infertile women with adenomyosis treated by means of conservative surgery and GnRHa or with GnRHa alone. They examined the cumulative pregnancy rate 3 years following the treatment.[10,11] The other two studies compared infertile women with adenomyosis treated with the use of long-term GnRHa before IVF treatment and those without GnRHa treatment. All the studies showed an increase in pregnancy rates following treatment of adenomyosis.[13,14]

## IMPACT OF TREATMENT OF ADENOMYOSIS ON ART RESULTS

### Effect of GnRHa Pretreatment before IVF

Niu Z et al. studied the effect of long-term GnRHa pretreatment on patients of adenomyosis undergoing frozen embryo transfer after preparation of the endometrium with hormone replacement therapy so they included 339 patients with adenomyosis out of which 194 received long-term GnRH agonist plus hormone-replacement therapy (HRT) (downregulation plus HRT) and 145 received HRT. On the day of progesterone administration, mean endometrial thickness and serum progesterone level were significantly greater in HRT patients. In downregulation plus HRT group, clinical pregnancy, implantation and ongoing pregnancy rates were 51.35%, 32.56% and 48.91% respectively, significantly higher than that of HRT group (24.83%, 16.07% and 21.38% respectively). So they concluded that in frozen embryo transfer long-term GnRHa pretreatment significantly improves pregnancy outcomes in patients with adenomyosis.[13]

### Effect of Focal versus Diffuse Adenomyosis on IVF

Benaglia L et al. carried a study to see the difference in the effects of focal and diffuse adenomyosis on IVF outcome. Adenomyosis was identified by using TVS at the initial workup and classified into focal and diffuse types. The IVF outcomes were also subanalyzed according to the adenomyotic region.

The pooled results gave an odd ratio of 1.36 favoring focal adenomyosis over diffuse adenomyosis.

### Effect of GnRHa Pretreatment before Fresh Embryo Transfer and Frozen Embryo Transfer

Park CW et al. conducted a retrospective study to determine the preferred regimen for women with adenomyosis undergoing IVF.[14]

They compared the IVF outcomes of fresh embryo transfer cycles with or without GnRHa pretreatment and of frozen-thawed embryo transfer (FET) cycles following GnRH agonist treatment.

This retrospective study included 241 IVF cycles of women with adenomyosis. Fresh ET cycles without (147 cycles, group A) or with (105 cycles, group B) GnRH agonist pretreatment, and FET cycles following GnRH agonist treatment (43 cycles, group C) were compared. The result of their study suggested that GnRH agonist pretreatment increased the stimulation duration and total dose of gonadotropin which resulted in a significantly higher number of retrieved oocytes in group B than in group A. Controlled ovarian stimulation for freezing resulted in a significantly higher number of retrieved oocytes with a lower dose of gonadotropin in group C than in group B. The clinical pregnancy rate in group C (39.5%) tended to be higher than those in groups B (30.5%) and A (25.2%) but without a significant difference.

## ■ DISCUSSION

It is found that the presence of any feature of adenomyosis is associated with a reduction in the chance of success with assisted conception. Also, adenomyosis on ultrasound presents with a multitude of features and the cumulative impact of these features on IVF–ET outcome has not been examined before. It is found that severity of adenomyosis, expressed as a score to represent accumulation of ultrasonic features, is associated with increasing chance of failed IVF–ET independent of age and ovarian reserve. Several authors have suggested the concept of adenomyosis as a continuum that becomes clinically significant when a threshold of severity is reached. Levguret et al. and Cirpan et al. (2008) showed that women with clinically significant dysmenorrhea have higher numbers of adenomyotic foci in histopathology specimens. Naftalin et al. (2016) demonstrated a correlation between number of adenomyosis features on ultrasound and severity of dysmenorrhea. Mild forms of adenomyosis have limited impact while more severely affected women have poorer outcomes.

## ■ CONCLUSION

Adenomyosis in infertile women has been encountered more frequently in recent years, owing to an improved diagnostic test with the use of high-resolution ultrasound as well as to the increasing age of women seeking fertility treatment. Yet the diagnosis of adenomyosis is often overlooked and not taken into consideration when planning an IVF treatment. It seems reasonable to suggest screening for adenomyosis in patients of unexplained infertility and recurrent implantation failure before embarking in medically assisted reproductive procedures. TVS should be preferred for screening because of its low cost and ubiquitous availability whereas MRI should be reserved for selected circumstances when TVS report is unconvincing or patient is to be taken up for surgery.

The diagnosis of adenomyosis should be standardized according to internationally agreed criteria, with the objective of selecting definite populations in terms of disease severity.

Women with lower number of adenomyotic lesions can be reassured while those with a higher number can be warned about the higher risk of treatment failure.

The IVF protocols include the use of long-term GnRHa before IVF treatment, long protocol, short protocol, and antagonist protocol. Long-term GnRHa treatment and long protocol might have a therapeutic effect on adenomyosis and improve the IVF outcome.[15]

Patients with more severe degree of adenomyosis than those whose uterus contains microscopic adenomyosis only are detected with TVS/MRI. They suffer from clinically relevant adenomyosis. They are the women whom we see in daily practice. In the context of infertility and IVF, treatment is indicated for women with symptomatic as well as asymptomatic adenomyosis. These women may benefit from prolonged GnRHa treatment or long protocol. In addition, more research is needed on the potential consequences of adenomyosis in terms of major obstetrical syndromes, such as spontaneous late miscarriage, preterm birth, intrauterine growth restriction, pre-eclampsia and obstetric hemorrhages.

## KEY POINTS

- Adenomyosis should be looked for in patients with unexplained infertility and recurrent implantation failures.
- Adenomyosis should be ruled out in patients with endometriosis before proceeding with treatment as both may coexist.
- MRI evaluation of junctional zone thickness is the best negative predictive factor of implantation failure and implantation failure was found to be high when the average junctional zone was greater than 7 mm.
- Conservative surgery or combination treatment in subfertile women with adenomyosis is more effective for increasing the pregnancy rates compared to GnRH analogs alone.
- Segmental transfer of embryo after treatment of adenomyosis with GnRH analogs has a better pregnancy rate than fresh embryo transfer cycle.

## REFERENCES

1. Leyendecker G, Herbertz M, Kunz G, et al. Endometriosis results from the dislocation of basal endometrium. Hum Reprod. 2002;17:2725-36.
2. Kunz G, Leyendecker G. Uterine peristaltic activity during the menstrual cycle: characterization, regulation, function and dysfunction. Reprod Biomed Online. 2002;4(Suppl 3):5-9.
3. Ota H, Tanaka T. Stromal vascularization in the endometrium during adenomyosis. Microsc Res Tech. 2003;60:445-9.
4. van Voorhis BJ, Heuttner PC, Clark MR, et al. Immunohistochemical localization of prostaglandin H synthase in the female reproductive tract and endometriosis. Am J Obstet Gynecol. 1990;163(1 Pt 1):57-62.

5. Fischer CP, Kayisili U, Taylor HS. HOXA10 expression is decreased in endometrium of women with adenomyosis. Fertil Steril. 2011;95:1133-6.
6. Younes G, Tulandi T. Effects of adenomyosis on in vitro fertilization treatment outcomes: a meta-analysis. Fertil Steril. 2017;108:483-90.
7. Vercellini P, Consonni D, Barbara G, et al. Adenomyosis and reproductive performance after surgery for rectovaginal and colorectal endometriosis: a systematic review and meta-analysis. Reprod Biomed Online. 2014;28(6):704-13.
8. Martinez-Conejero JA, Morgan M, Montesinos M, et al. Adenomyosis does not affect implantation, but is associated with miscarriage in patients undergoing oocyte donation. Fertil Steril. 2011;96:943-50.
9. Mavrelos D, Holland TK, O'Donovan O, et al. The impact of adenomyosis on the outcome of IVF-embryo transfer. Reprod Biomed Online. 2017;35(5):549-54.
10. Al Jama FE. Management of adenomyosis in subfertile women and pregnancy outcome. Oman Med J. 2011;26:178-81.
11. Wang PH, Fuh JL, Chao HT, et al. Is the surgical approach beneficial to subfertile women with symptomatic extensive adenomyosis? J Obstet Gynaecol Res. 2009;35:495-502.
12. Khan KN, Kitajima M, Hiraki K, et al. Cell proliferation effect of GnRH agonist on pathological lesions of women with endometriosis, adenomyosis and uterine myoma. Hum Reprod. 2010;25:2878-90.
13. Niu Z, Chen Q, Sun Y, et al. Long term pituitary downregulation before frozen embryo transfer could improve pregnancy outcomes in women with adenomyosis. Gynecol Endocrinol. 2013;29:1026-30.
14. Park CW, Choi MH, Yang KM, et al. Pregnancy rates in women with adenomyosis undergoing fresh or frozen embryo transfer cycles following gonadotropin-releasing hormone agonist treatment. Clin Exp Reprod Med. 2016;43:169-73.
15. Dueholm M. Uterine adenomyosis and infertility, review of reproductive outcome after in vitro fertilization and surgery. Acta Obstet Gynecol Scand. 2017;96:715-26.

CHAPTER
18

# Prevention of Complications in ART

*Praveena Pai, Pratap Kumar*

## ■ INTRODUCTION

Assisted reproductive technology (ART) is defined as any procedure that involves the handling of sperms, eggs or both outside the body. It includes in vitro fertilization (IVF), with or without intracytoplasmic sperm injection (ICSI), with fresh or frozen embryos and IVF with donor oocytes, sperms or donor embryos. Some organizations consider even intrauterine insemination (IUI) under ART.

Assisted reproductive technology has progressed by leaps and bounds over the years. However, as with any other branch of medicine it has its own share of problems. This chapter will deal with the prevention of complications arising during the process of IVF-ICSI as highlighted in Table 1.

| Table 1: Complications of in vitro fertilization-intracytoplasmic sperm injection (IVF-ICSI). | |
|---|---|
| Associated with COH | OHSS—thromboembolism, adnexal torsion, rupture |
| TVS-guided OPU | • Bleeding—vaginal, intraperitoneal<br>• Infection (PID)<br>• Perforation of bowel—especially with DIE<br>• Anesthetic complications |
| Pregnancy associated | • Multiple pregnancies<br>• Fetal reduction<br>• Ectopic pregnancy<br>• Heterotopic pregnancy<br>• Higher risk pregnancies—preeclampsia, diabetes, preterm, FGR, LBW, LGA babies |
| Rare complications | • Imprinting disorders<br>• Congenital malformations and chromosomal aberrations<br>• Neurological sequelae, cognitive development?<br>• Multiple cycles of IVF—cancer risk? |

(COH: controlled ovarian hyperstimulation; TVS: transvaginal scan; OHSS: ovarian hyperstimulation; FGR: fetal growth restriction; LBW: low birth weight; LGA: large for gestational age)

Ethical dilemmas and complications arising from advanced procedures such as ovarian tissue cryopreservation or uterine transplantation are outside the remit of this chapter and will not be discussed.

## PREVENTION OF COMPLICATIONS

### Ovarian Hyperstimulation Syndrome

Ovarian hyperstimulation syndrome (OHSS) is not so uncommon complication of IVF, characterized by enlargement of the ovaries, fluid retention, and weight gain. The main pathophysiological change is the increased capillary permeability leading to leakage of fluid from the vascular compartment with third-space fluid accumulation and intravascular dehydration. The release of vasoactive substances from the ovary, in particular vascular endothelial growth factor (VEGF), under the influence of hCG trigger (human chorionic gonadotropin) has emerged as the main culprit. The clinical presentations range from hypotension, tachycardia, renal and liver dysfunction, peritoneal and pleural collections, enlarged, fragile ovaries that may bleed or tort, thromboembolism and rarely death.

Some important risk factors associated with OHSS are:
- Young age
- Low body mass index (BMI)
- Polycystic ovary syndrome (PCOS)
- Agonist protocol of stimulation
- Higher doses of gonadotropins
- High absolute estradiol level/rapid rise in estradiol
- Previous OHSS.

Awareness of these risk factors and individually *tailored gonadotropin regimen* play an important role in preventing this complication. In women with PCOS, use of antagonist protocol and starting with low doses of gonadotropins is advisable. The starting dose is usually 75 IU of recombinant gonadotropins but some clinicians prefer starting even as low as 37.5 IU and increase it in a step-wise manner. Both step-up and step-down protocols have been found to decrease the risk of OHSS.[1]

Minimal stimulation IVF or natural cycle IVF are additional methods whereby the oocyte yield can be controlled, minimizing the OHSS and multiple birth risk.[2,3]

*Pretreatment with metformin* is known to decrease the risk of OHSS in women with PCOS and is highly recommended in those who are particularly at high risk such as low BMI or hyper-responders during ovulation induction.[4]

A Cochrane review in 2011[5] concluded that the use of *antagonist protocol* had a definite advantage over the agonist, in reducing OHSS rates. A more recent meta-analysis[6] concluded that the combined mild and moderate OHSS rates were reduced with antagonist protocol but there was no significant difference in the severe OHSS rates when agonists were compared with antagonists.

However, antagonist protocols have the added advantage of allowing the use of a gonadotropin releasing hormone (GnRH) agonist as a trigger for ovulation thus avoiding the use of hCG. This step, combined with *freezing the embryos* and resorting to a frozen embryo transfer (FET) later drastically reduces the risk of OHSS. With significant improvement in the embryo vitrification techniques, the live births are not affected when compared with fresh embryo transfers. In fact, by avoiding the embryo transfer during the excessively high estradiol levels generated during these cycles, there is a suggestion that the implantation rates may improve. A recent Cochrane review found similar pregnancy rates with fresh as well as FETs.[7]

OHSS is likely to occur despite these measures. Large number of follicles, fluid in peritoneum and high estradiol levels on the day of hCG trigger are good predictors of likely OHSS. Another good predictor is the hematocrit levels.[8] As highlighted in this study a rapid rise in hematocrit levels between the day of hCG trigger and oocyte retrieval is good risk factor for OHSS. Serial monitoring of hematocrit along with hemoglobin, white cell count, serum electrolytes and the renal and liver functions help manage and mitigate the effects of OHSS.

In addition to embryo freezing, a few additional measures decrease the risk of severe OHSS.

*Dopamine receptor agonists* such as bromocriptine, cabergoline and quinagolide inactivate the receptors and prevent the increase in capillary permeability. A recent Cochrane review[9] concludes that these drugs reduce the incidence of moderate or severe OHSS without affecting the pregnancy outcomes, should a fresh embryo transfer take place. Gastrointestinal side-effects were not uncommon particularly with quinagolide. A common practice is to give cabergoline 0.5 mg daily for 8 days after oocyte retrieval.

Use of *plasma expanders* is on the decline with the use of antagonists and elective freezing of embryos. However some clinicians still find these quite useful to prevent third space collections. A recent Cochrane[10] (based on only a few trials) suggested that plasma expanders (human albumin, hexaethyl starch or mannitol) reduce the rates of moderate and severe OHSS in high risk women. Albumin was found to reduce pregnancy rates but not the other two. It ultimately advised their use in selected women only and not as routine practice.

Low dose aspirin (100 mg) daily from the beginning of ovarian stimulation was shown to decrease the risk of severe OHSS in a randomized trial in 2009.[11] It acts by decreasing the platelet hyperstimulation associated with OHSS. More recent evidence for the same is lacking. The authors do not routinely use this in their practice.

Thromboembolism is a potentially life-threatening complication of severe OHSS. Women at high risk should be started on low molecular weight heparin (LMWH) which should be continued at least till the end of first trimester if she becomes pregnant.[12,13] LMWH is preferred to unfractionated heparin due to ease of administration and lack of monitoring required.

## Ovarian Torsion

Ovarian torsion is a complication of enlarged, hyperstimulated ovaries. In the presence of OHSS, the large cysts serve as a lead point for twisting on a vascular pedicle especially in the presence of pelvic ascites.[14] The incidence of ovarian torsion in IVF pregnancies is around 0.8%, which jumps to 7.5% in the presence of OHSS. Moreover, the OHSS patients who become pregnant are at a much higher risk of ovarian torsion than those who do not become pregnant (16 vs 2.3%).[15] The clinical presentation can be nonspecific but this possibility should be strongly considered and actively ruled out in any IVF patient presenting with severe abdominal pain. Timely intervention is needed to salvage the ovary and possibly the pregnancy. Gangrene of the ovary can lead to peritonitis and death in some cases. Preventive measures include all steps discussed above to reduce the occurrence of OHSS. Avoidance of sexual intercourse and any high impact activities in the event of OHSS are also recommended.

## Rupture and Bleeding

*Rupture and bleeding from hyperstimulated and fragile ovaries* is another rare complication. Vaginal examinations and ultrasound scans should be kept to a minimum and performed gently. Should paracentesis be needed (as in cases of significant symptomatic ascites), ultrasound guidance should be used to avoid trauma to the ovaries.

## Complications of Oocyte Retrieval

Oocyte retrieval is a fairly safe procedure when done by skilled persons under ultrasound guidance. These days it is done under short general anesthesia and the risks associated with anesthesia can be avoided by a thorough work-up before commencing IVF. Knowledge of the pelvic anatomy is the key to avoiding complications during oocyte retrieval particularly *intraperitoneal bleeding*. Internal iliac vessels run very close to the stimulated ovaries and in cross-section may appear like follicles. It is imperative to visualize the peripheral follicles in particular in both axes by turning the probe, to avoid puncturing a vessel. Sometimes, peritoneal bleed might result from the punctures on the surface of the ovary. This can be avoided by aspirating as many follicles as possible without withdrawing the needle tip from the ovary. Gentle manipulation of the needle and proper visualization of the needle tip at all times is important. Avoiding multiple jabs in the vagina can avoid excessive vaginal bleeding after the procedure. Vaginal bleeding usually responds to compression. Occasionally a tampon may need to be left for 2–4 hours or a stitch maybe required for a spurting vessel. Rarely the needle entry maybe through the cervix, especially in cases of previous surgery. Even the cervical bleeding usually responds to compression.

*Infections leading to ovarian abscesses or peritonitis* are rare complications of oocyte retrieval. Meticulous cleaning of the vagina with normal saline prior to the retrieval and use of prophylactic a broad spectrum antibiotic is recommended. Ovarian abscesses are more likely in the event of puncturing an ovarian endometrioma during follicular aspiration. Meticulous ultrasound to detect any small endometriomas and steering clear of these during follicular aspiration will help avoid this complication.

*Bowel perforation* is again a rare complication. It is more likely in cases of deeply infiltrating endometriosis (DIE) that distorts anatomy. This can go unnoticed at the time of oocyte retrieval only to present with peritonitis and sepsis later. Meticulous mapping of the ovaries before ovarian stimulation, establishing access to the ovaries through transvaginal route and rarely laparoscopic adhesiolysis to make them easily accessible are some of the recommended measures.

## Pregnancy Associated Complications

*Multiple pregnancies,* common with assisted conception increase the risk of maternal mortality, pregnancy induced hypertension, anemia, uterine atony, dystocia, increased operative deliveries, and postpartum hemorrhage.[16] Prematurity and low fetal growth restriction are common. Compared to spontaneously conceived twins, ART twin pregnancies have a higher risk of miscarriages, placenta praevia and vasa praevia though the risk of congenital anomalies is no different.[17] Monozygotic twins are more common after ART and have higher perinatal morbidity. Clearly the monitoring during such pregnancies is rigorous adding to the emotional and financial burden.

As mentioned earlier, minimal or mild stimulation IVF helps reduce the incidence of multiple births.[2,3] Another key strategy in preventing this is the adoption of *single embryo transfer.* Transfer of 2 embryos as against 3 is now accepted worldwide except in patients with repeat IVF failures or advanced maternal age. Recent data suggests that single embryo transfer with subsequent FET yields similar cumulative live birth rates as a double embryo transfer.[16] This should be the way forward but the additional cost of FET and couple preferences will have a bearing on this.

Another strategy is *multifetal reduction* that reduces triplet or higher order pregnancies to twins. These can be done in first or second trimester. First trimester reductions can be done early (8–10 weeks) or late (11–12 weeks). The latter are preferred to allow time for spontaneous reductions and performance of nuchal translucency (NT) for Down's screening. This procedure is associated with a miscarriage rate of 0.2–0.5% and additional risks such as anencephaly, limb amputation or the KCl (potassium chloride) causing retinal damage.[18] A recent paper suggests transvaginal intracardiac puncture till asystole without the use of KCl as a potentially safer option.[18]

*Ectopic and heterotopic pregnancies* are more common with ART pregnancies than spontaneous conceptions. Any risk factor for ectopic is also a risk factor for heterotopic pregnancy. The crucial difference between the two is that whereas an ectopic is easier to diagnose due to an empty uterine cavity raising suspicion, a heterotopic pregnancy is easily missed due to the false reassurance provided by the presence of an intrauterine pregnancy. A systematic review on heterotopic pregnancies by Talbot et al.[19] in 2011 found risk factors in 71% of their cases. These included previous PID, endometriosis, pelvic surgery, previous ectopic pregnancy and ART.

Risk reduction measures hence start with thorough history taking. *Hydrosalpinges* if present should be removed or clipped not only to avoid the efflux of tubal contents into the uterine cavity, jeopardizing implantation but also to decrease the risk of ectopic pregnancy. *Restricting the number of embryos to 2 or less* also decreases the risk. Some studies have suggested that *FET* decreases the risk of ectopic compared to a fresh transfer.[20,21] The rationale for this is that COH disturbs the endometrial receptivity and the very high estradiol levels could cause a reverse migratory process of the transferred embryos.[22] The site of embryo transfer, pressure used for pushing the embryos and the volume of culture medium used during transfer are additional factors influencing risk of ectopic pregnancy. It is suggested that the transfer catheter should not touch the fundus as it may generate uterine contractions, propelling the embryos into the tubes. A similar problem may occur with large volumes of culture media.[22] Gentle pressure to expel the embryos will reduce the risk of these migrating into the tubes.

A comprehensive systematic review by Palomba et al.[23] concluded that "subfertile women who conceived after the use of high technology infertility treatments are at *increased risk of pregnancy complications,* and every single step or procedure can play an independent and crucial role." Good preconception counseling, optimizing the woman's health prior to any treatment and meticulous antenatal care can go a long way in reducing these complications.

Most babies born after ART are healthy. There is a slightly higher risk for congenital anomalies in children born from ART.[24,25] ICSI is associated with a slightly higher risk of genetic diseases and imprinting disorders though the absolute risk is small. With improving pregnancy rates with FET there is a trend toward elective freezing of embryos. The genetic and epigenetic risks of embryo cryopreservation are still under investigation. So are the biopsy risks in preimplantation genetic diagnosis (PGD).[26] A recent meta-analysis has shown decreased risks of small for gestational age, low birth weight and preterm delivery but an increased risks of large for gestational age and high birth weights with FET.[27] The evidence on cognitive development and behavioral aberrations in children born from ART has been reassuring.[25]

A Cochrane review in 2013[28] found a slightly higher risk for borderline ovarian tumors in subfertile women treated with IVF but there was no convincing correlation with invasive ovarian tumors. A more recent Cochrane review[29] concluded that "exposure to clomiphene citrate as an ovary-stimulating drug in subfertile women is associated with increased risk of endometrial cancer, especially at doses greater than 2,000 mg and high (more than 7) number of cycles." However this was attributed to "the underlying risk factors in women who need treatment with clomiphene citrate, such as PCOS, rather than exposure to the drug itself."

Reducing these risks entails keeping abreast with the latest evidence and thorough counseling of the couple and choosing a treatment modality that has the best risk-benefit ratio.

## KEY POINTS

- OHSS is the most well-known complication of ART. Use of antagonist protocol, GnRHa as a trigger, elective freezing of embryos and use of dopamine receptor agonists are a few of the established measures to reduce this risk.
- Complications at oocyte retrieval can be minimized with thorough knowledge of pelvic anatomy and good ultrasound skills.
- Multiple pregnancies are a major burden of ART and steps must be taken to reduce these.
- Long-term follow up of children born after ART is overall reassuring but a close watch needs to be kept on emerging evidence.

## REFERENCES

1. Thessaloniki ESHRE/ASRM-Sponsored PCOS Consensus Workshop Group. Consensus on infertility treatment related to polycystic ovary syndrome. Hum Reprod. 2008;23:462-77.
2. Nargund G, Datta AK, Fauser BC. Mild stimulation for in vitro fertilization. Fertil Steril. 2017;108(4):558-67.
3. Zhang JJ, Merhi Z, Yang M, et al. Minimal stimulation IVF vs conventional IVF: a randomized controlled trial. Am J Obstet Gynecol. 2016;214(1):96.e1-8.
4. Tso LO, Costello MF, Albuquerque LE, et al. Metformin treatment before and during IVF or ICSI in women with polycystic ovary syndrome. Cochrane Database Syst Rev. 2014;(11):CD006105.
5. Al-Inany HG, Youssef MA, Aboulghar M, et al. Gonadotrophin-releasing hormone antagonists for assisted reproductive technology. Cochrane Database Syst Rev. 2011;5:CD001750.
6. Pundir J, Sunkara SK, El-Toukhy T, et al. Meta-analysis of GnRH antagonist protocols: do they reduce the risk of OHSS in PCOS? Reprod Biomed Online. 2012;24:6-22.
7. Wong KM, van Wely M, Mol F, et al. Fresh versus frozen embryo transfers in assisted reproduction. Cochrane Database Syst Rev. 2017;3:CD011184.
8. Kaur T, Pai P, Kumar P. Hematocrit as a simple method to predict and manage ovarian hyperstimulation syndrome in assisted reproduction. J Hum Reprod Sci. 2015;8(2):93-7.

9. Tang H, Mourad S, Zhai SD, et al. Dopamine agonists for preventing ovarian hyperstimulation syndrome. Cochrane Database Syst Rev. 2016;11:CD008605.
10. Youssef MA, Mourad S. Volume expanders for the prevention of ovarian hyperstimulation syndrome. Cochrane Database Syst Rev. 2016;(8):CD001302.
11. Varnagy A, Bodis J, Manfai Z, et al. Low-dose aspirin therapy to prevent ovarian hyperstimulation syndrome. Fertil Steril. 2009;93:2281-4.
12. Nelson SM. Prophylaxis of VTE in women during assisted reproductive techniques. Thromb Res. 2009;123(Suppl. 3):S8-S15.
13. RCOG. [2006]. RCOG Guideline No. 5—the Management of Ovarian Hyperstimulation Syndrome. [online] Available from https://www.rcog.org.uk/globalassets/documents/guidelines/gtg5_230611.pdf. [Accessed February, 2018].
14. Baron KT, Babagbemi KT, Arleo EK, et al. Emergent complications of assisted reproduction: expecting the unexpected. Radiographics. 2013;33(1):229-44.
15. Mashiach S, Bider D, Moran O, et al. Adnexal torsion of hyperstimulated ovaries in pregnancies after gonadotropin therapy. Fertil Steril. 1990;53(1):76-80.
16. Bhattacharya S, Kamath MS. Reducing multiple births in assisted reproduction technology. Best Pract Res Clin Obstet Gynaecol. 2014;28(2):191-9.
17. Jauniaux E, Ben-Ami I, Maymon R. Do assisted-reproduction twin pregnancies require additional antenatal care? Reprod Biomed Online. 2013;26(2):107-19.
18. Gunasheela D, Rao S, Jain G, et al. Outcomes of transvaginal multifetal pregnancy reduction without injecting potassium chloride. Int J Reprod Contracept Obstet Gynecol. 2017;6(1):182-9.
19. Talbot K, Simpson R, Price N, et al. Heterotopic pregnancy. J Obstet Gynaecol. 2011;31:7-12.
20. Muller V, Makhmadalieva M, Kogan I, et al. Ectopic pregnancy following in vitro fertilization: meta- analysis and single-center experience during 6 years. Gynecol Endocrinol. 2016;32(Suppl 2):69-74.
21. Huang B, Hu D, Qian K, et al. Is frozen embryo transfer cycle associated with a significantly lower incidence of ectopic pregnancy? An analysis of more than 30,000 cycles. Fertil Steril. 2014;102(5):1345-9.
22. Refaat B, Dalton E, Ledger WL. Ectopic pregnancy secondary to in vitro fertilisation-embryo transfer: pathogenic mechanisms and management strategies. Reprod Biol Endocrinol. 2015;13:30
23. Palomba S, Homburg R, Santagni S, et al. Risk of adverse pregnancy and perinatal outcomes after high technology infertility treatment: a comprehensive systematic review. Reprod Biol Endocrinol. 2016;14(1):76.
24. Giorgione V, Parazzini F, Fesslova V, et al. Congenital heart defects in IVF/ICSI pregnancy: systematic review and meta-analysis. Ultrasound Obstet Gynecol. 2018;51(1):33-42.
25. Bergh C, Wennerholm UB. Obstetric outcome and long-term follow up of children conceived through assisted reproduction. Best Pract Res Clin Obstet Gynaecol. 2012;26(6):841-52.
26. Jiang Z, Wang Y, Xin J, et al. Genetic and epigenetic risks of assisted reproduction. Best Best Pract Res Clin Obstet Gynaecol. 2017;44:90-104.

27. Maheshwari A, Pandey S, Amalraj Raja E, et al. Is frozen embryo transfer better for mothers and babies? Can cumulative meta-analysis provide a definitive answer? Hum Reprod Update. 2018;24(1):35-58.
28. Rizzuto I, Behrens RF, Smith LA. Risk of ovarian cancer in women treated with ovarian stimulating drugs for infertility. Cochrane Database Syst Rev. 2013;(8):CD008215.
29. Skalkidou A, Sergentanis TN, Gialamas SP, et al. Risk of endometrial cancer in women treated with ovary-stimulating drugs for subfertility. Cochrane Database Syst Rev. 2017;3:CD010931.

CHAPTER

# 19

# Assisted Reproductive Technology in Elderly Women: Risks and Outcome

*Soma Singh, Astha Chakravarty, Indranil Saha*

## ■ INTRODUCTION

Globally there is an increasing population of women seeking assisted reproductive technology (ART) treatment due to age-related infertility. With increasing age, there is a decline in woman's fertility. Most women reach menopause by their early fifties, but biological infertility occurs about 10–12 years before menopause. However, there is no universal definition of an advanced reproductive age for women, in part because the effects of increasing age occur as a continuum rather than as a threshold effect, and declining fertility is an individual event that differs in each woman.

There are already existing recommendations [(NICE, 2004; American Society for Reproductive Medicine (ASRM), 2006a)] that women over 35 should be classed as having advanced reproductive age and referred more promptly for early investigations and active treatment. Since there is no consensus about "how old is too old" for ART, in this article we will consider women and men more than 40 years of age as "elderly" and discuss the risks and outcome of ART treatment in this group.

## ■ WHY THERE IS INCREASING NEED FOR ART IN ELDERLY?

Loss of fertility with female aging is the main reason for ART in elderly. The different mechanisms postulated to be responsible for such loss include:

### Decreasing Ovarian Reserve

The loss of oocytes from the ovaries is a continual process that begins in utero. Earlier research suggested that a more accelerated process of decline occurs in the last 10–15 years before menopause, beginning around the age of 38 years.[2] However, more recent data suggest that oocyte loss occurs at the same rate through the reproductive lifetime, with the slope of decline remaining fairly consistent until menopause.[3]

## Poor Oocyte Quality

The main cause of infertility is diminishing oocyte quality with age. Studies on in vitro fertilization (IVF) oocytes have shown that the rate of oocyte aneuploidy increases with age.

The rate is low in women less than age 35 (10%), but increases to 30% at the age of 40, to 40% at the age of 43, and to 100% in women more than age 45.[4] This correlates with the increase in chromosomally abnormal pregnancies and spontaneous abortions with age.

The decline in oocyte quality may be in the formation and function of the spindles, which appears to be more diffuse.[5] This may result in chromosomes being less tightly arranged and may therefore lead to meiotic errors. Other proposed mechanisms include cumulative damage to the oocyte with age and decreasing quality of granulosa cells.[6]

## Lower Embryo Implantation

According to the study done by US Society for Assisted Reproductive technology (SART) on 27,959 fresh donor oocyte IVF cycles, the implantation rate declines after the age of 44.[7] Age however does not affect the endometrium's response to hormonal stimulation. The uterine endometrium has the capacity to maintain a pregnancy throughout a woman's reproductive years and, with newer technologies such as egg donation, even beyond the natural reproductive years.[8]

## Altered Hormonal Environment

Altered hormonal environment resulting in ovulatory dysfunction.[9]

## Uterine Problems

One of the causes for lower fertility in elderly are reduced blood supply to endometrium and increased fibroid and/or endometriosis in older women.[10,11]

## Others

Other possible causes of unexplained infertility in older women can be lifestyle factors such as increase in BMI, decreased coital frequency, smoking and stress. However, women can be counseled about these causes and with life-style modifications the situation can change.

## ■ EFFECT OF AGING ON MALE FERTILITY

Although aging has adverse effects on male reproductive function, the impact of age is less obvious than it is in women. Semen quality and male fertility as well as androgen production and serum testosterone levels decrease very gradually as age increases.

# Assisted Reproductive Technology in Elderly Women: Risks and Outcome

- Semen volume, sperm motility, and the proportion of morphologically normal sperm, but not sperm concentration, decrease gradually as age increases.[12]
- The available evidence indicates that pregnancy rates decrease and time to conception increases as male age increases.[12]
- Increased paternal age has been associated with an increase in numerical and structural chromosomal abnormalities, with increased DNA fragmentation and higher frequency of point mutation.[2]

**Why Preconception Counseling is needed before ART in Elderly Population?**

Assisted reproductive technology is regarded as panacea for perimenopausal women seeking motherhood late in their reproductive lives. But even ART cannot make up for the reduction in fecundity by more than 30–50% associated with advanced age and the procedure has some inherent risks. Therefore preconception counseling regarding the risks of pregnancy with advanced maternal age, promotion of optimal health and weight, and screening for concurrent medical conditions such as hypertension and diabetes should be considered for women.

In addition to a medical screening, an extensive psychological evaluation is necessary to elucidate any potential deficiencies in the patient's mental capacity and any psychosocial adversity that may be harmful to the child.

The option of using a donor gamete especially egg should be discussed with them. The success rate and the risk of birth defects should be explained to them. Men more than age of 40 years and their partners who are seeking pregnancy should be counseled about the potential risks of abortion and autosomal dominant disease, although the risks remain small.

## ■ WHAT IS THE OUTCOME OF ART IN ELDERLY?

Age is perhaps the most important single variable influencing outcome in assisted reproduction. Success rates for ART treatment for women using their own eggs are directly linked to the age of the women and many women may not realize that older women are successful using ART to achieve pregnancy later in life only with donor eggs.

### Cycle Cancellation Rate

According to Centers for Disease Control and Prevention (CDC) ART report 2015, Percentage of cancellations for women using their own egg, before retrieval were 12.2% for women less than 35 years and 15.7% for women between 40 years and 42 years. Not surprisingly, 40% of self-cycles get cancelled in women more than 44 years.

### Clinical Pregnancy Rate

According to Human Fertilization and Embryology Authority (HFEA) 2014, clinical pregnancy rates (CPR) per fresh embryo transfer is around 43.7% for the age group 18–34 years. In sharp contrast, the clinical pregnancy rate for women of 40–42 years is only 21.3% and in women more than 42 years, CPR per fresh embryo transfer is only 9.4%. According to US National Summary of IVF for 2015, the pregnancy rate per transfer in women less than 35 years has been reported to be 57.8% and in women more than 40 years is 26.9%.

## Implantation Rate

Older women undergoing IVF demonstrate not only a diminished response to ovarian stimulation but also decreased implantation efficiency, the impaired implantation rates appear to be independent of the magnitude of ovarian response.[13]

The largest study to date examining the relationship between recipient age and pregnancy outcomes was published by Jason S et al.[7] and used SART data from 2008 to 2010. In an analysis of 27,959 fresh donor oocyte IVF cycles, recipients were segregated into five age cohorts: ≤34, 35 to 39, 40 to 44, 45 to 49, and ≥50 years. Cycles with recipient age ≤34 years reported an implantation rate of 46.5%, the highest among the entire study population. Values trended downward with increasing age, and the lowest implantation rate of 40.9% was reported by cycles with recipients aged ≥50 years old.

## Live Birth Rates

Live birth rates for IVF cycles in US in 2015 were 47.7% in women less than 35 years and 15% in women more than 40 years. The 2007 Canadian live birth rate after IVF was 37.4% for women less than 35 years of age, 26.5% for women aged 35–39 years, and 11.4% for women aged more than or equal to 40 years. So it is evident that live birth rate reduces with advancing age.

### Live Birth Rates with Donor

In the biggest study by Jason S[7] with donor-eggs, Live-birth rates were highest (56.7%) in the group less than or equal to 34 years and lowest in the oldest group at 56.7% for age 45–49 years and 48.6% in recipients of age more than or equal to 50. According to authors the live birth rates decreases after age of 44.

## Miscarriage Rate

The incidence of clinically recognized spontaneous miscarriage rises as age advances. Spontaneous miscarriage rates in natural conception cycles are generally low before age 30 (7–15%) and then rise only slightly for ages 30–34 (8–21%), but to a greater extent for ages 35–39 (17–28%) and ages 40 and older (34–52%).[14] The same pattern is observed in pregnancies resulting from ART. In the 2007, US National Summary of IVF outcomes, spontaneous miscarriage rates were less than 15% for women younger than age 35, approximately 30% at age 40, and greater than 50% for women age 44 and older. In study on donor

IVF cycles, a miscarriage rate of 16% was seen in the recipient of less than or equal to 34 years and 19% in more than or equal to 50 years.[7]

**Do available ovarian reserve tests (AFC, AMH, FSH) predict the outcome of ART in elderly?**

Ovarian reserve tests like antral follicular count (AFC), anti-Mullerian hormone (AMH) and follicle-stimulating hormone (FSH) performed before starting ART treatment may be useful for counseling, but they have a poor predictive power for egg quality and pregnancy.[15] Therefore, these tests should not be used to exclude women from ART treatment, and abnormal tests do not preclude the possibility of pregnancy.

## ■ HOW CAN WE IMPROVE THE OUTCOME OF ART IN ELDERLY?

### High-dose Gonadotropins

It is generally believed that the dose of gonadotropins should be adjusted upward in an attempt to overcome the age-related decline in ovarian response to FSH stimulation. A common starting dose would be at least 300 IU/day. Nevertheless, further dose increments are of limited effectiveness, and clinically meaningful improvements are only rarely obtained with doses less than 300 IU/day.[16]

### Role of Androgens/Dehydroepiandrosterone

A meta-analysis of controlled trials of androgen adjuvants, such as testosterone and dehydroepiandrosterone (DHEA), and androgen-modulating agents, such as letrozole, showed no significant difference in the number of oocytes retrieved or pregnancy/live birth rates with androgen supplementation or modulation compared with controls. The author further concluded that the current level of evidence on the effectiveness of DHEA is rather low and does not support its routine use in poor responders.[17]

### Use of Growth hormone

An updated meta-analysis focusing on use of human growth hormone (hGH) cotreatment in poor responders has shown that hGH addition increases the probability of clinical pregnancy and live birth.[18] However, it was mentioned that the total number of patients analyzed was small, and thus further randomized controlled trials (RCTs) are warranted to prove or disprove this finding. There is currently no well-established clinical role for adjuvant hGH in the treatment of poor responders. Further studies should be directed at defining the dose of hGH and determining if select populations may benefit from hGH cotreatment.

## Assisted Hatching

It is proposed that there may be a spontaneous zona hardening due to age-related endocrine changes and/or the absence of lysins from surrounding tissues, which may act on embryos in vivo.[19] A meta-analysis examining data from five RCTs (561 patients) revealed a 73% improvement in clinical pregnancy rate when assisted hatching was employed in individuals with recurrent implantation failure (RIF).[20] Unselected patients, however, do not seem to experience the same benefit.

## Preimplantation Genetic Screening

The main goal of preimplantation genetic screening (PGS), which is the biopsy of one or more cells from a preimplantation embryo followed by the ploidy analysis of these cells and finally transfer of those embryos deemed to be euploid.

The rationale for PGS results from a combination of—(1) an increasing number of aneuploidies in clinical miscarriages of women of advanced maternal age; (2) the fact that aneuploidies are also found in preimplantation embryos of these women after IVF. Biopsy is done at the blastocyst stage of development, following the assumption that this is less detrimental to the embryo and that this avoids the negative effect of mosaicism on efficacy. Ploidy status is now determined using CGH arrays and SNP arrays, allowing the analysis of all chromosomes. Blastocyst-based PGS has been suggested to improve the efficiency of IVF in older individuals (>40 years of age) undergoing IVF.[22] Another retrospective study claimed a benefit in implantations and live births when PGS was used in women aged 40–43 years with multiple prior IVF failures, with a live birth rate for PGS frozen embryo transfer (45.5%) being significantly greater than for fresh transfer without PGS (15.8%) or frozen transfer of non-PGS embryos (19.0%).[23]

## Number of Embryos to be Transferred

According to the latest ASRM Committee opinion, patients 41–42 years of age should plan to receive no more than four cleavage-stage embryos or three blastocysts. In cases where euploid embryos are available, a single-blastocyst transfer should be the norm.[21] In women more than 43 years of age, there are insufficient data to recommend a limit on the number of embryos to transfer when the patient uses her own oocytes. According to NICE Guidelines 2013, for women aged 40–42 years consider double embryo transfer. But where a top quality blastocyst is available, use single embryo transfer. Caution should be exercised as the risk associated with multiple pregnancy increases dramatically with advancing maternal age. In donor-oocyte cycles, the age of the donor should be used to determine the appropriate number of embryos to transfer.

## Assisted Reproductive Technology in Elderly Women: Risks and Outcome

**Is there any role of COH and IUI in elderly women?**

A small study of 130 cycles of COH with gonadotropins and IUI found a live birth rate of 6% for women aged 38 to 39, and only 2% for women more than 40. All live births happened within the first or second cycles. Older women may consider 1–2 cycles of COH if they do not want to try IVF as a first-line treatment, but they should move on to IVF quickly if they are unsuccessful within the first couple of cycles.

## ■ WHAT ARE THE RISKS OF ART IN ELDERLY?

### Obstetrics Complications

In vitro fertilization pregnancies as such are associated with significantly higher odds of perinatal mortality, preterm delivery and small for gestational age and the risk increases with age. Pregnancy in advanced age (>40 years) is associated with higher maternal and fetal morbidities.[24] Elderly women are at increased risk of pregnancy-induced hypertension (PIH) and gestational diabetes mellitus (GDM).

Donor oocyte pregnancy acts as an independent risk factor for pregnancy complications, including hypertensive disorders, small for gestational age, cesarean section and preterm delivery.[25]

### Risk of Aneuploidy

As already mentioned before in the chapter, the prevalence of aneuploid oocytes increases progressively after the age of 35 years. Sperm aneuploidy also rises with paternal aging but the risk is small, i.e. 1–2%. There is increased proportion of embryos likely to be aneuploid and there is a possibility that all embryos will be aneuploid, leaving no embryo for transfer. Trisomies are by far the most common abnormality observed, followed in incidence by polyploidies and monosomy X (45,X).[2] Discussing these data at the outset will help set reasonable expectations and allow for quick movement onto the next cycle or other forms of treatment if there is a failure.

### Risk of Miscarriage

As already discussed before in the chapter, women of advanced age group have higher miscarriage rates whether they use their own oocytes or donor oocytes.

### Congenital Birth Defect/Possible Deleterious Effects of ART Itself

Conflicting data exists about the risks of IVF on the developing embryo. Despite this controversy, there is a general consensus that IVF confers a small but measurable increased risk for a variety of congenital abnormalities including anatomic abnormalities and imprinting errors as compared to the general population.[26]

A number of studies have observed that advanced paternal age is associated with an increase in the prevalence of birth defects (e.g. neural tube defects, cardiac defects and limb defects) and congenital disease (e.g. Wilms tumor).[2] Advanced paternal age is associated with an increased in de novo mutations causing autosomal dominant diseases (Waardenburg, Crouzon, achondroplasia and Alpert) and X-linked diseases (hemophilia A and Duchenne muscular dystrophy). The absolute risk of these diseases is still very small (<1%) because these diseases are rare.[2]

**What Ethical Considerations Should We Take to Avoid Unnecessary Risk and Poor Outcome of ART in Elderly?**

### Using Own Eggs

Infertility treatment in the perimenopausal woman raises many ethical questions. What constitutes poor prognosis or futile treatment? If a woman can afford treatment that is associated with less than 5% chances of success, should it be offered? The answers to these questions are provided by the Ethics Committee of the ASRM, 2004. Futility was defined as a 0 or 1% or less chance of achieving a live birth, while "very poor prognosis" was used to describe very low but not nonexistent odds of achieving a live birth (>1% but about <5% per cycle). According to the ethical committee, in case of very poor prognosis it is ethical to treat, if the patient is fully informed of the prognosis and still wants to proceed. However, physicians may ethically refuse to accept or provide further treatment to patients with very poor prognosis provided that they follow evidence-based policies and the rules of their fertility centers.

### Using Donor Eggs

With the use of donor eggs, women 50 years of age and older are able to conceive with ART, so one should be diligent in screening older women for IVF because unfortunate cases in which older donor egg recipients die before their offspring reach adulthood will likely continue to stir ethical debates. Before giving ART to a couple of advanced reproductive age, special consideration needs to be given to the potential child so it is likely that at least one parent or contingent legal guardian will be available and responsible for the child until that child reaches adulthood.

## ■ FINANCIAL AND SOCIAL SUPPORT SYSTEM

Childbearing and childrearing are both long periods of emotional stress, which combined with the degenerative aging of a person's physical and mental health, can be detrimental to a child's welfare. Women of advanced reproductive age who seek infertility treatment may have a poor social support system. Given their age, many may not have family who can assist them, especially if they are seeking to have a first child. Thus, it is essential to identify potential caretakers and ensure that the patient has a support system of caretakers during the child's younger years.

## KEY POINTS

- Elderly couple going for ART should be informed that the risk of spontaneous pregnancy loss and chromosomal abnormalities increases with age. They should be well counseled and offered appropriate prenatal screening once pregnancy is established.
- No fertility treatment, with the exception of oocyte donation, has been associated with a live birth rate of more than 15% in perimenopausal women but this is not an option in many parts of the world, and efforts must be made to maximize each patient's potential to use her own oocytes.
- The concepts of futility and very poor prognosis of treatment must be entertained in every case, before a decision to treat is made while respecting patient autonomy.
- There is a need for large-scale randomized controlled trials (RCTs) to test the efficacy of interventions such as androgens and hGH supplementation to improve the outcome in women of advanced age group.
- If a sufficient number of oocytes and embryos can be obtained, aneuploidy screening by PGS could be considered.

## REFERENCES

1. Human Fertilization and Embryo Authority. The patients' guide to DI and IVF clinic. London: Human Fertilization and Embryo Authority; 1996.
2. Speroff L, Fritz MA. Clinical gynaecologic endocrinology and infertility, 8th edition. Philadelphia: Lippincott Williams and Wilkins; 2011.
3. Hansen KR, Knowlton NS, Thyer AC, et al. A new model of reproductive aging: the decline in ovarian non-growing follicle number from birth to menopause. Hum Reprod. 2008;23:699-708.
4. Pellestor F, Andreo B, Arnal F, et al. Maternal aging and chromosomal abnormalities: new data drawn from in vitro unfertilized human oocytes. Hum Genet. 2003;112:195.
5. Volarcik K, Sheean L, Goldfarb J, et al. The meiotic competence of in-vitro matured human oocytes is influenced by donor age: evidence that folliculogenesis is compromised in the reproductively aged ovary. Hum Reprod. 1998;13:154-60.
6. Warburton D. Biological aging and the etiology of aneuploidy. Cytogenet Genome Res. 2005;111(3-4):266-72.
7. Yeh JS, Steward RS, Dude M, et al. Pregnancy outcomes decline in recipients over age 44: an analysis of 27,959 fresh donor oocyte in vitro fertilization cycles from the Society for Assisted Reproductive Technology. Fertil Steril. 2014;101(5):1331-1336.e1.
8. Noci I, Borri P, Chieffi O, et al. I. Aging of the human endometrium: a basic morphological and immunohistochemical study. Eur J Obstet Gynecol Reprod Biol. 1995;63:181-5.

9. Hull MG, Fleming CF, Hughes AO, et al. The age-related decline in female fecundity: a quantitative controlled study of implanting capacity and survival of individual embryos after in vitro fertilization. Fertil Steril. 1996;65:783-90.
10. Huang LS, Lee MS, Cheng EH, et al. Recipient age and pulsatility index affect uterine receptivity in oocyte donation programmes. Reprod Biomed Online. 2008;17:94-100.
11. Ron-El R, Raziel A, Strassburger D, et al. Outcome of assisted reproductive technology in women over the age of 41. Fertil Steril. 2000;74:471-5.
12. Kidd SA, Eskenazi B, Wyrobek AJ. Effects of male age on semen quality and fertility: a review of the literature. Fertil Steril. 2001;75:237.
13. Zev Rosenwaks, Davis OK, Damario MA. The role of maternal age in assisted reproduction. Hum Reprod. 1995;10:165-73.
14. Hull MG, Fleming CF, Hughes AO, et al. The age-related decline in female fecundity: a quantitative controlled study of implanting capacity and survival of individual embryos after in vitro fertilization. Fertil Steril. 1996;65:783.
15. Broekmans FJ, Soules MR, Fauser BC. Ovarian aging: mechanisms and clinical consequences. Endocr Rev. 2009;30:465-93.
16. Weissman A, Howles CM, SK Sunkara. Treatment strategies in assisted reproduction for the poor-responder patient. In: Gardner's Textbook of Assisted Reproductive Techniques: Clinical perspectives, 5th edition. Boca Raton: CRC Press; 2017.
17. Sunkara SK, Coomarasamy A, Arlt W, et al. Should androgen supplementation be used for poor ovarian response in IVF? Hum Reprod. 2012;3:637-40.
18. Duffy JM, Ahmad G, Mohiyiddeen L, et al. Growth hormone for in vitro fertilization. Cochrane Database Syst Rev. 2010.
19. Tucker MJ, Morton PC, Wright G, et al. Enhancement of outcome from intracytoplasmic sperm injection: does coculture or assisted hatching improve implantation rates? Hum Reprod. 1996;11:2434-7.
20. Martins WP, Rocha IA, Ferriani RA, et al. Assisted hatching of human embryos: a systematic review and meta-analysis of randomized controlled trials. Hum Reprod Update. 2011;17:438-53.
21. Practice Committee of the American Society for reproductive Medicine. Guidance on the limits to the number of embryos to transfer: a committee opinion. Fertil Steril. 2017;107:901-3.
22. Fragouli E, Katz-Jaffe M, Alfarawati S, et al. Comprehensive chromosome screening of polar bodies and blastocysts from couples experiencing repeated implantation failure. Fertil Steril. 2010;94:875-87.
23. Lee HL, et al. In vitro fertilization with preimplantation genetic screening improves implantation and live birth in women age 40 through 43. J Assist Reprod Genet. 2015;32:435-44.
24. Nabukera S, Wingate MS, Alexander GR, et al. First time births among women 30 years and older in the United States: patterns and risk of adverse outcomes. Reprod Med. 2006;51:676-82.
25. Jeve YB, Potdar N, Opuku A, et al. Donor oocyte conception and pregnancy complications: a systematic review and meta-analysis. BJOG. 2016:235(9):1471-80.
26. Fortunato A, Tosti E. The impact of in vitro fertilization on health of the children: an update. Eur J Obstet Gynecol Reprod Biol. 2011;154(2):125-9.

# CHAPTER 20

# OHSS and Its Management

*Anuradha Chaudhary*

## ■ INTRODUCTION

Ovarian hyperstimulation syndrome (OHSS) is an uncommon but serious complication associated with assisted reproductive technology (ART). Though data about true incidence is lacking but moderate to severe OHSS occurs in approximate 1–5% of cycles. Among high-risk women, the incidence approaches 20%. It occurs almost exclusively during ART cycle, although OHSS might also occur during ovarian stimulation using clomiphene citrate and even in a spontaneous pregnancy. This condition is self-limiting and in patients, who do not conceive, typically resolves at the time of next menstrual period. In patients who do become pregnant, rising human chorionic gonadotropin (hCG) level continue to stimulate the ovaries and symptoms may extend through the end of the first trimester.

## ■ PATHOPHYSIOLOGY

Classic physiology of OHSS includes arteriolar vasodilation and an increase in capillary permeability that result in fluid shifting from intravascular to extravascular spaces. This fluid shift results in a state of hypovolemic hyponatremia. Vascular endothelial growth factor appears to be integral to the development of this condition and is involved in follicular growth, corpus luteum function, angiogenesis and vascular endothelial stimulation. In response to hCG, vascular endothelial growth factor (VEGF) appears to mediate the vascular permeability[1] of OHSS, as systemic hCG level positively correlate with severity of the disease. Other systemic and local vasoactive substances include interleukin-6 (IL-6), IL-1β, insulin-like growth factor 1, transforming growth factor β, angiotensin II are directly and indirectly involved in the pathogenesis of OHSS symptoms.

Symptoms are often qualified by their severity (mild, moderate, or severe) and by the timing of onset (early and late). OHSS represented by early and late as described by Lyons et al. Early OHSS (within 9 days of retrieval) is the most iatrogenic and can be predicted by history [young age, polycystic ovary syndrome (PCOS),[2] in vitro fertilization (IVF) for male or mechanical factors]. OHSS can also be predicted by the follicular response to gonadotropins and the level of serum E2 on the day of ovulation triggering.[3]

High-risk patients should be identified and preventive measures should be taken.

## ■ CLASSIFICATION OF OHSS SYMPTOMS

The classification of OHSS symptoms is described in Table 1.

## ■ MANAGEMENT

**Table 1:** Classification of OHSS symptoms

| OHSS stage | Clinical features | Laboratory features |
|---|---|---|
| Mild | Abdominal distension/discomfort | No important alterations |
| | Mild nausea/vomiting | |
| | Mild dyspnea | |
| | Diarrhea | |
| | Enlarged ovaries | |
| Moderate | Mild feature | Hemoconcentration (Hct >41%) |
| | Ultrasonographic evidence of ascites | Elevated WBC (>15,000 mL) |
| Severe | Mild and moderate feature | Severe hemoconcentration (Hct >55%) |
| | Clinical evidence of ascites | WBC >25,000 mL |
| | Hydrothorax | CrCl <50 mL/min |
| | Severe dyspnea | Cr >1.6 mg/dL |
| | Oliguria/anuria | Na$^+$ <1,235 mEq/L |
| | Intractable nausea /vomiting | K$^+$ >5 mEq/L |
| | | Elevated liver enzymes |
| | Low blood/ central venous pressure | |
| | Pleural effusion | |
| | Rapid weight gain (>1 kg in 24 hr) | |
| | Syncope | |
| | Severe abdominal pain | |
| | Venous thromboembolism | |

*Contd...*

*Contd...*

| OHSS stage | Clinical features | Laboratory features |
|---|---|---|
| Critical | Anuria/acute renal failure | Worsening finding |
| | Arrhythmia | |
| | Thromboembolism | |
| | Pericardial effusion | |
| | Massive hydrothorax | |
| | Arterial thrombosis | |
| | Adult respiratory distress syndrome | |
| | Sepsis | |

Symptomatic moderate or severe OHSS is a hypovolemic hyponatremic state. It usually involves fluid replacement to maintain intravascular perfusion and supportive care. Prophylactic anticoagulant is warranted in case of severe OHSS from the time of diagnosis through the first trimester of pregnancy. Both volume expander and paracentesis or culdocentesis for the management of OHSS in an outpatient setting (severe) are recommended.

## ■ OBSTETRIC OUTCOME AFTER OHSS

The obstetric outcome after OHSS is controversial.[4] OHSS would predispose to more frequent adverse pregnancy outcomes like miscarriages, pregnancy-induced hypertension (PIH), gestational diabetes mellitus (GDM) and low birth weight.[5-9]

## ■ PREVENTIVE MEASURES

- Evidence that PCOS, elevated AMH values, peak estradiol levels, multifollicular development and a high number of oocytes retrieved increase the risk of OHSS.
- Cut-off points are AMH values >3.4 ng/mL, AFC >24, development of ≥25 follicles. Estradiol value > 3,500 pg/mL or ≥ 24 oocytes retrieved are particularly associated with an increased risk of OHSS.
- Evidence supports the use of ovarian stimulation protocols using GnRH antagonists in order to reduce the risk of OHSS.
- There is insufficient evidence that clomiphene independently reduces OHSS risk.
- Aspirin reduces the incidence of OHSS.
- Metformin decreases the risk of OHSS in PCOS patient.
- Insufficient evidence to recommend coasting for the prevention of OHSS.
- Use of a GnRH agonist to trigger oocyte maturation prior to oocyte retrieval in order to reduce the risk of OHSS.
- Live-birth rates are lower in fresh autologous cycles after GnRH trigger, but not donor-recipient cycles.

- Reproductive outcomes are improved when a low dose of hCG is coadministered at the time of GnRH agonist trigger for luteal support.
- Dopamine agonist administration starting at the time of hCG trigger for several days reduce the incidence of OHSS.
- IV calcium infusion lower OHSS risk (10 mL of 10% calcium gluconate in 200 mL of normal saline is to be infused on the day of oocyte retrieval and day 1, 2, 3 after retrieval).
- Cryopreservation prevents OHSS.

## CONCLUSION

- Women at risk for OHSS should be identified prior to stimulation and protocol should be individualized to minimize the risk for OHSS (Antagonist cycle).
- Use GnRH agonist as a trigger.
- Use of cabergoline and cryopreservation of all embryos rather than transfer.

This segmentation model should be followed to make OHSS free Clinic. If preventive strategies are not effective and patient experiences severe OHSS, fluid resuscitation, supportive care, paracentesis and prophylactic anticoagulant are recommended.

The condition is self-limiting and in patients who do not conceived typically resolves at the time of next menstruation period. In patients who do become pregnant, rising hCG level continue to stimulate the ovaries and symptoms may extend through the end of the first trimester.

## REFERENCES

1. Goldsman MP, Pedram A, Dominguez CE, Ciuffardi I, Levin E, Asch RH. Increased capillary permeability induced by human follicular fluid: a hypothesis for an ovarian origin of the hyperstimulation syndrome. Fertil Steril. 1995;63:268-72.
2. Luke B, Brown MB, Morbeck DE, et al. Factors associated with ovarian hyperstimulation syndrome (OHSS) and its effect on assisted reproductive technology (ART) treatment and outcome. Fertil Steril. 2010;94:1399-404.
3. Kahnberg A, Enskog A, Brannstrom M, et al. Prediction of ovarian hyperstimulation syndrome in women undergoing in vitro fertilization. Acta Obstet Gynecol Scand. 2009;88:1373-81.
4. Geva E, Jaffe RB. Role of vascular endothelial growth factor in ovarian physiology and pathology. Fertil Steril. 2000;74:429-38.
5. Neulen J, Yan Z, Raczek S, et al. Human chorionic gonadotropin-dependent expression of vascular endothelial growth factor/vascular permeability factor in human granulosa cells: importance in ovarian hyperstimulation syndrome. J Clin Endocrinol Metab. 1995;80:1967-71.
6. Whelan JG 3rd, Vlahos NF. The ovarian hyperstimulation syndrome. Fertil Steril. 2000;73:883-96.

7. Delbaere A, Bergmann PJM, Gervy-Decoster C, et al. Increased angiotensin II in ascites during severe ovarian hyperstimulation syndrome: role of early pregnancy and ovarian gonadotropin stimulation. Fertil Steril. 1997;67:1038-45.
8. Johnson MD, Williams SL, Seager CK, et al. Relationship between human chorionic gonadotropin serum levels and the risk of ovarian hyperstimulation syndrome. Gynecol Endocrinol. 2014;30:294-7.
9. Bergh PA, Navot D. Ovarian hyperstimulation syndrome: a review of pathophysiology. J Assist Reprod Genet. 1992; 9:429-38

CHAPTER 21

# AMH-based Stimulation Protocols: Can it Prevent OHSS and Predict ART Outcome

*V Radha, N Sanjeeva Reddy*

## ■ INTRODUCTION

Anti-Müllerian hormone (AMH) is a member of transforming growth factor β superfamily. It is also called Müllerian inhibiting substance. It is secreted by granulosa cells of preantral and small antral follicles.

AMH acts by suppressing the cyclic recruitment of primordial follicles into the pool of growing follicles. It is an accurate and an early marker of ovarian aging. It starts declining after 30 years unlike follicle-stimulating hormone (FSH) which starts increasing only after 35 years. So AMH is a better marker of ovarian reserve.[1] It is established that serum AMH has significantly higher intercycle reproducibility when compared to other markers.

In assisted reproductive technology (ART), the response to ovarian stimulation to gonadotropins is variable in the same age groups. The risk of poor response and cycle cancellation is an unpleasant situation to both the patient and clinician. The risk of hyper-response and ovarian hyperstimulation syndrome (OHSS) is another fatal iatrogenic complication of ART, so identification of these patients potential to extremes of response is of great clinical value. The main objective of individualization of treatment in ART is to offer every woman the best treatment tailored to her characteristics. This can maximize the chance of pregnancy and eliminate the iatrogenic complications of controlled ovarian hyperstimulation (COH).

The initial step to personalize the treatment is to predict the response based on age, ovarian reserve markers, body mass index (BMI), features suggestive of polycystic ovarian syndrome (PCOS), previous response to stimulation and previous ovarian surgery and decide the stimulation protocol.[2]

## ■ AMH ASSAY

There has been an evolution in AMH assay from Diagnostic Systems Laboratory (DSL) and Immunotech Beckman Coulter (IBC) to Generation II assay and automated assays. The Gen II assay retains the cross species specificity of DSL and is calibrated to IBC assay. The values calculated with DSL assay can be converted to IBC assay by multiplying by 1.39,[3] the conversion factor for AMH is 1 ng/mL = 7.143 pmol/L. There are not many studies with the automated assay method.

## Poor Responders

According to Bologna criteria, to define poor response in IVF, at least 2 of the 3 features must be present—(1) advanced maternal age or any of the risk factor for poor ovarian response (POR), (2) previous POR, (3) abnormal ORT.[4]

The cut-off values vary with each assay method. Studies with older assay methods take the cut-off value as <1 ng/mL. With AMH Gen II assay the cut-off value is taken as 1.25 ng/mL.[5]

The cut-off value of AMH for predicting poor response to gonadotropin stimulation have been reviewed (Table 1).

## Hyper-responders

The criteria for hyper-responders based on oocytes retrieved vary with various authors from 15 to >20 following standard COH protocol. The prevalence rate in ART cycles is around 7% and is more in younger age group of <30 years. This helps in predicting the hyper-responders to COH as it is the main risk factor for OHSS.

Seifer et al. demonstrated that a high AMH level was associated with more number of oocytes retrieved. So basal AMH and antral follicle count (AFC) are good tools for counseling the patients.[8] However accurate assessment of AFC depends on the clinician's expertise, technical properties of the ultrasound machine used, inter cycle and inter observer variability. In contrast, AMH levels are obtained in the laboratory by objective measurements and are free from intra- and interobserver variability.

## Significance of AMH Levels Prior to ART (Fig. 1)[9]

Various studies support "AMH tailored protocol". In patients with AMH ≥ 1.26 ng/mL, the starting dose of gonadotropins is 150 IU, with AMH < 0.5 ng/mL, it

**Table 1:** Anti-Mullerian hormone (AMH) cut-off values for poor response.

| References (et al.) | Study design | N | Cut-off value (ng/mL) | Sensitivity % | Specificity % | AMH assay |
|---|---|---|---|---|---|---|
| Arce (2013)[6] | Retros* | 759 | 1.68 | 92 | 83 | AMH GenII |
| Polyzos (2013)[7] | Retros* | 210 | 1.37 | 74.1 | 77.5 | AMH GenII |
| Radha et al.[5] | Prosp** | 246 | 1.25 | 91.2 | 94.1 | AMH GenII |

(*Retrospective, **Prospective)

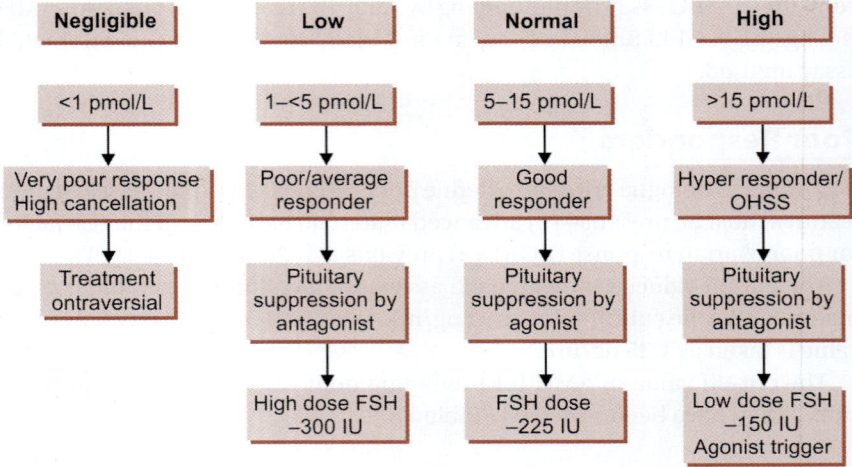

**Fig. 1:** Importance of anti-Müllerian hormone (AMH) levels prior to assisted reproductive technology (ART).[9]
(*1 ng/mL = 7.143 pmol/L)

is 375 ng/mL and they are counseled about the poor response irrespective of age.[10] AMH ≥0.5 ng/mL and ≤1.26 ng/mL, the starting dose is 300 IU. In women with AMH >6 ng/mL, the risk of OHSS is high, so the starting dose is 100 IU.

## Prediction of Ovarian Response based on AMH and AFC (Fig. 2)[11]

Ovarian reserve testing before the first ART cycle would permit to categorize patients as expected poor, normal or hyper-responders. Hence, the first-line protocol would be based on administration of low doses of FSH in a GnRH-antagonist-based scheme.[12]

## Modeling of Controlled Ovarian Stimulation based on Ovarian Reserve Markers (Fig. 3)[12,13]

Models have been used for the daily dose of gonadotropins which is tailored according to the pretreatment AMH levels independent of age and other characteristics of the patient. These have helped in adjusting the dose of gonadotropins and reduce the risk of OHSS.

It has also increased the pregnancy and live birth rates significantly.[13] The only limitation of these models is they were based on old DSL assay method and the value generated by the current AMH Gen II assay is 40% higher than old DSL method.[3]

There are nomograms for calculation of the starting dose of FSH based on age, serum AMH and FSH levels.[14] In this AMH was measured with IBS assay (Fig. 4).

# AMH-based Stimulation Protocols: Can it Prevent OHSS and Predict ART

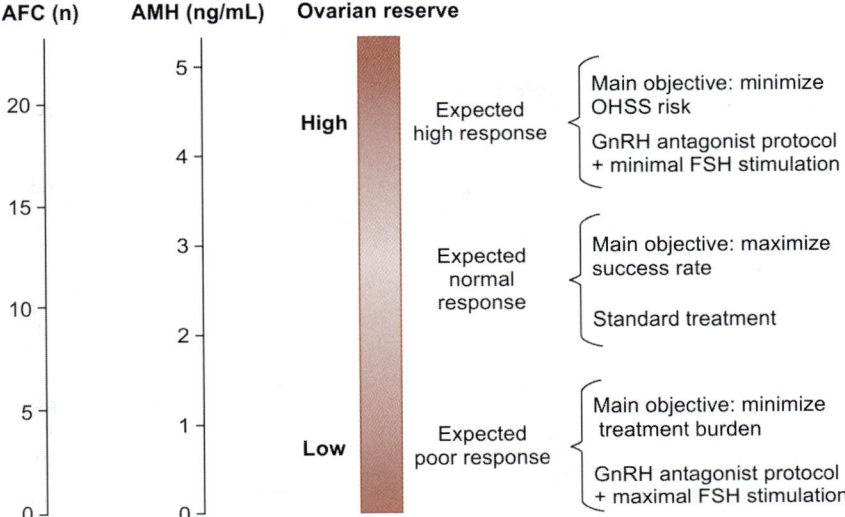

**Fig. 2:** Prediction of ovarian response based on anti-Müllerian hormone (AMH) and antral follicle count (AFC).[11]

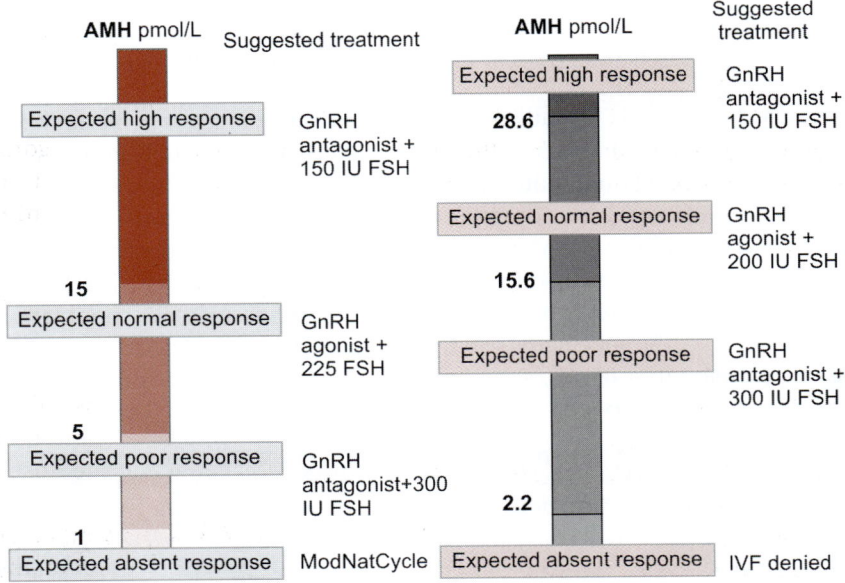

**Fig. 3:** Modeling of controlled ovarian stimulation based on ovarian reserve markers.[12,13]

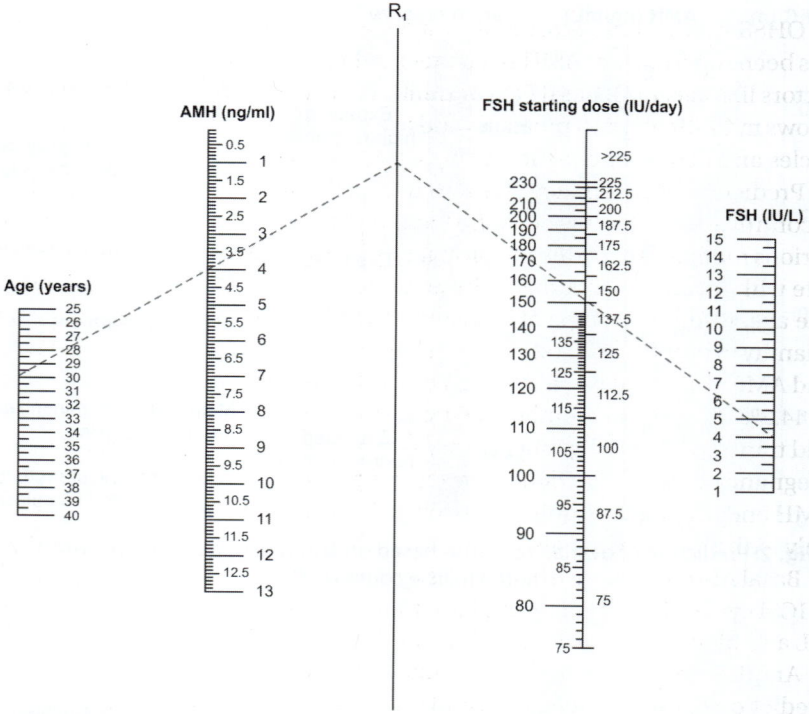

**Fig. 4:** Nomograms for calculation of the starting dose of follicle-stimulating hormone (FSH) based on age, serum anti-Müllerian hormone (AMH) and FSH levels.[14]

The AMH-tailored COH utilizing agonist and antagonist protocols has been reported as associated with improved IVF cycle. This may possibly improve the pregnancy prospects and reduce the cost. In patients anticipating extremes of response, GnRH antagonist protocol appears to be advantageous.

The cut-off values of AMH for hyper-response varied in various study designs (Table 2). The cut-off value with older assay methods was 3.5 ng/mL. But with recent assay methods it is 5.65 ng/mL in infertility population (sensitivity—86.4%, specificity—86.6%) whereas in non-PCOS, cut-off is 4.85 ng/mL (sensitivity—85.7%, specificity—89.7%), in PCOS, it is 6.85 ng/mL (specificity—66.7%, specificity—68.7%).[15]

**Table 2:** Anti-Müllerian hormone (AMH) cut-off values for hyper-response.

| References et al. | N | Study design | Cut-off value | Sensitivity % | Specificity % | AMH assay |
|---|---|---|---|---|---|---|
| Arce (2013)[6] | 759 | Retros* | 3.9 | 78 | 67 | AMH GenII |
| Polyzos (2013)[7] | 210 | Retros* | 3.52 | 89.5 | 83.3 | AMH GenII |
| Radha (2017)[15] | 246 | Prosp** (Non-PCOS) | 4.85 | 85.7 | 89.7 | AMH Gen II |

(*Retrospective, **Prospective)

OHSS is one of the most undesirable iatrogenic complications of COH. It has been reported that AMH is a better predictor of hyper-response than other factors like age, BMI, basal FSH or Inhibin B. Estimation of AMH prior to COH allows mild stimulation protocols and use of tailor treatment strategies for ART cycles and hence reduce the risk of OHSS.

Prediction of pregnancy rate and live birth rate by the serum AMH levels is controversial. This has been the focus of research for many years. There are various models to describe the probability of ongoing pregnancy and live birth rate with inconsistent results. These models included patient characteristics like age, BMI, cause, type of infertility, duration of infertility, the quality and quantity of oocytes, with recent models including AMH. A model including age and AMH predicted live birth rate with the sensitivity of 79.2% and specificity of 44.2%. In younger women, yield of more number of oocytes and embryos and transferring good quality embryos might be the reason for improving the pregnancy outcome. When the oocyte yield was excluded from the model, AMH and age were the only predictors of live birth. So AMH may be linked not only to the quantity but also the quality of female gametes.[16]

Basal AMH levels have been assessed as a marker of oocyte/embryo quality in ICSI cycles. The ongoing pregnancy rate was lowest when AMH is ≤ 0.89 ng/mL and highest in 2.89–4.83 ng/mL level.[17]

Another recent study showed that AMH is a fairly robust metric for the prediction of cycle cancellation and oocyte yield for Chinese women, but it is a relatively poor test for prediction of pregnancy outcomes. Patients with low levels of AMH still can achieve reasonable treatment outcomes and low AMH levels in isolation do not represent an appropriate marker for withholding fertility treatment.[18]

The pregnancy rate increased with concomitant increase in serum AMH, with a significant difference in AMH levels between pregnant and nonpregnant women of advanced age. So AMH seems to be useful clinically for predicting pregnancy as an independent predictor in advanced age women.[19]

The number of blastocyst available for fresh transfer and cryopreservation in all age groups also depends on serum AMH levels. If AMH is less than 1 ng/mL, there was significantly lower probability of successful supernumerary blastocyst for cryopreservation than those with AMH of 1–4 ng/mL.[20]

In a recent meta-analysis, AMH level was significantly higher in subjects who attained successful live birth compared with those who did not in fresh eSET cycles and that it showed weak to moderate predictive ability for live birth. However, AMH was not an independent predictor of live birth when age, BMI, FSH, number of oocytes retrieved and number of embryos transferred were included.[21]

## ■ CONCLUSION

- The baseline serum AMH level is a more reliable marker to predict ovarian response to COS.

- It also predicts the risk of OHSS prior to COS. In order to prevent OHSS, a mild, patient-friendly stimulation protocol may be applied in patients with a high basal serum AMH level.
- AMH values should be used for counseling the patient and should not deny treatment based on AMH values.
- Its ability to predict pregnancy rate and live birth rate is still controversial and further large studies are needed to confirm.

## REFERENCES

1. Vembu R, Nellepalli SR, Chandrasekar A, et al. Serum anti-Müllerian hormone levels: a better hormonal marker of ovarian reserve. Int J Med Res Health Sci. 2014;3(2):420-3.
2. Nelson SM, Yates RW, Lyall H, et al. Anti-Müllerian hormone-based approach to controlled ovarian stimulation for assisted conception. Hum Reprod. 2009;24:867-75.
3. Wallace AM, Faye SA, Fleming R, et al. A multicentre evaluation of the new Beckman Coulter anti-Müllerian hormone immunoassay (AMH Gen II). Ann Clin Biochem. 2011;48:370-3
4. Ferraretti AP, La Marca A, Fauser BC, et al. ESHRE consensus on the definition of poor response to ovarian stimulation for in vitro fertilization: the Bologna criteria. Hum Reprod. 2011;26(7):1616-24.
5. Vembu R, Nellepalli SR, Chandrasekar A, et al. Serum anti-Müllerian hormone levels: a predictor of ovarian response to controlled ovarian hyperstimulation in assisted reproductive technology. Asian J Obs Gyn. 2015;1(3);9-12.
6. Arce JC, La Marca A, Mirner Klein B, et al. Anti-Müllerian hormone in gonadotropin releasing-hormone antagonist cycles: prediction of ovarian response and cumulative treatment outcome in good-prognosis patients. Fertil Steril. 2013;99(6):1644-53.
7. Polyzos NP, Tournaye H, Guzman L, et al. Predictors of ovarian response in women treated with corifollitropin alfa for in vitro fertilization/intracytoplasmic sperm injection. Fertil Steril. 2013;100(2):430-7.
8. Seifer DB, Mac Laughlin DT, Christian BP, et al. Early follicular serum Müllerian-inhibiting substance levels are associated with ovarian response during assisted reproductive technology cycles. Fertil Steril. 2002;77(3):468-71.
9. Nelson SM, Yates RW, Fleming R. Serum anti-Müllerian hormone and FSH: prediction of live birth and extremes of response in stimulated cycles-implantations for individualization of therapy. Hum Reprod. 2007;22(9):2414-21.
10. Gnoth C, Schuring AN, Friol K, et al. Relevance of anti-Müllerian hormone measurement in a routine IVF program. Hum Reprod. 2008:23(6):1359-65.
11. Marca AL, Sunkara SK. Individualization of controlled ovarian stimulation in IVF using ovarian reserve markers: from theory to practice. Hum Reprod Update. 2014;20(1):124-40.
12. Nelson SM, Yates RW, Lyall H, et al. Anti-Müllerian hormone-based approach to controlled ovarian stimulation for assisted conception. Hum Reprod. 2009;24:867-75.

13. Yates AP, Rustamov O, Roberts SA, et al. Anti-Müllerian hormone-tailored stimulation protocols improve outcomes whilst reducing adverse effects and costs of IVF. Hum Reprod. 2011;26:2353-62.
14. La Marca A, Papaleo E, Grisendi V, et al. Development of a nomogram based on markers of ovarian reserve for the individualisation of the follicle-stimulating hormone starting dose in in vitro fertilisation cycles. BJOG. 2012;119:1171-9.
15. Vembu R, Reddy NS. Serum AMH level to predict the hyper response in women with PCOS and non-PCOS undergoing controlled ovarian stimulation in ART. J Hum Reprod Sci. 2017;10(2):91-4.
16. Marca AL, Nelson SM, Sighinolfi G, et al. Anti-Müllerian hormone-based prediction model for a live birth in assisted reproduction. Reprod Biomed Online. 2011;22:341-9.
17. Irez T, Ocal P, Guralp O, et al. Different serum anti-Müllerian hormone concentrations are associated with oocyte quality, embryo development parameters and IVF-ICSI outcomes. Arch Gynecol Obstet. 2011;284:1295-301.
18. Zheng H, Chen S, Du H, et al. Ovarian response prediction in controlled ovarian stimulation for IVF using anti-Müllerian hormone in Chinese women: a retrospective cohort study. Medicine. 2017;96(13):e6495.
19. Sahmay S, Oncul M, Tuten A, et al. Anti-Müllerian hormone levels as predictor of the pregnancy rate in women of advanced reproductive age. J Assist Reprod Genet. 2014;31:1469-74.
20. Kavoussi SK, Odenwald KC, Boehnlein LM, et al. Anti-Müllerian hormone as a predictor of good-quality supernumerary blastocyst cryopreservation among women with levels <1 ng/mL versus 1-4 ng/mL. 2015;104(3):633-6.
21. Tal R, Seifer DB, Wantman E, et al. Anti-Müllerian hormone as a predictor of live birth following assisted reproduction: an analysis of 85,062 fresh and thawed cycles from the Society for Assisted Reproductive Technology Clinic Outcome Reporting System database for 2012-2013. Fertil Steril. 2018;109(2):258-65.

CHAPTER 22

# Endometrial Scratch: Does It Work?

*Kamini Patel*

## ■ INTRODUCTION

According to a 2013 World Bank estimate, the drop in fertility started about 10 years ago in India, with a steady 17% decline from the year 2000. In Gujarat, there is a decline in the total fertility rate which is 2.5% seen in past few years according to the National Health Mission. The 2013 data for the Sample Registration Survey (SRS), conducted by the Registrar General of India, showed that the *total fertility rate*—the average number of children that will be born to a woman during her lifetime,[1] in eight States has fallen below two children per woman. Today, around 20% of the Indian population, both male and female, are known to be diagnosed as infertile (Haripriya, 2014). To overcome the problem more IVF and ICSI protocols were introduced in the country, however repetitive failures due to unidentified error causes burden to both patient and doctors.

Advancement in embryo culture conditions and transfer methods have been observed over recent decades, but increase in pregnancy and delivery rates are not observed.[2] Many factors affects pregnancy rates including woman's age, the indication for IVF, ovarian reserve, the treatment protocol employed, uterine pathology, immunological factors, number of embryos transferred, number of available embryos, embryo quality, embryo transfer technique, sperm quality, and luteal phase support (Milan et al., 2017). However the embryo quality and endometrial receptivity remains the major cause. Velez et al. (2014) predicts that despite advances made in ART techniques, implantation of embryo still remain to be a rate limiting step as even high quality embryo fails to implant which results in an implantation rate of approximately 25–30% per transferred embryo.[3]

## ■ ENDOMETRIAL SCRATCHING

The endometrial receptivity can be increased by a procedure introduced by Loeb et al. known as "Endometrial scratch". Endometrial scratching (or injury) is defined as intentional damage to the endometrium, such as by biopsy or curettage.[4] The procedure is sometimes referred to as an endometrial biopsy, as it involves taking a biopsy of the lining of the uterus, called the "endometrium", using a thin catheter (Pipille) that is passed through the cervix. No anesthetic is required, but patients are generally advised to take over-the-counter pain medication beforehand as it can cause some pain. An endometrial scratch is best performed in the week or so prior to the start of an IVF or frozen embryo transfer (FET) cycle (the luteal phase). Although the mechanism by which endometrial scratching increases the pregnancy rates remain unknown, hypotheses include: (1) that endometrial scratching during the previous cycle might induce decidualization, increasing the chance of implantation;[5] (2) that it induces a significant increase in the secretion of cytokines, interleukins, growth factors, macrophages and dendritic cells, all of which might be beneficial to embryo implantation,[6] and (3) that endometrial scratching might lead to better synchronicity between the endometrium and the transferred embryo.[7]

## ■ LITERATURE REVIEW

In order to find out the effectiveness of endometrial scratching on pregnancy rates, comparison is required to be made based on clinical outcomes. Over last decade, Barash et al.[8] (2003) described a link between endometrial scratching and increased chance of pregnancy in subsequent ART procedures. Nastri et al. in a Cochrane review concluded that endometrial injury before controlled ovarian stimulation, IVF/ICSI and fresh embryo transfer can improve live birth rate and clinical pregnancy rates without evidence of miscarriage or multiple pregnancy. However, endometrial injury on the day of oocyte retrieval seems to reduce clinical and ongoing pregnancy rates.

In a study carried out by Milan et al. shows implantation rates increases in women experiencing recurrent IVF failure when hysteroscopy is performed with local endometrium injury prior to ovarian stimulation. Similar study was carried out Mehmet et al. (2016)[9] on 345 patients with recurrent implantation failure showed endometrial scratching during diagnostic hysteroscopy enhances implantation as well pregnancy rates in comparison to diagnostic hysteroscopy alone. In the same year, Jennifer et al. also showed the same finding. Contrary to this Baum et al. reported that local injury to the endometrium by Pipille twice in follicular and luteal phase of preceding IVF cycle did not have any benefits in high-order RIF patients and that clinical outcomes in the intervention group were significantly lower than those in the control group.

## ■ CONCLUSION

Literature survey suggests endometrium scratching does increase the implantation rates in the patients with history of recurrent IVF failure than doing scratching during first IVF cycle. Thus it can be used as an add-on to improve the implantation rates. However, heterogeneity in the findings calls for the need to carry out the research on larger subject scale.

## REFERENCES

1. Arokiasamy P. International Institute for Population Sciences (IIPS). Mumbai. 2014.
2. Salehpour S, Zamaniyan M, Saharkhiz N. Does intrauterine saline infusion by intrauterine insemination (IUI) catheter as endometrial injury during IVF cycles improve pregnancy outcomes among patients with recurrent implantation failure?: An RCT. Int J Reprod BioMed. 2016;14(9):583.
3. Velez MP, Connolly MP, Kadoch IJ, et al. Universal coverage of IVF pays off. Hum Reprod. 2014;29(6):1313-9.
4. Nastri CO, Gibreel A, Raine-Fenning N, et al. Endometrial injury in women undergoing assisted reproductive techniques. Cochrane Database Syst Rev. 2012;7(CD009517).
5. Baum M, Yerushalmi GM, Maman E, et al. Does local injury to the endometrium before IVF cycle really affect treatment outcome? Results of a randomized placebo controlled trial. Gynecol Endocrinol. 2012;28(12):933-6.
6. Gnainsky Y, Granot I, Aldo PB, et al. Local injury of the endometrium induces an inflammatory response that promotes successful implantation. Fertil Steril. 2010;94(6):2030-6.
7. Li R, Hao G. Local injury to the endometrium: its effect on implantation. Curr Opin Obstet Gynecol. 2009;21(3):236-9.
8. Barash A, Dekel N, Fieldust S, et al. Local injury to the endometrium doubles the incidence of successful pregnancies in patients undergoing in vitro fertilization. Fertility and sterility. 2003;79(6):1317-22.
9. Seval MM, Şükür YE, Özmen B, et al. Does adding endometrial scratching to diagnostic hysteroscopy improve pregnancy rates in women with recurrent in-vitro fertilization failure? Gynecol Endocrinol. 2016;32(12):957-60.

# CHAPTER 23

# Near-miss Situations in Assisted Reproductive Technology

*Sadhana Gupta*

## ■ INTRODUCTION

Assisted reproductive technology (ART) is now considered a mainstream treatment for infertility of varying causes, severity and duration. There has been marked technological advancement in all fields of ART ranging from drugs, equipment and laboratory procedures. Despite it a generalized carry home baby rate after ART is still in range of 20–35% because of various individual reasons as well still present wide gaps in knowledge. However, a general concept and idea amongst patient, media as well doctors is that ART procedure can have failures but not any life-threatening risk to mother and babies. Fact is not the same, and during process of ART to delivery, there can be many life-threatening complications. It is prudent that we as doctors in *obstetrics* as well *ART practitioners* have adequate knowledge for these *near-miss situations* in process of ART for timely diagnosis and optimum management.

## ■ POSSIBLE LIFE-THREATENING SITUATIONS

There are some possible life-threatening situations in ART, which are discussed here.

### Selection of Couple

The couple especially women must have thorough medical, surgical and psychological evaluation before subjecting to ART. Uncontrolled hypertension, diabetes mellitus, obesity not only make process of ART difficult but also result in high rate of pregnancy complication. History of thromboembolism and myocardial infarction make use of hormones in ART highly risky. For these situations a multidisciplinary approach and careful selection or rejection should be made.

## Ovarian Hyperstimulation Syndrome

Ovarian hyperstimulation syndrome (OHSS) is now a well-known life-threatening complication associated with ART. It is characterized by massive transudation of protein rich fluid mainly albumin from vascular space into peritoneal, pleural and occasionally pericardial cavity.

The key to prevention of OHSS is individualized stimulation protocol and close monitoring of cycle with ultrasound and serum estradiol level. More than 20 follicle in each ovary, high estradiol value >3,000 pg/mL and steep rise of estradiol like doubling of values in couple of days are warning signs for impending OHSS. The preventive approaches are coasting of cycles, cancelling the hCG trigger, or trigger by GnRh agonist in antagonist cycle or with freeze all embryos in present cycle. Coasting effect the pregnancy rate adversely, freeze all policy is safe policy and should be considered and available in all ART centers. Use of dopamine agonist inhibits early onset of OHSS by inhibiting phosphorylation of VEGFR2 and preventing increased vascular permeability. Albumin or 6% hydroxyethyl starch administration at the day of oocyte pick up reduces incidence as well severity of OHSS.

Early recognition of OHSS is crucial. *Mild OHSS* require close observation and maintenance of hydration by the oral route. *Moderate grade OHSS* requires close observation and in most instances hospitalization. *Severe OHSS* requires immediate hospitalization and treatment. Large volume crystalloid infusion is recommended for restoration of the depleted intravascular volume. Mainstay of treatment is conservative and supportive. Albumin is proven to be advantageous. Prophylaxis with heparin should be added. Tension ascites with oliguria warrants paracentesis. Impending renal failure and unrelenting hemoconcentration require intensive care and possibly dopamine drip. Therapeutic termination of pregnancy may be life-saving when all other measures fail, yet this decision is very difficult for physician as well as woman and family.

## Surgical Emergencies in ART

### Ovarian Torsion

Enlarged ovaries during ovarian stimulation are prone to torsion. Ovarian torsion is a surgical emergency. Suspicion of ovarian torsion, timely confirmation of diagnosis by clinical and imaging modality and proper timely management of ovarian torsion is crucial to save life. Nowadays laparoscopic or open detorsion of ovary is mainstay of treatment of ovarian torsion, however if ovary appear badly necrosed, oophorectomy has to be done. Counseling of women for warning signs especially in polycystic ovaries is important for timely notification.

### Tension Ascites

In OHSS if there is tension ascites, ascites tapping has to be done.

## Ectopic Pregnancy

Incidence of *ectopic pregnancy* in ART is 1–3%. It is important to counsel the couple and family for possibility of ectopic pregnancy in ART procedure as a part of pregnancy complications. In ART beta hCG is closely followed if with increased hCG level there is no gestational sac visible in utero, possibility of ectopic pregnancy has to be kept in mind strongly and followed-up closely. Ectopic pregnancy can be managed medically by methotrexate or surgically by laparoscopic or open salpingectomy or salpingostomy depending upon availability of expertise and facility.

Late management or diagnosis of ectopic pregnancy is one of the life-threatening situations. It is psychological rejection of possibility of failure of ART, which causes delay on part of clinician as well women and family.

## Complications during Oocyte Pick up

During oocyte pick up there is possibility of injury to ovarian/pelvic vessels especially in difficult pick up and in learning phase. It is important to have a good preview of previous scan for site of ovaries, adherent ovaries, endometriosis or any tubo-adnexal mass. In case of any confusion use of color Doppler should be done to differentiate follicle from vessel. It is a good practice to look for any free fluid after completion of oocyte aspiration and check for any vaginal bleeding. Usually tight pressure is enough to check the bleeding, yet rarely it can result in hemoperitoneum and accordingly conservative or surgical management. Hypovolemia with increasing free fluid and unstable vitals warrants immediate management.

## Rupture of Ovarian/Endometriotic Cyst

Endometriotic cyst can accidentally punctured during oocyte pick up, likewise ovarian cyst or endometriotic cyst can rupture spontaneously. Possibility of rupture of ovarian or endometriotic cyst should be kept in mind if there is pain with disappearance of cyst noted in previous scan with free fluid in pelvis or peritoneal cavity. Watchful observation is first line if patient is stable, however in persistent symptoms and signs or acute abdomen surgical intervention is sometimes needed.

## Ovarian Abscess

Rarely after oocyte pick up there is septic foci in ovary especially in situation of aspiration of endometrioma and when bowel loops are present or adherent close to ovary. Prophylactic antibiotics are preferred before and after oocyte pick up, in high-risk cases patient should be counseled for warning sign of fever and pain. Usually it can be managed conservatively, rarely ovarian abscess has to be drained or managed surgically.

## Obstetric Complications in ART

### Multifetal Pregnancy

Assisted reproductive technology has been the key contributing factor in increase in multiple birth rates. Majority of ART related multiple gestations are thought to be dizygotic, many reports suggest increased monozygotic pregnancies as well. Complications and risk for both women and infants in multiple pregnancies are well recognized which include preterm birth, still birth, neonatal morbidity and mortality for babies and increased preeclampsia, gestational diabetes mellitus and operative intervention for mothers. Strategies to prevent multiple birth are adhering to mild and strict ovarian stimulation protocol, excess oocyte aspiration and vitrification, elective single embryo transfer in selected cases, coasting and freezing of embryos.

### Fetal Reduction

Fetal reduction involves elimination of one or more fetus in the multiple pregnancy iatrogenically in order to improve the perinatal outcome of the surviving fetuses. It is consequence of high order pregnancy, achieved in ART procedure or otherwise. The process has its own risk, the risk of complete pregnancy loss can be 1–2% that too in experienced hands. The pregnancy loss could be as a result of premature rupture of membrane, accidental entry of KCl into nontargeted sac or preterm labor. Besides there is risk of sepsis of varying degree, which in rare situation can lead to decision of termination of pregnancy.

*Multifetal pregnancy is now considered as adverse event in ART and all protocols right from mild stimulation to less embryo transfer should be applied in ART practices.*

### Prophylactic Cervical Cerclage in ART Pregnancy

It is a procedure which has not been found effective in improving outcome of pregnancy in any pregnancy if done without history or ultrasound guided indication. Rather the procedure itself can initiate uterine contractions, bleeding and sepsis.

### Fragmented Obstetric Care

It is today irony of Indian scenario where people get ART done at distant cities and fail to followup with good quality obstetric care. ART pregnancies are always considered as high-risk pregnancy and need careful maternal and fetal surveillance. Integration of ART and obstetric services are must for improving obstetric outcome in term of healthy mothers and babies.

## CONCLUSION

Assisted reproductive technology procedures have their own risk and limitation. Open minded discussion with patient and family goes a long way in having positive experience for technology irrespective of result. However, all preventive and curative measures have to be taken well in time from selection of patient for ART to delivery of baby and puerperium.

It is important to keep the expectation of family in realistic level and have all back up and referral facility in case of complications.

# CHAPTER 24

# Anesthesia in Assisted Reproductive Technology

*Namrata Biswas*

## ■ INTRODUCTION

Since Louise Brown, the first in vitro fertilization (IVF) baby, an estimated 6.5 million babies have been born with assisted reproductive technology (ART). Though many studies have been carried out, no consensus has yet been reached for the ideal anesthesia for ART. The various procedures for which anesthesia is needed in ART are:

1. *Transvaginal ovum retrieval (TVOR):* The process whereby a small needle is inserted through the vagina and guided via ultrasound into the ovarian follicles to collect the fluid that contains the eggs.
2. *Embryo transfer (ET):* The process whereby one or several embryos are placed into the uterus of the female with the intent to establish a pregnancy.
3. *Surgical sperm retrieval (SSR):* Where the reproductive urologist obtains sperm from the vas deferens, epididymis or directly from the testis in a short outpatient procedure.
4. *Gamete intrafallopian transfer (GIFT):* Wherein a mixture of sperms and eggs are placed directly into a woman's fallopian tubes using laparoscopy, following a TVOR.
5. *Reproductive surgery*, e.g. treating fallopian tube obstruction and vas deferens obstruction, or reversing a vasectomy by a reverse vasectomy.

Since many of these procedures require mainly pain relief, the ideal method would be one that is safe, providing adequate pain relief with minimal side effects and complications; easy to administer and monitor; short acting and easily reversible; and without deleterious effects on oocytes and embryos.

## ■ GENERAL CONSIDERATIONS

### Coexisting Illness

Patients may be suffering from any coexisting medical or surgical disorders. Special emphasis should be placed on known anticipated cause of infertility such as tuberculosis and thyroid disorders.

## Current Medications

Patients may be on anticoagulants, thyroid medications, antidepressants or anxiolytics like selective serotonin reuptake inhibitors (SSRI) tricyclics or trazodone, analgesics or antitubercular drugs.[1] These patients are often on aspirin or heparin so as to prevent the hypercoagulable state because of gonadotrophic injections.[2] Aspirin should be stopped 3 days prior to egg retrieval procedure. In case patient is on heparin, activated prothrombin time needs to be monitored.

## Special Considerations

Morbid obesity, severe renal, cardiac, pulmonary disease and diabetes need to be optimized before any surgical procedure. Cancer patients, in whom the oocyte retrieval is usually performed prior to chemotherapy or radiotherapy, need special care.[3]

## Monitoring

Existing guidelines identify the need for pulse oximetry, electrocardiography (ECG), and automated noninvasive arterial pressure monitoring in all patients.[4] Clinical and instrumental monitoring, to a degree relevant to the patient's medical status and the sedation method should be used wherever indicated. Regular communication with the patients not only puts them at ease, but additionally allows for monitoring of the level of sedation. If verbal communication is lost, the patient requires the same level of care as for general anesthesia. Monitoring should be continued through recovery until the discharge criteria are met.[5]

Respiratory depression may occur during the use of intravenous (IV) sedatives and opioid analgesic drugs. Oxygen supplementation should be administered. However, while administration of oxygen prevents hypoxia, it might mask hypoventilation. The monitoring of ventilation with continuous waveform capnography should be considered, particularly where

- Deep sedation is used
- Ventilation cannot be directly observed [e.g. during magnetic resonance imaging (MRI) or computed tomography (CT)]
- Multiple anesthetic drug techniques are used
- Preassessment highlights increased clinical risk.

## Setting

It is important to recognize the limitations of working in the relative "isolation" of the nontheater or nonhospital setting, where the skilled assistance of an operating department practitioner/operating department assistant (ODP/ODA) and familiar equipment may be lacking. Staffing and equipment must meet the needs of both the technique (including monitoring) and its possible complications. Appropriate recovery facilities and discharge criteria relevant to the patient's destination are necessary. Resuscitation equipment must be checked, maintained and must include all the drugs necessary for life support. The management of sedation related complications and medical emergencies should be regularly rehearsed as a team.

## ■ ART ANESTHESIA TECHNIQUES

Oocyte retrieval for IVF is usually performed transvaginally under ultrasound guidance. ET, SSR, GIFT and office hysteroscopy are relatively brief outpatient procedures. This necessitates a short-acting anesthetic approach with minimal side effects.[6] The various anesthetic modalities used for these procedures include
1. Monitored anesthesia care (MAC) and conscious sedation
2. General anesthesia (GA)
3. Regional anesthesia, i.e. epidural or subarachnoid block
4. Local anesthetic injections such as paracervical block (PCB) and preovarian block (POB)
5. Total IV anesthesia (TIVA)
6. Patient-controlled analgesia (PCA)
7. Alternative therapies such as acupuncture and electroacupuncture.

## Monitored Anesthesia Care and Conscious Sedation

Monitored anesthesia care is relatively easy to deliver; drugs are well-tolerated and best suited in day care settings. It avoids the potentially harmful effects of anesthetic drugs on oocytes. Singhal H et al. did a cross-sectional study on patient experience with conscious sedation.[7] They found that when the duration of the procedure was more than 12 min, immediate postprocedure pain score was significantly higher compared to those where the procedure duration was less than 12 min. There was no correlation between pain score and the number of oocytes retrieved and transmyometrial passage of needle. According to the updated Cochrane review conducted in 2013, the various approaches for MAC and conscious sedation used for IVF appear to be equally acceptable and were associated with a high degree of satisfaction. It was found that simultaneous use of more than one method of sedation and analgesia resulted in better pain relief than one modality alone.[6]

## General Anesthesia

It is preferred when egg retrieval is done laparoscopically and for other laparoscopic procedures, e.g. for blocked tubes, etc. Most of the anesthetic agents being used in GA have been found in the follicular fluid.[8] The duration of GA should be kept to a minimum to avoid detrimental effects of these drugs on oocytes.[9]

## Regional Anesthesia

Spinal anesthesia is also an effective technique used for ART.[10] Martin et al., in 1998, combined low dose hyperbaric 1.5% lidocaine (45 mg) with low dose fentanyl (10 mcg) for egg retrieval and found it suitable for egg retrieval.[11] Tsen compared low dose bupivacaine and fentanyl with lidocaine and fentanyl for oocyte retrieval and did not find either of the two combinations superior to the other.[12] Epidural anesthesia in ART also forms a viable option but does not demonstrate any advantage over intravenous sedation. Hormonal response to follicular puncture is fully attenuated by regional anesthesia while it is only partially attenuated by techniques using sedation.[11]

## Local Anesthesia

In paracervical block, a local anesthetic is injected at 2–6 sites, at a depth of 3–7 mm into the vaginal fornices and alongside the vaginal portion of the cervix. In a comparatively newer technique, the preovarian block (POB), the local anesthetic is infiltrated in the vaginal wall under ultrasound guidance, between the vaginal wall and peritoneal surface near the ovary.

## Patient-controlled Analgesia

This is an alternative technique of analgesia, allowing women control over their drug administration, thereby achieving a higher level of patient satisfaction. However, Bhattacharya et al. have concluded that although intraoperative PCA with fentanyl is an effective alternative to physician-administered techniques in terms of patient comfort and satisfaction, gynecologists preferred the latter.[13]

## Alternative Therapies

### *Acupuncture*

It is a traditional Chinese, nontoxic and relatively affordable therapy with possible indications as an adjunct in assisted reproduction, with some beneficial effects. It has been shown to be sympathoinhibitory, antidepressant and anxiolytic, has a neuroendocrine effect on the hypothalamic-pituitary-ovarian axis and increases uterine blood flow and beta endorphin levels.[14]

### *Electroacupuncture*

It has been used with along with paracervical block for analgesia during oocyte retrieval. Various conscious sedation regimens have been used along with electroacupuncture to enhance analgesia for oocyte retrieval.[15,16]

## ■ DRUGS USED IN ART ANESTHESIA

## Propofol and Thiopental

Propofol and thiopentone are being used extensively in IVF.[17] It has been shown that when TIVA is maintained with continuous propofol infusion; a gradual, time dependent, linear increase of its concentration is observed in follicular fluid (Christiaens et al., 1999).[18] Interestingly, no possible biological effects on the oocytes were detected. Various other studies have demonstrated that there is no detrimental effect of the rising concentrations of follicular fluid propofol on oocyte quality.[19] Additionally, there is no evidence that the administration of propofol during the procedure of embryo transfer has a negative impact on the embryos, as measured by probability of a clinical pregnancy or implantation rates.[18] Propofol has the added advantage of having antiemetic properties along with faster recovery time. Therefore, propofol anesthesia is useful while dealing with a difficult ET.

## Etomidate

Heytens et al. observed a sharp decrease in the plasma concentration of 17 beta-estradiol, progesterone, 17-hydroxyprogesterone-progesterone, and testosterone within 10 min after induction of anesthesia with etomidate (0.25 mg/kg), which was followed by a gradual return to the baseline levels thereafter.[20] He concluded that that etomidate could interfere with the endocrine function of the ovary.

## Dexmedetomidine

Dexmedetomidine is an effective sedative and analgesic in ART procedures. It offered not only a shorter PACU stay without significant side effects, but also better overall patient satisfaction scores.[21]

## Local Anesthetic Agents

Bupivacaine compared favorably to xylocaine in all aspects except that it increased the time for postoperative micturition and discharge by 30 minutes.[22] Schnell et al. in their study demonstrated that the local anesthetics lidocaine (L), chloroprocaine (C), and bupivacaine (B), adversely affect mouse IVF and embryo development in the order of C>L>B.[23]

### Opioids

Various opioids (fentanyl, alfentanil, remifentanil, and pentazocine) have been used safely for anesthesia in ART.[24]

## Benzodiazepines

Midazolam is the most commonly used benzodiazepine for ART procedures.[25] Although a minimal amount of this benzodiazepine is found in the follicular fluid, no deleterious effects have been demonstrated on the oocyte quality.[26]

## Ketamine

A combination of midazolam and ketamine has been found to be a good alternative to general anesthesia.[27]

## Nitrous Oxide

Nitrous oxide is one of the most widely used anesthetic gases but its effect on IVF outcome still remains questionable. Some studies have found a significant lower clinical pregnancy rate. $N_2O$ deactivates methionine synthase thereby reducing the amount of thymidine available for DNA synthesis in dividing cells.[28] However, this effect is minimal as the inactivation of the enzyme proceeds slowly in the human liver. Moreover, the low solubility of $N_2O$ exposes the oocytes to this gas for a short duration. Contrary to this, some studies have demonstrated that $N_2O$ increases the success rate of IVF by lowering the concentration of other potentially toxic and less diffusible anesthetic drugs.[27,29,30] Therefore the role of nitrous oxide in ART still remains controversial.

## Volatile Halogenated Agents

Most of the studies have demonstrated a deleterious effect of halogenated fluorocarbons on IVF outcomes.[28,31] Postoperative nausea and vomiting (PONV) is a common problem after IVF procedures under anesthesia with inhalation gases and its frequency is related to peak plasma level of estradiol and previous history of PONV.[31,32]

## Postoperative Nausea and Vomiting, and Antiemetic Agents

Strategies recommended to reduce PONV include: avoidance of general anesthesia and use of regional anesthesia; preferential use of propofol infusions; avoidance of nitrous oxide and volatile anesthetics; use the 5-hydroxytryptamine (5-HT3) receptor antagonists (ondansetron, etc.); minimization of perioperative opioids; and adequate hydration. Metoclopramide-induced hyperprolactinemia impairs ovarian follicle maturation and corpus luteum function and should be avoided.[33]

## Bromocriptine

Bromocriptine, a potent dopamine agonist, given before anesthesia, can suppress transient, anesthesia-induced hyperprolactinemia, and have a positive influence on embryonic development.[34]

## Nonsteroidal Anti-inflammatory Drugs

Mialon et al. compared two analgesic protocols: Paracetamol and alprazolam combination versus nefopam and ketoprofen combination on IVF outcomes. They found that both groups had similar IVF outcomes and nefopam with ketoprofen protocol enhanced patient comfort without jeopardizing the IVF success rates.

## CONCLUSION

The role of the anesthetist in IVF is to provide adequate comfort and pain relief to the patients during oocytes retrieval and embryo transfer procedures. The modality of providing the same should depend on patient cooperation. If the patient is comfortable, conscious sedation is a good option. However, in some cases, regional or GA may be requested. Different studies have explored the effect of anesthesia on IVF outcome but have yielded contradictory findings. These differences may be attributed to the differences in study design and randomization, the anesthetic drugs used or the anesthetic technique performed. Attention must be paid to comorbidities including those contributing to infertility and the drugs that the patient is taking. Furthermore, the anesthesia should be given for the shortest duration required.

## REFERENCES

1. Hashemi S, Simbar M, Ramezani-Tehrani F, et al. Anxiety and success of in vitro fertilization. Eur J Obstet Gynecol Reprod Biol. 2012;164:60-4.
2. Fleming T, Sacks G, Nasser J. Internal jugular vein thrombosis following ovarian hyperstimulation syndrome. Aust N Z J Obstet Gynaecol. 2012;52:87-90.
3. Barton SE, Missmer SA, Berry KF, et al. Female cancer survivors are low responders and have reduced success compared with other patients undergoing assisted reproductive technologies. Fertil Steril. 2012;97:381-6.
4. Ghisi D, Fanelli A, Tosi M, et al. Monitored anesthesia care. Minerva Anestesiol. 2005;71(9):533-8.
5. Smith I, Taylor E. Monitored anesthesia care. Int Anesthesiol Clin. 1994;32(3):99-112.
6. Kwan I, Bhattacharya S, Knox F, et al. Pain relief for women undergoing oocyte retrieval for assisted reproduction. Cochrane Database Syst Rev. 2013;1:CD004829.
7. Singhal H, Premkumar PS, Chandy A, et al. Patient experience with conscious sedation as a method of pain relief for transvaginal oocyte retrieval: a cross sectional study. J Hum Reprod Sci. 2017;2:119-23.
8. Hammadeh ME, Wilhelm W, Huppert A, et al. Effects of general anesthesia vs sedation on fertilization cleavage and pregnancy rates in an IVF program. Arch Gynecol Obstet. 1999; 263:56-9.
9. Hayes MF, Sacco AG, Savoy-Moore RT, et al. Effect of general anesthesia on fertilization and cleavage of human oocytes in vitro. Fertil Steril. 1987;48:975-81.
10. Endler G, Magyar D, Hayes M, et al. Use of spinal anesthesia in laparoscopy for in vitro fertilization. Fertil Steril. 1985;43:809-10.
11. Martin R, Tsen L, Tzeng G, et al. Anesthesia for in vitro fertilization: the addition of fentanyl 1.5% lidocaine. Anesth Analg. 1999;88:523-6.
12. Tsen L, Schultz R, Martin R, et al. Intrathecal low dose bupivacaine versus lidocaine for in vitro fertilization procedures. Reg Anesth Pain Med. 2000;26:52-6.
13. Bhattacharya S, MacLennan F, Hamilton MP, et al. How effective is patient-controlled analgesia? A randomized comparison of two protocols for pain relief during oocyte recovery. Hum Reprod. 1997;12:1440-2.

14. Han JS. Acupuncture: neuropeptide release produced by electric stimulation of different frequencies. Treends Neurosci. 2003;26:17-22.
15. Humaidan P, Stener-Victorin E. Pain relief during oocyte retrieval with a new short duration electro-acupuncture technique—an alternative to conventional analgesic methods. Hum Reprod. 2004;19:1367-72.
16. Stener-Victorin E, Waldenström U, Wikland M, et al. Electro-acupuncture as a preoperative analgesic method and its effects on implantation rate and neuropeptide Y concentrations in follicular fluid. Hum Reprod. 2003;18:1454-60
17. Endler GC, Stout M, Magyar DM, et al. Follicular fluid concentrations of thiopental and thiamylal during laparoscopy for oocyte retrieval. Fertil Steril. 1987;48:828-33.
18. Christiaens F, Janssenswillen C, Verborgh C, et al. Propofol concentrations in follicular fluid during general anaesthesia for transvaginal oocyte retrieval. Hum. Reprod. 1999;14:345-8.
19. Ben-Shlomo I, Moskovich R, Golan J, et al. The effect of propofol anesthesia on oocyte fertilization and early embryo quality. Hum Reporɗ. 2000;15:2197-9.
20. Heytens L, Devroey P, Camu F, et al. Effects of etomidate on ovarian steroidogenesis. Hum Reprod. 1987;2:85-90.
21. Elnabtity AM, Selim MF. A Prospective Randomized Trial Comparing Dexmedetomidine and Midazolam for Conscious Sedation During Oocyte Retrieval in An In Vitro Fertilization Program. Anesth Essays Res. 2017;11(1):34-9.
22. Tummon I, Newton C, Lee C, et al. Lidocaine vaginal gel versus lidocaine paracervical block for analgesia during oocyte retrieval. Hum Reprod. 2004;19:1116-20.
23. Schnell VL, Sacco AG, Savoy-Moore RT, Ataya KM, Moghissi KS. Effects of oocyte exposure to local anesthetics on in vitro fertilization and embryo development in the mouse. Reprod Toxicol 1992; 6:323-7.
24. Ben-Shlomo I, Moskovich R, Katz Y, et al. Midazolam/ketamine sedative combination compared with fentanyl/propofol/isoflurane anesthesia for oocyte retrieval. Hum Reporɗ. 1999;14:1757-9.
25. Chapineau J, Bazin JE, Terrisse MP, et al. Assay for midazolam in liquor follicular during in vitro fertilization under anaesthesia. Clin Pharm. 1993;12:770-3.
26. Hadimioglu N, Titz T, Dosemeci L, et al. Comparison of various sedation regimes for traps vaginal oocyte retrieval. Fertil Steril. 2002;78:648-9.
27. Gonen O, Shulman A, Ghetler Y, et al. The impact of different types of anesthesia on in vitro fertilization-embryo transfer treatment outcome. J Assist Reprod Genet. 1995;12:678-82.
28. Chetkowski RJ, Nass TE. Isofluorane inhibits early mouse embryo development in vitro. Fertil Steril. 1988;49:171-3.
29. Handa-Tsutsui F, Kodaka M. Effect of nitrous oxide on propofol requirement during target-controlled infusion for oocyte retrieval. Int J Obstet Anesth. 2007;16:13-6.
30. Palot M, Harika G, Visseaux H, et al. Use of nitrous oxide in general anaesthesia for oocyte retrieval. Ann Fr Anesth Reanim. 1989;8:R147.
31. Matt DW, Steingold KA, Dastvan CM, et al. Effects of sera from patients given various anesthetics on preimplantation mouse embryo development in vitro. J In Vitro Fert Embryo Transf. 1991;8:191-7.

32. Kauppila A, Leinonen P, Vihko R, et al. Metoclopramide-induced hyperprolactinemia impairs ovarian follicle maturation and corpus luteum function in women. J Clin Endocrinol Metab 1982; 54:955-60.
33. Sopelak VM, Whitworth NS, Norman PF, et al. Bromocriptine inhibition of anesthesia-induced hyperprolactinemia: effect on serum and follicular fluid hormones, oocyte fertilization, and embryo cleavage rates during in vitro fertilization. Fertil Steril. 1989;52:627-32.
34. Mialon O, Delotte J, Lehert P, et al. Comparison between two analgesic protocols on IVF success rates. J Gynecol Obstet Biol Reprod (Paris) 2011;40:137-43.

CHAPTER
25

# Surgery before ART: Does it Improve Outcomes?

*Laxmi Shrikhande, Bhushan Shrikhande*

## ■ INTRODUCTION

As there is no guarantee that assisted reproductive technology (ART) will result in pregnancy, various strategies have been elucidated to improve its success rate. Surgery before ART is one of these; however, whether it really improves the outcome is a big debate. Clinicians have to consider various other issues like financial costs, surgical and anesthesia-related risks, degree of improvement and the chances of recurrence before considering any surgery prior to ART. Here we discuss the various surgeries that can be done prior to ART:

- *Laparoscopic surgeries:* Ovarian cyst, endometriosis, myomectomy, surgery for hydrosalpinx.
- *Hysteroscopic surgeries:* Correction of uterine septum, T-shaped cavity, removal of polyps, fibroids, and synechiae.
- *Surgery in male:* Varicocelectomy.

## ■ LAPAROSCOPIC SURGERIES

### Ovarian Cyst

Cochrane authors have investigated the effectiveness and safety of cyst aspiration before ovarian stimulation versus a conservative approach (no aspiration) in women undergoing in vitro fertilization (IVF) or intracytoplasmic sperm injection (ICSI). Three randomized controlled trials were included involving 339 women of reproductive age who required IVF treatment due to tubal factor infertility, anovulation, male factor infertility, endometriosis or fertility of unknown cause. These studies compared the outcome of IVF cycles in women whose cyst was drained versus the outcomes when the cyst was not drained.

There is insufficient evidence to determine whether drainage of functional ovarian cysts prior to controlled ovarian hyperstimulation influences rates of live birth, clinical pregnancy, number of follicles recruited, or number of oocytes collected in women with a functional ovarian cyst. The findings of this review do not provide supportive evidence for this approach, particularly in view of the requirement for anesthesia, extra cost, psychological stress and risk of surgical complications.

This review highlights the need for well powered, well designed randomized controlled trials (RCTs) to further evaluate the role of cyst aspiration in women undergoing IVF treatment. Future trials need to be rigorous in design and delivery and with subsequent reporting to include high quality descriptions of all aspects of methodology to enable appraisal and interpretation of results. Current evidence lacks data on live birth rates and adverse events related to aspiration of ovarian cysts. Research conducted in the future should report these outcomes to maximize the care of women undergoing IVF in whom ovarian cysts are detected.[1]

## Surgery for Hydrosalpinx

Laparoscopic unilateral or bilateral salpingectomy has been the first and most studied surgical technique proposed. Although several observational and retrospective studies have been published, only five RCTs (of which one published only in abstract form) concerning the potential benefit of prophylactic laparoscopic salpingectomy before ART in case of hydrosalpinx were conducted. Despite potential bias due to small sample size and lack of blind randomization, data analysis in all trials showed a clear advantage in terms of implantation rate, pregnancy rate and ongoing pregnancy rate in treated patients compared to untreated controls.[2,3]

The derived data encouraged the scientific community to recommend tubal removal or tubal occlusion for hydrosalpinx prior to ART.[4] Though these recommendations may be of use in the management of evident hydrosalpinx, controversy persists regarding the ideal management of smaller unilateral or bilateral hydrosalpinx due to the potential detrimental effects of surgery on the ovarian reserve.

## Fibroids

All fibroids do not produce infertility. A detected fibroid sometimes gets undeserved attention and surgical treatment which is costly, time-consuming and not risk-free for patients who have a narrowing timeline to successful pregnancy. Therefore, the challenge is to distinguish between fibroids that do not affect the results, those that can marginally affect the results and those that deserve surgical management before proceeding to IVF.

If the fibroid is found to distort the uterine cavity on hysteroscopy, implantation rate is affected. In such patients with an abnormal uterine cavity, surgical treatment should be considered prior to IVF due to the reduced implantation rate.[5] However, some studies have also reported that intramural fibroids, which supposedly lack an intrauterine component, may have a deleterious effect on IVF results. As a result, excision of such fibroids should be considered. This conclusion remained controversial and is not confirmed by others.[6]

Considering that the uterine wall is no more than 2 cm in thickness, it is possible that all the intramural fibroids that are larger than 5 cm have some submucous component and therefore deserve surgical consideration. On the other hand, it is not advisable to perform myomectomy on intramural fibroids that are smaller than 5 cm and definitely not on those smaller than 3 cm. The final decision on these cases remains at the discretion of the treating physician and the patient, based on personal experience with IVF, his/her surgical skills in myomectomy, and the kind of pregnancy failure that they are experiencing.

Despite few RCTs, a provisional summary of the literature permits one to conclude that fibroids that impinge on the uterine cavity may lower implantation rates, and thus myomectomy prior to IVF might solve the problem. Conversely, the effect of intramural fibroids not encroaching on the uterine cavity warrants further investigation.[7]

## Endometrioma

The studies on IVF–ICSI cycles in women with ovarian endometriosis are limited by the fact that, in most cases, only one gonad is involved. This limitation is important and poorly considered. Patients with a single ovary do not in general have a reduced fertility potential to conceive through IVF treatment. In women with unilateral disease, the contralateral intact gonad may adequately compensate for the reduced function of the affected ovary.[8]

The presence of endometriomas *per se* may negatively influence ovarian function and may impose difficulties and risks during oocyte retrieval. The magnitude of the negative effect on ovarian reserve is unknown. On the other hand, there are no definite data clarifying whether the treatment of endometriomas increases (or decreases) the chances of success using IVF.

Results from large randomized trials are needed to elucidate whether or not ovarian endometriomas should be treated before undergoing an IVF–ICSI cycle and which treatment is more suitable. In the meantime, physicians should pursue a comprehensive and personalized approach in the decision-making process to identify the best option for the couple. At least five points have to be considered; the age of the woman, the presence/absence of pain, the number of previous interventions, ovarian reserve and the possibility of occult malignancy. In conclusion, although the optimal treatment cannot presently be proposed, there is insufficient evidence to support a strategy of systematic surgical treatment of endometriomas before IVF–ICSI cycles.

## ■ HYSTEROSCOPIC SURGERIES

## Fibroids

According to the American Society for Reproductive Medicine (ASRM, 2008) hysteroscopic myomectomy is indicated for intracavitary myomas and submucous myomas having at least 50% of their volume within the uterine cavity.[9]

A recent Cochrane review tried to assess the effects of the hysteroscopic removal of submucous fibroids in women with otherwise unexplained subfertility or prior to intrauterine insemination, IVF, or ICSI. In women with otherwise unexplained subfertility and submucous fibroids, there is no evidence of benefit with hysteroscopic myomectomy compared to regular fertility-oriented intercourse during 12 months for clinical pregnancy [odds ratio (OR) 2.4, 95% confidence interval (CI) 0.97 to 6.2, and / = 0.06, 94 women] and miscarriage (OR 1.5, 95% CI 0.47 to 5.0, and / = 0.47, 94 women). Nonetheless, the quality of the evidence considered was very low.[10]

Pritts et al. (2009) published a systematic literature review and meta-analysis of existing controlled studies regarding the effect of fibroids on fertility and of myomectomy in improving outcomes. They concluded that fertility outcomes are decreased in women with submucosal fibroids and removal seems to confer benefit in terms of pregnancy rates.[11]

## Polyp

A recent Cochrane review tried to assess the effect of hysteroscopic polypectomy on the results of intrauterine insemination (IUI). Apparently, the hysteroscopic removal of polyps prior to IUI increases the odds of clinical pregnancy compared to diagnostic hysteroscopy and polyp biopsy only (OR 4.4, 95% CI 2.5 to 8.0, and / < 0.00001).[10]

Implantation and clinical pregnancy rates were statistically significantly increased after hysteroscopic polypectomy in a group of women with recurrent implantation failure after IVF.[12] In conclusion, it appears that polypectomy prior to IUI or IVF (even in cases with previous implantation failure) increases the chances of pregnancy.

## Septum

Most studies of metroplasty for a septate uterus combine women with recurrent miscarriage and infertility, and no study has been published that randomizes infertile women to treatment versus no treatment. For this reason controversy exists as to whether infertile women should undergo metroplasty. Hysteroscopic metroplasty in women with septate uterus and unexplained infertility could improve clinical pregnancy rate and live birth rate in patients with otherwise unexplained infertility.[13,14]

## T-shaped Cavity

In the case of uterine dysmorphism, infertility and obstetric complications are believed to be more common compared with those with a normal uterine cavity.[15] In a study published in BJOG, 21 women (72.4%) became pregnant after the metroplasty. Thirteen women gave birth to 16 live infants. Nine of them delivered 12 viable term neonates. Among these 13 women, one woman with primary infertility gave birth to two live infants. These results are in accordance with other studies using hysteroscopic metroplasty. This is the largest series to date (with the longest follow up) which details the reproductive performance of patients with hypoplastic uterus after hysteroscopic metroplasty.[16]

The results show that hysteroscopic metroplasty seems to be an operation that improves the rate of live births for women with a hypoplastic uterus and a history of primary infertility and/or recurrent abortion and/or preterm delivery.

## Synechiae

Pace et al. reported that in women with Asherman's syndrome, pregnancy rate varied from 28.7% before surgery to 53.6% after hysteroscopic treatment.[17] In a study of women with two or more previous unsuccessful pregnancies, the operative success as measured by live birth rate improved from 18.3% preoperatively to 68.6% postoperatively.[18] In the literature, the pregnancy rate after hysteroscopic lysis of intrauterine adhesions in women who wanted to have a child has been about 74%, which is much higher than found in untreated women (46%). The pregnancy rate after treatment in women with infertility is about 45.6%; the successful pregnancy rate after treatment in severe cases is reported to be consistently lower at 33%. For women with previous pregnancy wastage, both the pregnancy rate and the live birth rate after treatment are reasonably high—89.6% and 77.0% respectively. Women who conceive after treatment of Asherman's syndrome still have a high risk of pregnancy complications, including spontaneous abortion, premature delivery, abnormal placentation, intrauterine growth restriction (IUGR) and uterine rupture during pregnancy or delivery.

## Office Hysteroscopy

The clinical value of hysteroscopic removal of uterine cavity abnormalities to increase fertility rates in subfertile women remains unknown. The limited evidence at present shows that hysteroscopy may improve the odds of a clinical pregnancy. Removing polyps and other uterine cavity abnormalities via hysteroscopy in women with unexplained infertility may increase their chances of becoming pregnant. Certain analyses show the practice is associated with important increases in pregnancy rates or at least a benefit trending toward increased fertility, but the evidence is limited and additional, larger studies are needed.[10]

A systematic review comparing the outcome of IVF treatment performed in patients who had an outpatient hysteroscopy in the cycle preceding their IVF treatment with a control group in which hysteroscopy was not performed was conducted. The results of these five studies showed evidence of benefit from outpatient hysteroscopy in improving the pregnancy rate in the subsequent IVF cycle.[19-21]

The role of hysteroscopy in the management of the infertile female remains under debate. Although a variety of studies demonstrate that the procedure is well tolerated and effective in the treatment of intrauterine pathologies, there is no consensus on the effectiveness of hysteroscopic surgery in improving the prognosis of subfertile women. There are not enough prospective randomized trials to clearly demonstrate that surgical removal of all intrauterine abnormalities improves fertility or IVF outcomes. However, published observational results suggest a benefit for resection of submucosal leiomyomas, adhesions, and at least a subset of polyps in increasing pregnancy rates. More randomized controlled studies with adequate controls are needed to substantiate the effectiveness of the hysteroscopic removal of suspected endometrial polyps, submucous fibroids, uterine septum, or intrauterine adhesions in women with unexplained subfertility or prior to assisted reproductive technology (IUI, IVF, or ICSI).

## ■ SURGERY IN MALE

### Varicocelectomy

A varicocele is a pathologic dilation of the pampiniform venous plexus of the spermatic cord, one of three venous drainage pathways of the testicle. Clinically, the dilated venous plexus is graded by size: subclinical (detected by ultrasound only), grade I, grade II, or grade III.

Overall, the literature examining the effectiveness of IUI after varicocelectomy is suboptimal, with all existing studies being retrospective and underpowered. No meta-analysis has specifically examined the efficacy of IUI after varicocelectomy, owing to the dearth of studies and the poor quality of existing studies, as noted by Kirby et al. in a 2016 meta-analysis examining the effect of ART on pregnancy and live birth rates after varicocele repair.[21]

Within the existing literature, after varicocele correction, the per couple pregnancy rate after IUI ranges from 7.7% to 50%, making it a challenge to establish the true rate, and most of the studies that compare IUI success in men with treated versus untreated varicocele fail to find a statistically significant difference.

The current literature is inadequate to draw any firm conclusion regarding the impact of varicocele repair on IUI success. Future large scale studies are necessary to determine if the correction of a varicocele affects IUI pregnancy success rates.

### IVF/ICSI after Varicocoelectomy in Men with Oligospermia

In the most recent and the largest retrospective study to date, 306 infertile couples undergoing IVF/ICSI, 168 men underwent varicocelectomy before

IVF/ICSI and 138 men had untreated varicocele. The two groups were similar in male and female ages, proportion of women with concurrent infertility diagnosis, and proportions of varicocele grades. Couples with men who had undergone varicocelectomy had a higher pregnancy rate compared with those with uncorrected varicocele (62.5% vs 47.1%; P <0.01). Live birth rates were also higher in couples with men who had undergone varicocele repair (47.6% vs 29.0%; P <.001).[22] Though retrospective, these large studies convincingly suggest that varicocoelectomy improves IVF/ICSI pregnancy rates.[23]

## KEY POINTS

- Evidence is in favor of salpingectomy or tubal clipping in cases of hydrosalpinx as it improves the reproductive outcome.
- Submucus fibroids and intramural fibroids which impinge on the endometrial cavity can be considered for myomectomy. It is best not to disturb other fibroids unless they are very large.
- There is no consensus on the effectiveness of hysteroscopic surgery in improving the prognosis of subfertile women but evidence is in favor of hysteroscopy in repeated implantation failures. It should always be a "see and treat" approach.
- Evidence suggests that varicocelectomy improves IVF/ICSI pregnancy rates.
- Reproductive outcome should not be the only concern before deciding for a surgery. Cost and risks involved should also be taken into account.

## REFERENCES

1. McDonnell R, Marjoribanks J, Hart RJ. Ovarian cyst aspiration prior to in vitro fertilization treatment for subfertility. Cochrane Database Syst Rev. 2014;CD005999.
2. Kontoravdis A, Makrakis E, Pantos K, et al. Proximal tubal occlusion and salpingectomy result in similar improvement in in vitro fertilization outcome in patients with hydrosalpinx. Fertil Steril. 2006;86:1642-9.
3. Moshin V, Hotineanu A. Reproductive outcome of the proximal tubal occlusion prior to IVF in patients with hydrosalpinx (Abstracts of the 22nd Annual Meeting). Prague, Czech Republic: ESHRE; 2006.
4. Johnson N, van Voorst S, Sowter MC, et al. Tubal surgery before IVF. Hum Reprod Update. 2011;17:3.
5. Eldar-Geva T, Meagher S, Healy DL, et al. Effect of intramural, subserosal, and submucosal uterine fibroids on the outcome of assisted reproductive technology treatment. Fertil Steril. 1998;70(4):687-91.
6. Donnez J, Jadoul P. What are the implications of myomas on fertility? A need for a debate? Hum Reprod. 2002;17(6):1424-30.
7. Pritts EA, Parker WH, Olive DL. Fibroids and infertility: an updated systematic review of the evidence. Fertil Steril. 2009;91(4):1215-23.
8. Lass A. The fertility potential of women with a single ovary. Hum Reprod Update. 1999;5:546-50.
9. The Practice Committee of American Society for Reproductive Medicine in collaboration with Society of Reproductive Surgeons. Myomas and reproductive function. Fertil Steril. 2008;90(5):S125-S130.

10. Bosteels J, Kasius J, Weyers S, et al. Hysteroscopy for treating subfertility associated with suspected major uterine cavity abnormalities. Cochrane Database of Syst Rev. 2013;CD009461.
11. Pritts EA, Parker WH, Olive DL. Fibroids and infertility: an updated systematic review of the evidence. Fertil Steril. 2009;91(4):1215-23.
12. Stamatellos I, Apostolides A, Stamatopoulos P, et al. Pregnancy rates after hysteroscopic polypectomy depending on the size or number of the polyps. Arch Gynecol Obstet. 2008:277(5):395-9.
13. Mollo A, de Franciscis P, Colacurci N, et al. Hysteroscopic resection of the septum improves the pregnancy rate of women with unexplained infertility: a prospective controlled trial. Fertil Steril. 2009;91(6):2628-31.
14. Bakas P, Gregoriou O, Hassiakos D, et al. Hysteroscopic resection of uterine septum and reproductive outcome in women with unexplained infertility. Gynecol Obstet Invest. 2012;73(4):321-5.
15. Heininen PK, Saarikoski S, Pystynen P. Reproductive performance of women with uterine anomalies: an evaluation of 182 cases. Acta Obstet Gynecol Scand. 1982;61:157-62.
16. Barranger E, Gervaise A, Doumerc S, et al. Reproductive performance after hysteroscopic metroplasty in the hypoplastic uterus: A study of 29 cases. BJOG. 2002:109:1331-4.
17. Pace S, Stentella P, Catania R, et al. Endoscopic treatment of intrauterine adhesions. Clin Exp Obstet Gynecol. 2003;30:26-8.
18. Katz Z, Ben-Arie A, Lurie S, et al. Reproductive outcome following hysteroscopic adhesiolysis in Asherman's syndrome. Int J Fertil Menopausal Stud. 1996;41:462-5.
19. Lorusso F, Ceci O, Bettocchi S, et al. Office hysteroscopy in an in vitro fertilization program. Gynecol Endocrinol. 2008;24(8):465-9.
20. Karayalcin R, Ozcan S, Moraloglu O, et al. Results of 2500 office-based diagnostic hysteroscopies before IVF. Reprod BioMed Online. 2010;20(5):689-93.
21. Kirby EW, Wiener LE, Rajanahally S, et al. Undergoing varicocele repair before assisted reproduction improves pregnancy rate and live birth rate in azoospermic and oligospermic men with a varicocele: a systematic review and meta-analysis. Fertil Steril. 2016;106:1338-43.
22. Gokce A, Demirtas A, Ozturk A, et al. Association of left varicocoele with height, body mass index and sperm counts in infertile men. Andrology. 2013;1:116-9.
23. Kirby EW, Wiener LE, Rajanahally S, et al. Undergoing varicocele repair before assisted reproduction improves pregnancy rate and live birth rate in azoospermic and oligospermic men with a varicocele: a systematic review and meta-analysis. Fertil Steril. 2016;106:1338-43.

# CHAPTER 26

# Recurrent Implantation Failure

*Kanthi Bansal*

## ■ INTRODUCTION

Recurrent implantation failure (RIF) refers to failure to achieve a clinical pregnancy after transfer of at least four good-quality embryos in a minimum of three fresh or frozen cycles in a woman under the age of 40 years. No universal consensus about the definition, most accepted definition is proposed by Coughlan et al.[1] Since, the introduction of ART, it has achieved major progress in optimizing stimulation protocols, fertilization procedures and embryo culture conditions. However, the success rates and the rate of implantation and pregnancy still need to be enhanced. For successful implantation we need to depend on two main components, a healthy embryo with potential to implant and a receptive endometrium that should enable implantation. This "cross-talk" between the embryo and the endometrium during the window of implantation that allows apposition, attachment and invasion of embryos is necessary for successful implantation and subsequent normal placentation. Implantation failure may be a consequence several factors including embryo or endometrial factors. Therefore, in assessing RIF thorough evaluation should be carried out to ascertain the underlying cause of the condition.

## ■ ETIOLOGY

Recurrent implantation failure is mutlifactorial and can occur due to abnormality in embryo, endometrium, and immune system and other factors.

### Embryo

Embryo is the most important factor in implantation. The quality of embryo decides the rate of success. One-third of RIF is due to abnormalities in embryo. The abnormality of embryos can be due to genetic abnormality, oocyte quality, sperm quality and parental chromosomal abnormalities. This abnormality can be due to the abnormality in embryo itself or due to poor quality of oocytes and sperms. Quality of oocyte reduces with age due to increased mitochondrial

DNA damage and these results in aneuploid embryos.[2] Even poor ovarian response, higher number of immature oocytes, advanced age can leads to poor oocyte quality and reduced fertilization rates and poor embryo formation rates. Even sperms can equally contribute for poor quality of embryo. One important cause is sperm DNA damage which has shown association with failure to achieve conception. DNA fragmentation seems to affect embryogenesis and embryo viability resulting in poor implantation in both spontaneous and assisted conception. Meta-analysis by Collins et al.[3] suggested that sperm DNA damage has a modest impact on pregnancy rates following IVF treatment. Increased incidence of chromosomal inversions, translocations and deletions has been reported in patients with RIF. Balanced translocation in parents may lead to gametes with chromosomal aberrations that may fail to implant or be aborted. Increased sperm chromosomal abnormality is also reported in patients with RIF with normal karyotype, especially in cases of severe oligoasthenozoospermia and azoospermia due to testicular failure.[4]

### *Zona Hardening*

Blastocyst hatching through the zona pellucida is an important step proceeding implantation. Abnormality in hatching due to increased thickness or hardening of zona may lead to failed implantation.

### *Suboptimal Culture Conditions*

Even morphologically defined good quality embryos may cease to develop in utero and fail to reach up to blastocyst stage which can be due to suboptimal culture conditions.

## Uterine Factor

Initial step in evaluation of RIF patients include assessment of the uterus. Intact and functional uterine cavity is an important pre-requisite for successful implantation. Congenital or acquired anatomical malformation of uterus may interfere with normal implantation. Congenital uterine anomalies such as septate or bicornuate may impair endometrial receptivity, manifesting as infertility or recurrent pregnancy loss. These poor outcomes are not only due to disturbances of cavity but also impaired blood supply such as in case of septate uterus. Acquired intracavitary lesions such as submucous fibroids, endometrial polyps, and intrauterine adhesions may lead to RIF. Fibroids such as submucous or intramural cause the mechanical obstruction as well as lead to increased uterine contractility, deranged cytokine profile, abnormal blood supply and chronic endometrial inflammation. Meta-analysis by Pritts et al.[5] concluded that women with submucous and intramural fibroids have reduced implantation rates. There is evidence to suggest that submucosal and intramural fibroids that distort the endometrial cavity are associated with decreased pregnancy and implantation rates in women who attempt to conceive spontaneously or who are proceeding with IVF treatment. There is controversy as to whether or not non-cavity distorting intramural fibroids adversely affect IVF outcome. Some studies suggest an adverse effect of noncavity distorting fibroids on implantation and pregnancy rates in women undergoing IVF, particularly with large fibroids >4 cm, whereas others fail to demonstrate such an association. Mechanism by which polyps affect the implantation can be related to mechanical interference of the sperm transport, implantation of embryos and abnormal expression of markers of implantation. Adhesions affect the endometrial receptivity and prevent implantation by interfering with the attachment of embryo to the luminal surface of endometrium. Intrauterine adhesions often occur following curettage of the gravid uterus to terminate an unwanted pregnancy or in cases of retained products of conception after a pregnancy or miscarriage. Intrauterine surgery or intrauterine infection of the nongravid uterus may also lead to the formation of intrauterine adhesions. Successful implantation depends on adequate growth of endometrium. Studies have shown that implantation rate and clinical pregnancy rates are higher in patients with thickness more than 9-10 mm.[6] Thin endometrium is related to the high impedance to blood flow, and decreased expression of angiogenic factors such as vascular endothelial growth factor (VEGF), resulting in decreased blood supply to endometrium. Studies have shown that adenomyosis affects the female fertility.[7] It has been suggested to reduce the endometrial receptivity similar to endometriosis. The prevalence of adenomyosis in women with RIF is likely to be underestimated as it may not always be detected by transvaginal ultrasonography (TVS). The condition may appear in two forms, diffuse and focal, and the posterior uterine wall appears to be predominantly affected. Adenomyosis almost always affects the junctional zone of the uterus which is just beneath the endometrium. Acute and chronic endometritis affect implantation due to possible effect of microbial products on endometrial receptivity. Acute endometritis is mostly caused by bacteria while chronic endometritis can be due to bacterial, viral and parasitic agents. In developing countries, genital TB is the most frequent cause of chronic pelvic inflammatory disease (PID). Dysregulation of expression of adhesion molecules such as cytokines, interleukins (IL-12, 15, 18), integrins, etc. has been associated with failed implantation. Both inherited and acquired thrombophilia have been mainly related with recurrent pregnancy loss, however several reports suggest an association with RIF as well. Probable mechanism responsible for implantation failure is disturbed blood flow to endometrium, which hampers endometrial receptivity.[8]

## Multifactorial Factors

### Hydrosalpinges

Presence of hydrosalpinges has been found to be associated with implantation failure. This adverse effect can be related to the negative effect on endometrial receptivity as well as a direct embryotoxic effect due to the presence of cytokines, prostaglandins and other inflammatory compounds in hydrosalpinx fluid. The expression of leukemia inhibitory factor, a cytokine essential for successful implantation, was reduced in the presence of hydrosalpinges.

### *Suboptimal Ovarian Stimulation*

Supraphysiological levels of steroids in COH cycles alter endometrial receptivity due to premature expression of pinopodes and integrins, which results in premature luteal transformation of endometrium.

## ■ EVALUATION AND MANAGEMENT

Treatment of RIF should be targeted to find out the underlying cause and its correction. Approach for the assessment and treatment of RIF can be described as given in Flowchart 1.[9]

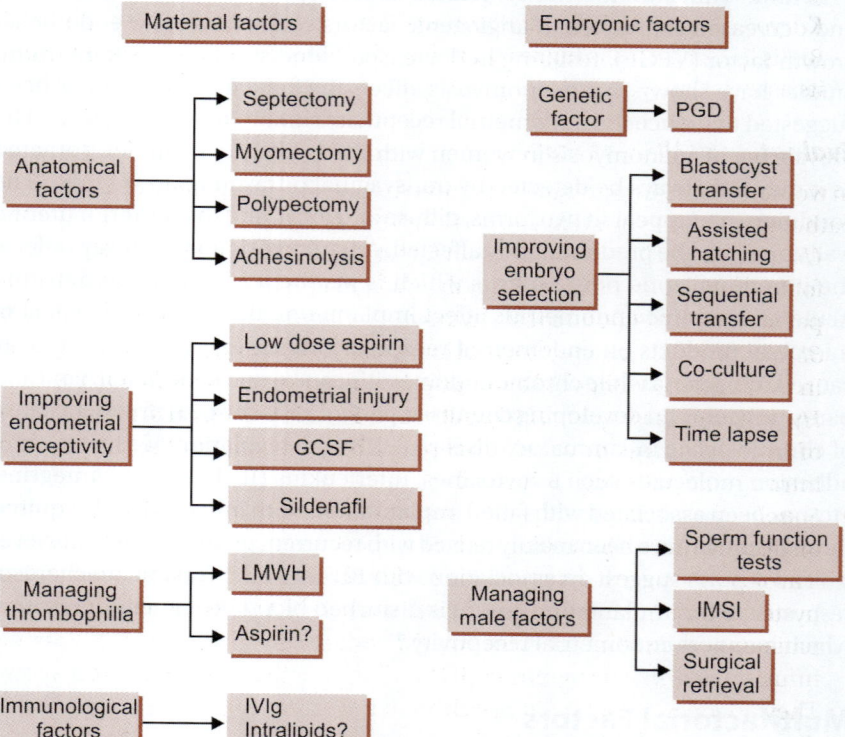

**Flowchart 1:** Evaluation and management of recurrent implantation failure.

(GCSF: granulocyte colony-stimulating factor; PGD: preimplantation genetic diagnosis; LMWH: low molecular-weight heparin; IMSI: intracytoplasmic morphologically selected sperm injections; IVIg: intravenous immunoglobulin)

## Evaluation

- Complete history and evaluation of previous records, if any may give some insight into the problem
- A complete examination (general and pelvic)
- Endocrinological evaluation: Includes thyroid function test, prolactin, blood sugars as association has been seen with uncontrolled hypothyroidism and diabetes mellitus with RIF.

### Evaluation of Embryo Factors

- *Ovarian function tests:* Such as basal follicle-stimulating hormone (FSH), anti-müllerian hormone (AMH) and antral follicle count to rule out any significant compromise of ovarian function.
- *Sperm DNA integrity tests:* Several tests are used to measure sperm DNA fragmentation such as Terminal deoxynucleotidyl transferase dUTP nick end labeling (TUNEL), comet assay, sperm chromatin structure assay (SCSA), etc.
- *Karyotyping:* Although, the chances of abnormal karyotype in couples with RIF is low (2.5%), it is higher than that of general population. This suggests its association with RIF.

### Evaluation of Uterine Factors

In women with RIF thorough evaluation should be done to rule out any uterine pathology. This assessment can be done as follows:

- *Ultrasonography:* Pelvic scan is an integral part of IVF treatment to monitor follicle growth and endometrial development. It also throws light on other pathologies like endometriosis, hydrosalpinx, fibroids and endometrial polyps.
- *3D ultrasound* is an effective tool for assessment of endometrium as well as in evaluation of congenital and acquired uterine cavity anomalies.
- *Hysterosalpingography (HSG):* Although HSG is a useful test for detection of hydrosalpinges or other tubal pathology, its value in the detection of intrauterine pathology is limited.
- *Sonohysterography:* It is the radiographic visualization of uterine cavity after instillation of contrast media such as saline. It has advantage over the HSG as it avoids exposure to radiation and iodine contrast and it is less invasive than hysteroscopy. Study conducted by Shokeir and Abdelshaheed,[10] included patients with at least previous two IVF failures and performed TVS, saline infusion sonohysterogram (SHG) and then HSG prior to hysteroscopy. They concluded that in comparison to hysteroscopy, SHG offered similar diagnostic capabilities, is less invasive and costly.
- *Hysteroscopy:* It is the gold standard to diagnose intrauterine pathology and is one of the most important investigations in women with RIF. Incidence of abnormal hysteroscopic findings in women with recurrent IVF failures varies

between 25% and 50%.[11] Apart from diagnostic use, it also allows therapeutic procedures to be carried out simultaneously at the time of diagnosis.

- *Combined laparoscopy and hysteroscopy:* In women with congenital uterine anomaly diagnosed on the basis of USG, SSG or HSG, further investigation like 3D USG, MRI or combined hysteroscopy and laparoscopy is required to confirm the diagnosis. The later is considered to be the gold standard as it allows for direct visualization of the internal and external contour of the uterus and enables the clinician to diagnose and treat concurrently.

### Evaluation of Thrombophilia

Evaluation includes assessment of anticardiolipin antibodies and lupus anticoagulant for acquired factors and factor V Leiden mutation, protein C and S deficiencies, antithrombin III and methylenetetrahydrofolate reductase (MTHFR) mutation for inherited thrombophilias.

## Management

Management of RIF is a multidisciplinary approach which includes an experienced fertility specialist, a senior embryologist and, if possible a reproductive counselor.

### Managing Embryonic Factors

*Preimplantation genetic diagnosis:* There is significant evidence that implantation failure especially in elderly women is closely related to aneuploidy. Preimplantation genetic diagnosis (PGD) has been developed for the detection of these genetic abnormalities. Embryo biopsy taken as polar body biopsy, blastomere biopsy on day 3 and trophectoderm biopsy. By selecting only the chromosomally normal embryos for transfer, PGD was initially presumed to significantly increase the implantation rates; however its role in RIF is controversial. A recent review by Donoso et al.[12] highlighted mosaicism of blastomeres as the major source of misdiagnosis in PGD and concluded that it should not be implemented on a routine basis in women with RIF. However study by Fragouli et al.[13] suggest that an approach combining blastocyst biopsy and comprehensive chromosome screening using CGH or microarray CGH may represent the optimal approach for PGD.

Considering above points, it is recommended that PGD/PGS should not currently be offered in routine clinical care. "It should, if at all, only be offered to patients as a part of randomized controlled trial (RCT) with proper informed consent pending evidence of effectiveness."[14]

*Blastocyst transfer:* In vitro fertilization (IVF) success can be improved by prerequisite to identify the embryos with higher implantation potential. By extending culture of embryos till blastocyst stage, we can get the initiation. In human embryos genomic activation occurs at 8–10 cell stage, i.e. day 3 of culture. The embryos that grow in culture after day 3 and progress to blastocyst stage are assumed of having higher implantation potential, as these are no longer dependent on maternal genomic control.

A recent Cochrane review by Blake et al.[15] also supported the rationale that blastocyst transfer improves implantation rates by enabling better selection of embryos and with better synchronicity between the embryo and endometrium.

*Assisted hatching:* Abnormalities of the hatching process may be a contributing factor in failed implantation. This is supported by the early reports that observed a significant improvement in human embryo implantation rates when assisted hatching was attempted. Since then use of assisted hatching has been incorporated the in efforts to improve clinical outcomes. However, American Society for Reproductive Medicine (ASRM)[16] practice committee in 2008 concluded that the published evidence currently available does not support the routine or universal application of assisted hatching in all IVF cycles. Nonetheless, assisted hatching may be clinically useful in patients with a poor prognosis, including those with more than 2 failed IVF cycles and poor embryo quality, and in woman of an advanced age ($\geq$38 years of age). In 2014, Committee opinion on AH concluded that "there is good evidence that AH slightly improves CPR in poor prognosis patients, including those with prior failed IVF cycles and who have a poor prognosis (Level A)."[17]

*Sequential transfer:* Blastocyst culture and transfer improves selection and decreases the risk of multiple pregnancies. However, it is possible that no blastocyst forms during culture increasing the risk of cycle cancellation. To overcome these problems, day-3 and day-5 sequential transfer has been proposed. It ensures transfer on day 3, thereby reducing risk of cancellation and provides the option of blastocyst transfer when it is developed.

The rationale is that, during the first transfer, the embryos may induce an increase in endometrial receptivity, thereby creating a better endometrial environment for the second transfer on day 5.

Study by Madkour et al.[18] suggests that day-3 and day-5 sequential transfer can improve the clinical pregnancy (37.8% vs 21.9%), and implantation rates (17.1% vs 10.5%) compared to conventional day 3 transfer in patients with repeated IVF–ET failures.

*Co-culture conditions:* Despite improvement in culture conditions in women with RIF even good quality embryos fail to implant, probably due to intrinsic factors. Co-culture of embryos has been suggested as a means of improving culture conditions and subsequent implantation rates. Possible benefits of co-cultures to the embryo include secretion of trophic factors such as nutrient substrates, growth factors and cytokines, and the removal of potentially toxic substances by feeder cell layers. The most promising co-culture method seems to be homologous endometrial cells.

Although previous randomized controlled studies failed to demonstrate a significant benefit for such conditions in unselected patient populations undergoing IVF–ET, recent studies have shown that co-culture was found to be highly beneficial for patients with RIF.[19]

*Metabolomics:* Since the selection of embryos for transfer is mainly based on morphological assessment of embryos at various stages of development. To improve the selection, metabolomic changes in the culture medium of embryos and oocytes (exometabolomics) may be measured determining what the embryo consumes or secretes (e.g. amino acids, proteins and oxygen consumption) and these parameters have been shown to correlate with embryo viability. These methods improve the selection of embryos thus improving the implantation rate. However, its application in women with RIF has yet to be confirmed.[20]

*Time-lapse monitoring:* The current scoring system for morphological assessment analyzes the fertilized egg and the embryo at a few predefined time points, thus missing all the events that occurred between these points. Continuous image monitoring of the cultured embryo through time lapse is a noninvasive method which provides a complete picture of the developmental kinetics that the embryo undergoes.

Meseguer et al.[21] identified the morphokinetic parameters specific to embryos that were capable of implanting, and proposed a multivariable model to classify embryos according to their probability of implantation. They concluded that image acquisition and time lapse analysis makes it possible to determine exact timing of embryo cleavage in clinical setting.

### Management of Abnormal Male Factor

Several studies have suggested that low sperm quality due to abnormalities in chromatin arrangements and compactions in the sperm, as well as increased DNA fragmentation, can lead to failure of implantation. Several treatment options may be considered for such cases.

*Antioxidants:* First, medical treatment in particular, oral antioxidant may be used to improve sperm quality and to reduce the incidence of sperm DNA fragmentation.

*Annexin-V:* A number of techniques have been proposed, to select spermatozoa with low levels of DNA damage from the ejaculated semen samples, such as use of annexin-V columns which has been shown to significantly reduce the percentage of spermatozoa with DNA fragmentation as measured by the TUNEL test and a sperm selection method incorporating sperm hyaluronic acid binding.

*Intracytoplasmic morphologically selected sperm (IMSI):* It is the refined form of ICSI which utilizes spermatozoa selected under high-power magnification (6000X) with a defined set of morphological criteria. Rationale behind the use is that routine sperm cell assessment identifies normal spermatozoa using low magnification. However, some hidden anomalies can only be detected at higher magnification.

A meta-analysis by Souza Setti et al.[22] comparing ICSI and IMSI outcome demonstrated a statistically significant improvement in implantation and pregnancy rates and a significant decrease in miscarriage rates with use of IMSI. However further randomized controlled studies are required to confirm the superiority of IMSI over ICSI.

*Surgical retrieval of sperms:* Studies have observed that sperm DNA damage is lower in the seminiferous tubules as compared with the cauda epididymis and ejaculated spermatozoa.[23] So in men with high levels of DNA damage in ejaculated spermatozoa, surgical removal of sperms from the testis for ICSI is recommended. This method of using testicular spermatozoa in couples with repeated implantation failure associated with high sperm DNA fragmentation in semen has been reported to result in a significant increase in pregnancy rate[24] and reduction of miscarriage rate, but further studies are required to confirm the benefit.

## Managing Uterine Factors

*Hysteroscopic correction of cavity pathologies:* It improves the clinical pregnancy rate and in addition to correction, hysteroscopy results in release of cytokines and growth factors secondary to endometrial injury thus helps in implantation. Following corrective procedures should be done:
- *Myomectomy:* Performance of hysteroscopic removal of submucous fibroids distorting the cavity is recommended. Resection of a solitary submucous fibroid less than 5 cm in diameter and with little intramural extension should not pose significant difficulties. However, a submucous fibroid more than 5 cm in diameter or more than 50% embedded in the intramural part of the uterus may require removal in two stages (Pritts et al.).
- *Septum resection:* Ban-Frangez et al.,[25] found that small and large septae had similar adverse impact, with significant increase in miscarriage rate in women undergoing IVF/ICSI treatment and recommended removal of septae regardless of the size.
- *Endometrial polyp:* As endometrial polyps affect the implantation; these should be removed in women with RIF.
- *Intrauterine adhesions:* It is accepted that intrauterine adhesions interfere with the implantation process and adversely affect the implantation rate and so, if present in women with RIF, should be removed. The procedure should be carried out by an experienced reproductive surgeon to minimize complications. Special measures including the use of antiadhesion barrier, intrauterine balloon, antibiotic therapy and high-dose estrogen in the postoperative period to promote regeneration of the endometrium should be considered.

## Managing Thin endometrium

The endometrium and its ability to provide, an environment suitable for embryo implantation is an important factor for implantation. RIF may sometimes be associated with a thin endometrium usually described as thickness less than 7 mm. Following approaches are advised for managing a thin endometrium.

*Hysteroscopic examination:* Hysteroscopic examination of the uterine cavity is recommended to rule out intrauterine adhesions or Asherman's syndrome.

*Vaginal sildenafil:* Sildenafil which is a phosphodiesterase-5 inhibitor augments the vasodilatory effects of nitric oxide. Thus it increases endometrial blood flow, which then leads to an increase in endometrial function.

*Low-dose aspirin:* For the management of the patients with thin endometrium, aspirin administration was shown to increase embryo implantation rate. Possible mechanism of aspirin is through improving the resistance of uterine blood flow in the peri-implantation period by shifting local production of thromboxane toward prostacyclin.[26]

*Endometrial perfusion with granulocyte colony-stimulating factor:* A recent study by Gleicher et al.,[27] reported the successful use of endometrial perfusion with granulocyte colony-stimulating factor in four women with inadequate development of endometrium and previously resistant to the use of estrogens and vasodilators. However, this novel approach requires further investigation to confirm its usefulness.

*Endometrial injury:* The possibility that local injury of the endometrium in the cycle preceding IVF treatment increases the success rate of implantation was proposed by Barash et al. The mechanism is that endometrial injury would induce up regulation of inflammatory cytokines, chemokines and growth factors which facilitate the process of implantation.

A recent systematic review of published literature and meta-analysis by Neelam Poddar et al.[28] provided strong evidence that endometrial injury done in the cycle before ovarian stimulation and IVF/ET increased the pregnancy rate in RIFs patients.

*Cryopreservation of embryos:* Another approach is to freeze all embryos, when thickness is less than 7 mm, and to transfer them in a natural cycle or alternatively, in an artificially prepared cycle, while applying increased dosages of estradiol, for as long as 3 weeks before progesterone is added.

*Endometrial reconstruction from stem cells:* Because of their ability to reconstruct endometrial tissues in vivo, adult stem cells have been identified in human endometrium. The identification of specific markers for endometrial mesenchymal stem cells and candidate markers for epithelial progenitor cells enables the potential use of endometrial stem/progenitor cells in reconstructing endometrial tissue in Asherman's syndrome and intrauterine adhesions.[29]

## Management of Thrombophilias

Treatment with low molecular weight heparin has been shown to significantly improve implantation, as well as the clinical pregnancy rate in patients with RIF, diagnosed with thrombophilia, in subsequent IVF attempts.[30] In patients with RIF who have prothrombotic disorder heparin treatment is beneficial, but for those without this abnormality empiric treatment with heparin is not justifiable.[31]

So, it is recommended that patients diagnosed with RIF should be investigated for acquired as well as hereditary thrombophilia disorders and be treated accordingly.

## Management of Immunological Factors

Role of immunological factors in implantation and maintenance of pregnancy has been described by several studies. Following treatment options have been proposed:

- *Paternal leukocyte immunization:* Previously used paternal leukocyte immunization is no longer recommended due to its possible side effects for mother and fetus because of its unpredicted immune response to either autologic or allogenic blood components[32].
- *IV immunoglobulin (IVIg):* Its administration is found beneficial in patients with RIF who share human leukocyte antigen (HLA) alleles with their partners. However due to higher cost of both HLA testing and IVIg treatment, it is recommended that assessment of immune system's contribution in RIF should be done in last, when other causes are ruled out.[33]
- *Intralipid (20%):* Intralipid has recently reported to improve outcome in women with RIF, especially in patients with elevated TH1 cytokine response. Intralipid is a fat emulsion which suppresses abnormal NK cytotoxic activity in peripheral NK cells both in vivo and in vitro.[34] However, large scale studies are recommended to prove the efficacy of intralipids.

## Managing Multifactorial Factors

*Hydrosalpinges:* Good evidences are available to recommend that removal of hydrosalpinges improve the implantation and live birth rate in patients undergoing IVF. In a meta-analysis, Johnson et al.[35] concluded that pregnancy and live birth rates doubled following prophylactic salpingectomy.

However, precautions should be taken to use diathermy or incision as close to fallopian tube as possible and far away from ovary to avoid disruption of blood supply. Other methods described for managing hydrosalpinges are salpingostomy, USG-guided drainage, or occlusion of proximal fallopian tube. However recommended treatment for hydrosalpinges in women with RIF is either salpingectomy or salpingostomy in cases with severe tubo-ovarian adhesions when surgical morbidity is increased hysteroscopic occlusion of tubes.

*Tailoring the stimulation protocols:* Luteal phase defect associated with the COH results in advanced endometrial histological maturity and decreased concentration of cytoplasmic progesterone receptors. Use of milder protocols has been demonstrated to improve implantation due to improved endometrial and embryo quality due to low E2.

*Improving embryo transfer techniques:* Since the difficult embryo transfer has been shown to affect pregnancy rate, atraumatic embryo transfer is recommended. Techniques used to reduce the trauma are, USG-guided ET, filling the bladder in women with acute anteversion and anteflexion, and use of soft tip catheters, etc.

Recently use of oxytocin antagonist atosiban has been tried in patients with RIF, before embryo transfer. A recent study[36] found that atosiban reduced the number of uterine contractions in these patients and also increased the implantation and pregnancy rates.

## ■ CONCLUSION

Recurrent implantation failure is distressing both to the patient as well as treating clinician. Since the etiology of RIF is ill understood and treatment options are vague, efforts should be put to ascertain the underlying cause of the condition and a multidisciplinary approach should be adopted in the management of RIF. Evaluation of cases of RIF is the most important aspect. The management is decided on the factor which is detected on evaluation. Management is a challenge in many cases as the cause of RIF may not be clear. Methods to improve results in all cases of RIF are yet to be established.

## ■ REFERENCES

1. Coughlan C, Ledger W, Wang Q, et al. Recurrent implantation failure: definition and management. Reprod Biomed Online. 2014;28(1):14-38.
2. Wang LY, Wang DH, Zou XY, et al. Mitochondrial functions on oocytes and preimplantation embryos. J Zhejiang Univ Sci B. 2009;10:483-92.
3. Collins JA, Barnhart K, Schlegel PN. Do sperm DNA integrity tests predict pregnancy with in vitro fertilization? Fertil Steril. 2008;89:823-31.
4. Rubio C, Gil-Salom M, Simon C, et al. Incidence of sperm chromosomal abnormalities in a risk population: relationship with sperm quality and ICSI outcome. Hum Reprod. 2001;16:2084-92.
5. Pritts EA, Parker WH, Olive DL. Fibroids and infertility: an updated systematic review of the evidence. Fertil Steril. 2009;91:1215-23.
6. Richter KS, Bugge KR, Bromer JG, et al. Relationship between endometrial thickness and embryo implantation, based on 1294 cycles of in vitro fertilization with transfer of two blastocyst stage embryos. Fertil Steril. 2007;87:53-9.
7. Maheshwari A, Gurunath S, Fatima F, et al. Adenomyosis and subfertility: a systematic review of prevalence, diagnosis, treatment and fertility outcomes. Hum Reprod Update. 2012;18:374-92.
8. Azem F, Many A, Ben Ami I, et al. Increased rates of thrombophilia in women with repeated IVF failures. Hum Reprod. 2004;19:368-70.
9. Simon A, Laufer N. Assessment and treatment of repeated implantation failure (RIF). J Assist Reprod Genet. 2012;29(11):1227-39.
10. Shokeir T, Abdelshaheed M. Sonohysterography as a first-line evaluation for uterine abnormalities in women with recurrent failed in vitro fertilization-embryo transfer. Fertil Steril. 2009;91:1321-2.

11. Makrakis E, Pantos K. The outcomes of hysteroscopy in women with implantation failures after in-vitro fertilization: findings and effect on subsequent pregnancy rates. Curr Opin Obstet Gynecol. 2010;22:339-43.
12. Donoso P, Staessen C, Fauser BC, et al. Current value of preimplantation genetic aneuploidy screening in IVF. Hum Reprod Update. 2007;13:15-25.
13. Fragouli E, Alfarawati S, Daphnis D, et al. Cytogenetic analysis of human blastocysts with the use of FISH, CGH and aCGH: Scientific data and technical evaluation. Hum Reprod. 2011;26:480-90.
14. Mastenbroek S. One swallow does not make a summer. Fertil Steril. 2013; 99(5):1205-6.
15. Glujovsky D, Blake D, Bardach A, et al. Cleavage stage versus blastocyst stage embryo transfer in assisted reproductive technology. Cochrane Database Syst Rev. 2013;6:CD002118.
16. Practice Committee of Society for Assisted Reproductive Technology; Practice Committee of American Society for Reproductive Medicine. The role of assisted hatching in in vitro fertilization: a review of the literature. A committee opinion. Fertil Steril. 2008;90(5 Suppl):S196-8.
17. Practice Committee of the ASRM. Role of assisted hatching in in vitro fertilization: a guideline. Fertil Steril. 2014;102:348-51.
18. Wael A, Madkour I, Noah B. Does sequential embryo transfer improve pregnancy rate in patients with repeated implantation failure? A randomized control study. Middle East Fertil Soc. 2015;20(4):255-61.
19. Eyheremendy V, Raffo FG, Papayannis M, et al. Beneficial effect of autologous endometrial cell coculture in patients with repeated implantation failure. Fertil Steril. 2010;93:769-73.
20. Scott L, Berntsen J, Davies D, et al. Symposium: innovative techniques in human embryo viability assessment. Human oocyte respiration-rate measurement--potential to improve oocyte and embryo selection? Reprod Biomed Online. 2008;17(4):461-9.
21. Meseguer M, Herrero J, Tejera A, et al. The use of morphokinetics as a predictor of embryo implantation. Hum Reprod. 2011;26:2658-71.
22. Souza Setti A, Ferreira RC, Paes de Almeida Ferreira Braga D. Intracytoplasmic sperm injection outcome versus intracytoplasmic morphologically selected sperm injection outcome: a meta-analysis. Reprod Biomed Online. 2010;21:450-5.
23. Greco E, Scarselli F, Iacobelli M, et al. Efficient treatment of infertility due to sperm DNA damage by ICSI with testicular spermatozoa. Hum Reprod. 2005;20:226-30.
24. Weissman A, Horowitz E, Ravhon A, et al. Pregnancies and live births following ICSI with testicular spermatozoa after repeated implantation failure using ejaculated spermatozoa. Reprod Biomed Online. 2008;17:605-9.
25. Ban-Frangez H, Tomazevic T, Virant-Klun I. The outcome of singleton pregnancies after IVF/ICSI in women before and after hysteroscopic resection of a uterine septum compared to normal controls. Eur J Obstet Gynecol Reprod Biol. 2009;146:184-7.

26. Hsieh YY, Tsai HD, Chang CC, et al. Low-dose aspirin for infertile women with thin endometrium receiving intrauterine insemination: a prospective, randomized study. J Assist Reprod Genet. 2000; 17(3):174-7.
27. Gleicher N, Vidali A, Barad DH. Successful treatment of unresponsive thin endometrium. Fertil Steril. 2011;95(2123):e13-7.
28. Potdar N, Gelbaya T, Nardo LG. Endometrial injury to overcome recurrent embryo implantation failure: a systematic review and meta-analysis. Reprod Biomed Online. 2012;25(6):561-71.
29. Gargett CE, Ye L. Endometrial reconstruction from stem cells. Fertil Steril. 2012;98(1):11-20.
30. Qublan H, Amarin Z, Dabbas M, et al. Low-molecular weight heparin in the treatment of recurrent IVF-ET failure and thrombophilia: a prospective randomized placebo-controlled trial. Hum Fertil (Camb). 2008;11:246-53.
31. Seshadri S, Sunkara SK. Low-molecular-weight-heparin in recurrent implantation failure. Fertil Steril. 2011;95:e29.
32. Tanaka T, Umesaki N, Nishio J, et al. Neonatal thrombocytopenia induced by maternal anti-HLA antibodies: a potential side effect of allogenic leukocyte immunization for unexplained recurrent aborters. J Reprod Immunol. 2000;46:51-7.
33. ElramT, Simon A, Israel S, et al. Treatment of recurrent IVF failure and human leukocyte antigen similarity by intravenous immunoglobulin. Reprod Biomed Online. 2005;11:745-9.
34. Ndukwe G. Recurrent embryo implantation failure after in vitro fertilisation: improved outcome following intralipid infusion in women with elevated T Helper 1 response. Hum Fertil (Camb). 2011;14(2):21-2.
35. Johnson N, van Voorst S, Sowter MC, et al. Surgical treatment for tubal disease in women due to undergo in vitro fertilisation. Cochrane Database Syst Rev. 2004;(3):CD002125.
36. Lan VT, Khang VN, Nhu GH, et al. Atosiban improves implantation and pregnancy rates in patients with repeated implantation failure. Reprod Biomed Online. 2012; 25(3):254-60.

# CHAPTER 27

# Empty Follicle Syndrome: Myth or Reality?

*K Jayakrishnan, Niranjana Jayakrishnan*

## ■ INTRODUCTION

The failure to recover any oocytes from mature-size ovarian follicles during oocyte retrieval was first described 25 years ago by Coulam et al.[1] and is now known as "empty follicle syndrome (EFS)". The etiology remains enigmatic, and the very existence of this syndrome has been questioned.

The prevalence of EFS has been reported to vary between 0.6% and 7%. Stevenson and Lashen described two types of EFS in 2008. Cases of EFS can be subdivided into "false" (F-EFS) or "genuine" (G-EFS).

False-empty follicle syndrome is rigorously defined as instances in which no oocytes are retrieved in the setting of undetectable serum or urine levels of beta-human chorionic gonadotropin ($\beta$-hCG), suggesting either a human or pharmaceutical error. G-EFS is defined as cases in which no oocytes are retrieved, despite appropriate levels of $\beta$-hCG. In a review of EFS by Stevenson et al. 33% of EFS cases were labeled as genuine and 67% as false. Regardless of the etiology, EFS is a condition that may cause substantial stress and anxiety for both the patient and physician during assisted reproductive technology (ART).[2]

A subset of patients have appropriate serum $\beta$-hCG levels at the time of oocyte retrieval and report receiving the medication at the appropriate time, but despite adequate follicle size and vigorous follicle aspiration, no oocytes are recovered. Furthermore, there are recurrent cases of EFS in the same patient,[3] suggesting the existence of a problem other than hCG administration. Notably, patients with repeated EFS have a significantly reduced likelihood of pregnancy that ranges from 0% to 6.25% per cycle. Even more intriguing, instances of repeated G-EFS have been reported in sisters or in the setting of a chromosomal anomaly, suggesting a genetic basis for the syndrome. While a genetic etiology seems likely in some cases, the prevalence of the condition is reported to vary widely.

## POSSIBLE THEORIES

Several possible causes of G-EFS have been proposed. Some reports propose an error in folliculogenesis or premature apoptosis of the oocytes that still continued follicular growth.[4] Other investigators suggest that in rare cases follicles may need longer exposure to hCG to undergo cumulus expansion and separate from the follicular wall. It is worth noting that EFS has been reported with immature oocytes that were zona-free or that had a zona that was lacking in oocytes, which suggests that abnormal oocytes may cause some cases.

Another possibility is a yet-to-be discovered genetic cause of the syndrome. Possible candidate genes include genes shown in studies of knockout mice to be required for folliculogenesis and fertility. Luteinizing hormone (LH)-dependent cumulus expansion requires communication between the mural granulosa cells and the cumulus complex involving amphiregulin, epiregulin, and beta-cellulin. These growth factors induce expression of prostaglandin synthase 2 (*Ptgs2*), tumor necrosis factor alpha-induced protein (*Tnfaip 6*), and hyaluronan synthase 2 (*Has2*), which in turn are necessary for cumulus expansion and subsequent oocyte release. It remains to be determined whether G-EFS is accompanied by altered expression of genes regulating cumulus expansion, but studies in mice support the possibility of such a mechanism.[5]

## PREDICTING EMPTY FOLLICLE SYNDROME

Optimal serum concentrations of hCG to predict EFS and a successful yield of mature oocytes are still not unequivocally defined. Various authors have reported various levels of serum β-hCG as the threshold cut-off value on the day of OR; a serum hCG levels less than 10 mIU/mL as reported by Ndukwe et al. could predict EFS with a sensitivity and specificity of 100%.[6] Driscoll et al. reported a median serum hCG concentration of 117.1 IU/L (range: 48–249) after R-hCG 250 µg and 83.6 IU/L (range: 32–99) with 5,000 IU urinary hCG due to the immunoassays used to measure serum hCG. Urinary hCG may contain dissociated and oxidized subunits that would be detected by immunoassay but may have no biological activity. R-hCG, due to the absence of contaminant urinary proteins and the exacting standards applied during the production process, may make it possible to predict the risk of unsuccessful or more accurately.

## THERAPEUTIC APPROACH

Patients with EFS present a challenge to the treating physician. No single treatment is universally effective. Some authors, relying on the low frequency of recurrence, recommend repeating the standard ART cycle, regardless of the treatment protocol. Since in most EFS cases, downregulation was achieved by GnRH agonist (possibly presenting the higher prevalence of agonist over antagonist in ART cycles), shifting from an agonist to antagonist protocol was suggested. In cases where no oocytes are aspirated[7] from one ovary and hCG levels are low, some have suggested readministering hCG from a different batch and aspirating the second ovary or even reaspirating the same follicles. Others suggested changing the hCG from a urinary to a recombinant preparation.

## ■ GnRH AGONIST FOR TRIGGERING FINAL OOCYTE MATURATION

Human chorionic gonadotropin has long been used as a surrogate for the LH surge. Later on, it was demonstrated that ovulation triggering may be achieved by GnRH agonist. Among the possible advantages of GnRH agonist for final oocyte maturation is the simultaneous induction of a follicle-stimulating hormone (FSH) surge. The role of the natural mid-cycle FSH surge is not fully clear. FSH was reported to induce LH receptor formation in luteinizing granulosa cells, promote oocyte nuclear maturation and cumulus expansion.[8] FSH also has a role in keeping the gap junctions open between the oocyte and cumulus cells and thus may have an important role in signaling pathways. FSH stimulates plasminogen activator activity within granulosa cells, which results in production of plasmin in the follicular fluid. Plasmin, in turn, generates active collagenase which disrupts the follicular wall. Expansion and dispersion of the cumulus cells allows the oocyte–cumulus cell mass to detach from the follicular wall before ovulation. This process involves synthesis of hyaluronic acid matrix, which is stimulated by FSH. Adding FSH at the time of the hCG trigger enhances oocyte recovery and improves fertilization. GnRH receptors have been identified in a wide variety of human tissues including preovulatory granulosa cells. Mammalian oocytes remain at prophase of first meiosis from birth until the gonadotropin surge at puberty. During this long period, intraoocyte cAMP and cGMP prevents oocyte meiosis resumption. The cGMP level decreases in response to LH and meiosis resumes. It was demonstrated that peripheral GnRH receptor activation leads to a decrease in the intracellular cAMP level. GnRH induces transcription of several genes that are involved in follicular rupture and oocyte maturation. The FSH surge and the direct action of the agonist on the ovarian GnRH receptor might explain the favorable results in the eighth cycle in our patient. One can speculate that, for an unknown reason, the LH path is blocked in the patient and the GnRH agonist activates a different path.

## ■ DUAL TRIGGER

The concept being a "dual trigger" combines a single dose of the GnRH agonist with a reduced or standard dosage of hCG at the time of triggering. The use of a GnRH agonist with a reduced dose of hCG in high responders demonstrated luteal phase support with improved pregnancy rates, similar to those after conventional hCG and a low risk of ovarian hyperstimulation syndrome (OHSS). The administration of a GnRH agonist and a standard hCG in normal responders, demonstrated significantly improved live-birth rates and a higher number of embryos of excellent quality, or cryopreserved embryos. The concept of the "double trigger" represents a combination of a GnRH agonist and a standard hCG, when used 40 hr and 34 hr prior to ovum pick-up, respectively. The use of the "double trigger" has been successfully offered in the treatment of empty follicle syndrome and in patients with a history of immature oocytes retrieved or with low/poor oocytes yield. Further prospective studies are required to confirm the aforementioned observations prior to clinical implementation.

## ■ PROLONGING THE INTERVAL BETWEEN OVULATION TRIGGERING AND OVUM PICK-UP

In a natural cycle, the onset of LH surge occurs 34–36 hr prior to follicular rupture. Similarly, administering exogenous hCG causes follicular rupture after approximately 37 hr (Edwards and Steptoe, 1975). Resumption of meiosis begins 18 hr after the onset of the LH surge. LH concentration must be maintained above a threshold for 14–27 hr in order to maximize oocyte maturation. Follicular rupture and oocyte maturation are time-dependent processes, with different times needed in different patients. It might be hypothesized that cumulus expansion which allows the oocyte to detach from the follicular wall also requires longer time periods in certain patients. In these cases, EFS may result when aspiration takes place 34 hr after hCG administration.

## ■ CONCLUSION

Implantation may be impaired in patients with sporadically occurring EFS. Additionally, those patients with recurrent cycles of EFS are likely to have advanced age, poor response, dropped cycles, and diminished pregnancy rate, so that oocyte donation might be their best option for conception.

Whatever the underlying cause of an EFS cycle, patients with an EFS cycle should be counseled regarding the possibility of recurrence of such an event in future cycles. Care should also be taken, during future oocyte retrievals from these patients, to aspirate some of the follicles initially and, if no oocyte-cumulus complex (OCC) are noted, then proceed with a another retrieval attempt following administration of a second dose of hCG as previously reported by several authors.

## ■ KEY POINTS

- Prevalence of 0.6–7%
- Two types of EFS: False and genuine
- Optimal concentrations of hCG may be used to detect EFS
- Dual trigger used successfully to retrieve oocytes in EFS
- Recurrence in future cycles, a possibility.

## REFERENCES

1. Coulam CB, Bustillo M, Schulman JD. Empty follicle syndrome. Fertil Steril. 1986;46:1153-5.
2. Ben-Shlomo K, Schiff E, Levran D, et al. Failure of oocyte retrieval during in vitro fertilization: a sporadic event rather than a syndrome. Fertil Steril. 1991;53:324-7.
3. Awonuga A, Govindbhadi ZS, Schnauffer K. Continuing the debate on empty follicle syndrome: can it be associated with normal bioavailability of β-human chorionic gonadotrophin on the day of oocyte recovery? Hum Reprod. 1998;13:1281-4.
4. Desai N, Austin C, Abdel Hafez F, et al. Evidence of "genuine empty follicles" in follicular aspirate: a case report. Hum Reprod. 2009;24:1171-5.
5. Ashkenazi H, Cao X, Matola S, et al. Epidermal growth factor family mediators of the ovulatory response. Endocrinology. 2005;146:77-84.
6. Ndukwe G, Thornton S, Fishel S, et al. Curing empty follicle syndrome. Hum Reprod. 1997;12:21-3.
7. Reichman DE, Hornstein MD, Jackson KV, et al. Empty follicle syndrome-does repeat administration of hCG really work? Fertil Steril. 2010:94:375-7.
8. Humaidan P, Kol S, Papanikolaou E. The Copenhagen GnRH Agonist Triggering Workshop Group. GnRH agonist for triggering of final oocyte maturation: time for a change of practice? Hum Reprod Update. 2011;17:510-24.

# CHAPTER 28

# Luteinized Unruptured Follicle Syndrome: A Mystery

*Gita Khanna, Kalika Dubey, Farhat Kazim, Arti Gupta*

## ■ INTRODUCTION

During the last stage of puberty, the hypothalamic-pituitary-ovarian axis acquires the ability to respond to high levels of estradiol; this results in a sharp increase in the pituitary output of luteinizing hormone (LH). It is believed that within a mature follicle, the LH surge triggers a complex set of events that results in two apparently independent phenomena: ovulation and luteinization. The term ovulation will imply rupture of the follicular wall and release of an oocyte, whereas luteinization will imply the morphologic and biochemical shift in the granulosa cells toward the production of progesterone.

Ovulation is associated with significant hormonal changes, and the process is primarily under the control of LH. This is the hormone that rises in the mid-cycle, surge occurs about 36 hours before ovulation and is the basis for home ovulation predictor kits. During this process, cellular chemicals called prostaglandins and proteolytic enzymes weaken the wall of the follicle, resulting in an opening, or rupture, through which the oocyte is released. It then enters the fallopian tube where it awaits fertilization. The cells left behind in the follicle undergo a hormonal change called luteinization and produce progesterone, the hormone that prepares and maintains the uterine lining for implantation. This structure is now called a corpus luteum. If pregnancy does not occur, the activity of the corpus luteum declines. As estrogen and progesterone levels fall, menstruation follows.

When a woman has regular cycles, in more than 95% of cases it is the sign of regular ovulation. Most tests that are used to confirm ovulation document only the hormonal changes. Serial ultrasound studies can be used to follow the growth of the follicle and its collapse following ovulation. In a small percentage of normal women, the dominant follicle will occasionally undergo the luteinization process without rupture following the mid-cycle surge. As a result of the increased progesterone secretion, the uterine lining develops its normal characteristic changes following ovulation, but no oocyte is released and conception cannot occur. This phenomenon is called the luteinized unruptured follicle (LUF) (Fig. 1).

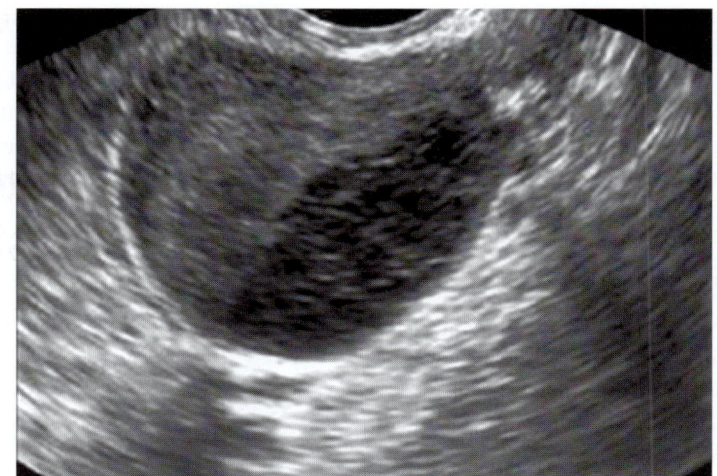

**Fig. 1:** Ultrasound of a luteinized unruptured follicle.

## ■ DEFINITION

Luteinized unruptured follicle syndrome, also known as *trapped egg syndrome,* is defined as a failure of ovulation, in which despite the absence of follicular rupture and release of the oocyte, the unruptured follicle undergoes luteinization under the action of LH. LUF can also be defined as failure of the ovulatory follicle to rupture on ultrasound examination performed daily from day 10 to 20 of the cycle despite normal indices of ovulation.

## ■ HISTORY OF LUF

Interest in the diagnosis of LUF as a pathologic distinctive entity was sparked by two reports published in 1978 in the same issue of fertility and sterility. Marik and Hulka[1] as well as Koninckx et al.[2] reported independently the absence of ovulatory stigmata during laparoscopy in a group of infertile women during the early luteal phase. This leads to further studies in diagnosing and solving the mystery of LUF.

## ■ INCIDENCE

The true incidence of this problem in both the fertile and infertile population was thought to be low until recently. With new improved diagnostic tools such as B-mode ultrasonography (USG) rise in the incidence of LUF is seen. It is thought, but not proven, that women with 'unexplained' infertility may experience this phenomenon a bit more often than fertile women.

LUF is seen in 10% of menstrual cycles of normal fertile females.[3] The incidence of LUF has been reported to be 25–43% in infertile women. The recurrence of LUF increases from 25% in first cycle to 78.6% and 90% in second and third cycle,[4] respectively, so an increased tendency to recur in subsequent cycles is observed.

Yun et al.[5] reported that more than half of LUF cycles had luteal phase shorter than 11 days, suggesting inadequate luteal functions presenting in LUF cycle. There is evidence that the incidence of LUF in ovulation cycles were higher than that in natural cycle.[6] In a study, the incidence of LUF was reported 58.9% in ovulation induction cycle (clomiphene citrate cycle).[7]

## ■ DISEASES ASSOCIATED WITH LUF

- Polycystic ovaries [polycystic ovarian disease (PCOD)]
- Endometriosis
- Pelvic inflammatory disease
- Hyperprolactinemia
- Pelvic adhesions
- Genital tuberculosis.

## ■ ETIOPATHOGENESIS OF LUF

The mechanism of LUF is attributed to the following factors.

### Endocrinal Factors

These refer to the internal environmental factors leading to ovulation disorders, such as elevated level of cyclic adenosine monophosphate due to insufficient secretion of LH, reduced secretion of progesterone, lowered activity of profibrinolysin activators, decreased fibrinolysis and autolysis of the wall of the ovaries leading to disorders in the maturation of follicles, cleavage and discharge of oocytes.[8]

### Mechanical Factors

Luteinized unruptured follicle cycles might also result from defects as collagen, which usually lead to lowered progesterone level.[9,10] The later condition is also known as "false LUF". It is usually caused by adhesion, thickening of pelvic soft tissues resulting from infarction of fallopian tube, endometriosis, pelvic surgeries or inflammation.[11]

### Role of Prostaglandins

Prostaglandin E2 (PGE) stimulates the production of plasminogen activator by granulosa cells, although PGF 2α does not. Plasminogen activator catalyzes a reaction that produces plasmin, an enzyme capable of weakening follicle wall strips in vitro. Morphologic studies in the rabbit and human ovarian surface epithelium immediately before ovulation have demonstrated the presence of lysosomes after administration of human chorionic gonadotropin (hCG).[12,13]

PGF 2α makes the lysosome more labile, a mechanism by which it may play role in ovulation. Thus any factor decreasing prostaglandin concentration will lead to decrease in ovulation.

In a recent provocative double-blind crossover study, placebo or a prostaglandin synthetase inhibitor was administered to normal volunteers undergoing sonographic follicular monitoring.[14] The spontaneous incidence of LUF was 10.7%. All eight patients receiving periovulatory indomethacin and 5 of 10 azapropazone treated cycles, had evidence of LUF. Early luteal (day 7) progesterone concentrations were lower in LUF cycles, when compared in the same patient with ovulatory or pharmacologically induced LUF cycles. Thus LUF cycles are evident in females using certain nonsteroidal anti-inflammatory drugs (NSAIDs), such as mezolin, meloxicam, etc.[15,16]

## ■ DIAGNOSIS

The diagnosis of LUF has been made in the past by laparoscopically with direct visualization of the ovaries, by hormonal profiles of the peritoneal fluid, and by USG. B-mode USG is the standard tool used nowadays to diagnose LUF. A study on ovarian blood flow by USG, demonstrated that intraovarian resistance indexes (RI) of LUF cycles was similar to those of anovulatory cycles but was much higher as compared with the ovulatory cycles.[17,18] The high impedance of flow was partially caused by the defective corpus luteum formation and angiogenesis.[19]

## ■ DIAGNOSTIC CRITERIA OF LUF

The diagnostic criteria of LUF on USG are:[20,21]
- Continuous growth in size of the follicle with a thickened follicular wall and increased internal resonance; meanwhile, extensive intrafollicular bright spots would be detected after 2–4 days
- Rapid enlargement of the size of follicle to 30–35 mm in diameter with strong internal resonance, persistent till the next cycle or even longer.
- The presence of lowered cervical score, biphase of BBT, elevated serum LH, E2 and P level at the time together with the above findings establish the diagnosis of LUF. The serum P levels are more than 3 ng/mL (9.5 nmol/L) in LUF cycles.[22]

## ■ SIGNS AND SYMPTOMS OF LUF

### A "Silent" Problem

Luteinized unruptured follicle is a "silent" problem and because it does not cause any symptoms or signs, it is very easy to miss the diagnosis as well! Diagnosis is made on the basis of imaging. The only symptom of LUF is that conception does not occur.

## PREVENTION OF LUF

There is no clear prevention for LUF to happen. On the other hand, the quality of alimentation has quite great impact on hormonal balance of the body, including progesterone production. Proper supplementation with fatty acids may help to maintain the progesterone balance within the body and prevent luteal defect to happen, thus reducing the chances of LUF.

## MANAGEMENT OF LUF

Once the diagnosis of LUF is made which is statistically more frequent in women with unexplained infertility, the goal is to achieve ovulation. Various studies have been done with different ovulation induction protocols to overcome this problem.

### Clomiphene Citrate-HMG versus Letrozole-HMG

Ovulation induction can be done by clomiphene citrate which is a selective estrogen receptor modulator, administrated orally in doses of 100 mg/day from day 2 to 6 of menstrual cycle. Another category of drug used for ovulation induction is aromatase inhibitor—letrozole given in a dose of 5 mg/day from day 3 to 7 of the menstrual cycle. Then HMG 75 IU/day is administered intramuscularly on day 8 of the menstrual cycle and the dose is adjusted based on ovarian response. Transvaginal sonography is performed on day 10 or 11 of the menstrual cycle in order to monitor follicular growth.

A randomized control single blinded clinical study was done in Department of Reproduction and Infertility, Mirza Kouchak Khan Women's Hospital, Tehran University of Medical Sciences, Tehran, Iran in 2014 by Azra et al.[23] A total number of 196 subjects were taken. Comparison was done by making two groups on the above two ovulation induction protocols. Ovulation was determined based on the complete collapse of the preovulatory follicle or the shrinkage of it to at least 50% of its primary size with or without free fluid in the pouch of Douglas and serum mid-luteal progesterone more than or equal to 10 ng/mL. LUF was diagnosed when none of the follicles ruptured and mid-luteal progesterone level more than 3 ng/mL. Serum β-hCG was measured 1 week after the missed period in order to confirm a biochemical pregnancy. Luteal phase support by progesterone was given to none of the patients. All hormonal assays were conducted by ELISA. The outcome was compared between the two medication groups. There was significant difference between clomiphene-HMG and letrozole-HMG in LUF ($p = 0.021$) and pregnancy rates ($p = 0.041$). Thus, letrozole with a lower incidence of LUF is more effective than clomiphene citrate for induction of ovulation. This is because clomiphene citrate has an estrogenic structure and downregulates estrogen receptors in the hypothalamus. It seems that a central antiestrogenic effect and a longer half-life (2 weeks) of clomiphene citrate leads to unexpulsion of the oocyte, but letrozole has a shorter half-life (45 hours) and does not reduce estrogen receptors.

## hCG Trigger

Since LH is responsible for inducing follicular rupture, LUF can be treated by giving an injection of hCG in a dose of 10,000 IU intramuscularly, when the lead follicle reaches 18–20 mm in diameter. Ultrasound is used to document ovulation. It takes about 36–40 hours for the oocyte to be released after the injection. Intercourse or insemination should be timed accordingly. If it still does not take place, the dose of the hCG injection can be increased. If ovulation still cannot be achieved even with an increased dose of 20,000 IU, then IVF is the best solution.[7]

## ■ LUF AND INFERTILITY

There is no agreement, however, as to whether LUF is only a contributing factor (causing *subfertility*) or an entity important enough to cause infertility by itself.

The LUF must meet one of these conditions in order to be considered as a factor causing infertility:

- It must be significantly more common in infertile women.
- It must be a recurrent phenomenon or, in other words, occur in a significant proportion of the menstrual cycles of any particular infertile patient diagnosed as having the syndrome.
- It must be associated with lower pregnancy rates than in similar ovulatory women.

Various studies have done worldwide and showed a significant association of LUF and subfertility.

## ■ LUF AND PELVIC ADHESIONS

It is seen that in cases where pelvic adhesions are present the incidence of LUF increases. In a study, Devroey et al.[24] examined the ovaries laparoscopically and collected peritoneal fluid in 26 infertile women 3 days after the LH peak. Eighteen women had visible corpora lutea, 10 of them had LUF (38%), and 8 had a luteinized ruptured follicle (LRF). In eight patients, the corpus luteum could not be identified due to adhesions localized exclusively in the periovarian region. The volume of peritoneal fluid was significantly higher in LRF than in LUF; likewise, the volume in LUF patients was significantly higher than in the volume in patients with periovarian adhesions. E2 levels were higher in LRF than in LUF cases. Since serum progesterone did not differ in these groups and the endometrium was secretory in all cycles, Devroey et al.[24] concluded that ovarian adhesions impair ovulation but not luteinization. Similarly, in Marik and Hulka's study[25] the incidence of LUF in patients with adhesions (71%) was higher than in patients with normal pelvis (33%).

## LUF AND ENDOMETRIOSIS

Women with severe endometriosis have significantly higher incidence of LUF diagnosed at laparoscopy as compared to the females without the disease. This has been proven in various studies done over the years. In one such study Brosens and colleagues[26] found LUF in 1 (6.3%) of 16 infertile women undergoing laparoscopy and in 23 (79%) of 29 patients with endometriosis. The authors acknowledged that the laparoscopic inspection of the ovaries in patients with endometriosis was not always complete. Nevertheless, the same conclusion persisted when control infertile women were compared with a set of 13 patients with mild endometriosis. Ten of these women (77%) presented with LUF. Thus, it shows that endometriosis has a strong correlation with LUF.

## CONCLUSION

Without release of an oocyte, it is impossible for a woman to get pregnant in the "old fashion" way, meaning that LUF significantly reduces the fertility potential of a woman. Yet luteinized unruptured follicles syndrome is not affecting every ovulation so it may "just" take significantly longer time to get pregnant.

To conclude, LUF is a silent problem that needs to be investigated and searched upon thoroughly in order to diagnose it as soon as possible and relieve the female of her anxiety!

## KEY POINTS

- LUF is a silent problem.
- Incidence of LUF increases in subsequent cycles.
- LUF is associated with other disorders like PCOD, endometriosis, PID and genital TB.
- USG is the standard diagnostic modality for LUF.
- Letrozole is associated with decrease incidence of LUF as compared to clomiphene citrate.
- hCG trigger to an increased dose of 20,000 IU has shown a positive outcome in LUF.

## REFERENCES

1. Marik J, Hulka J. Luteinized unruptured follicle syndrome: a subtle cause of infertility. Fertil Steril. 1978;29:270.
2. Koninckx PR, Heyns WJ, Corvelyn PA, et al. Delayed onset of luteinization as a cause of infertility. Fertil Steril. 1978;29:266.
3. Killick S, Elstein M. Pharmacologic production of luteinized unruptured follicles by prostaglandin synthetase inhibitors. Fertil Steril. 1978;47:773-7.
4. Wang L, Qiao J, Liu P, et al. Effect of luteinized unruptured follicle cycles on clinical outcomes of frozen thawed embryo transfer in Chinese women. J Assist Reprod Genet. 2008;25(6):229-33.

5. Yun F, Zijiang C, Zhongli Y. Luteinized unruptured follicle syndrome: clinical analysis of 30 cases. Acta Academic Medicine Shandong. 1994;32:236-8.
6. Giannopoulos T, Sherriff E, Croucher C. Follicle tracking of women receiving clomiphene citrate for ovulation induction. J Obstet Gynaecol. 2005;25:169-71.
7. Qublan H, Amarin Z, Nawasreh M, et al. Luteinized unruptured follicle syndrome: incidence and recurrence rate in infertile women with unexplained infertility undergoing intrauterine insemination. Hum Reprod. 2006;21:2110-3.
8. Gumen A, Wiltbank MC. Length of progesterone exposure needed to resolve large follicle anovular condition in dairy cows. Theriogenology. 2005;63:202-18.
9. Gottsch ML, Van Kirk EA, Murdoch WJ. Tumour necrosis factor alpha up-regulates matrix metalloproteinase-2 activity in periovulatory ovine follicles: metamorphic and endocrine implications. Reprod Fertil Dev. 2000;12:75-80.
10. Murdoch WJ, Gottsch ML. Proteolytic mechanisms in the ovulatory folliculo-luteal transformation. Connect Tissue Res. 2003;44:50-7.
11. Hamilton CJ, Wetzels LC, Evers JL, et al. Follicle growth curves and hormonal patterns in patients with the luteinized unruptured follicle syndrome. Fertil Steril. 1985;43:541-8.
12. Bjersing L, Cajander S. Ovulation and the role of the ovarian surface epithelium. Experimentia. 1975;31:60.
13. Okamura H, Takenaka A, Yajima Y, et al. Ovulatory changes in the wall at the apex of the human Graafian follicle. J Reprod Fertil. 1980;58:153.
14. Killick S, Elstein M. Pharmacologic production of luteinized unruptured follicles by prostaglandin synthetase inhibitors. Fertil Steril. 1978;47:773.
15. Salhab AS, Amro BI, Shomaf MS. Further investigation on meloxicam contraceptivity in female rabbits: luteinizing unruptured follicles, a microscopic evidence. Contraception. 2003;67:485-9.
16. Stone S, Khamashta MA, Nelson-Piercy C. Nonsteroidal anti-inflammatory drugs and reversible female infertility: is there a link? Drug Safety. 2002;25:545-51.
17. Dal J, Vural B, Caliskan E, et al. Power Doppler ultrasound studies of ovarian, uterine, and endometrial blood flow in regularly menstruating women with respect to luteal phase defects. Fertil Steril. 2005;84:224-7.
18. Merce LT, Garces D, Barco MJ, et al. Intraovarian Doppler velocimetry in ovulatory, dysovulatory and anovulatory cycles. Ultrasound Obstet Gynecol. 1992;2:197-202.
19. Abulafia O, Sherer DM. Angiogenesis of the ovary. Am J Obstet Gynecol. 2000;182:240-6.
20. Check JH, Adelson HG, Dietterich C, et al. Pelvic sonography can predict ovum release in gonadotrophin-treated patients as determined by pregnancy rate. Hum Reprod. 1990;5:234-6.
21. Jie Q, Meizhi L. Analysis of the factors related with luteinized untrupture follicle syndrome of patients with polycystic ovarian syndrome after ovulation induction. Chin J Clin Obstet Gynecol. 2000;1:137-40.
22. Coulam CB, Hill LM, Breckle R. Ultrasonic evidence for luteinization of unruptured preovulatory follicles. Fertil Steril. 1982;37:524-9.
23. Azmoodeh A, Manesh MP, Asbagh FA, et al. Effects of letrozole-HMG and clomiphene-hmg on incidence of luteinized unruptured follicle syndrome in

infertile women undergoing induction ovulation and intrauterine insemination: a randomised trial. Global J Health Sci. 2016;8(4):1-9.
24. Devroey P, Temmerman M, Naaktgeboren N, et al. Ovarian adhesions impair ovulation. Acta Eur Fertil. 1985;16:183.
25. Marik J, Hulka J. Luteinized unruptured follicle syndrome: a subtle cause of infertility. Fertil Steril. 1978;29:270.
26. Brosens A, Koninckx PR, Corveleyn PA. A study of plasma progesterone, oestradiol-17β, prolactin and LH levels, and of the luteal phase appearance of the ovaries in patients with endometriosis and infertility. Br J Obstet Gynaecol. 1978;85:246.

# CHAPTER 29

# Poor Responders

*GA Ramaraju*

## ■ INTRODUCTION

After Gracia et al. in 1983 published the first study on poor responders, a lot of research done. It is the 34th years in the area of diagnosis, pathogenesis, characterization and possible treatment. In in vitro fertilization (IVF) the incidence of poor ovarian responder varies from 10–20%. The prevalence also depends on the age of the population as per clinical observation. Lower prevalence is seen in women below 34 years and higher prevalence is seen in women as they age closer to 40 years and beyond.[1]

## ■ DEFINITION

In the initial decades of IVF there was lot of confusion what constitutes a poor response until ESHRE stepped in to create the Bologna consensus statement on poor responders. Like polycystic ovary Rotterdam criteria this will improve with time and fine tune research in the right direction. There should be a word of caution in interpretation of poor responder and hyporesponder. Poor responder is a state whatever you do the number of eggs will not increase. Whereas a hyporesponder is a lady with appropriate dose and understanding of LH polymorphism will improve the number of oocyte yields in the subsequent cycle (Fig. 1).

## ■ BOLOGNA CRITERIA

Following the introduction of Bologna Criteria there certain amount of clarity is coming and recently another group named Poseidon group have come up with another classification called Poseidon classification.[2,3] The basic difference between both the groups are one involves age of 40 years (Bologna) and another involves age of 35 years and additional subset called hyporesponder.

At least two of the following three features must be present: Two episodes of POR after maximal stimulation are sufficient to define a patient as poor responder in the absence of advanced maternal age or abnormal ORT.

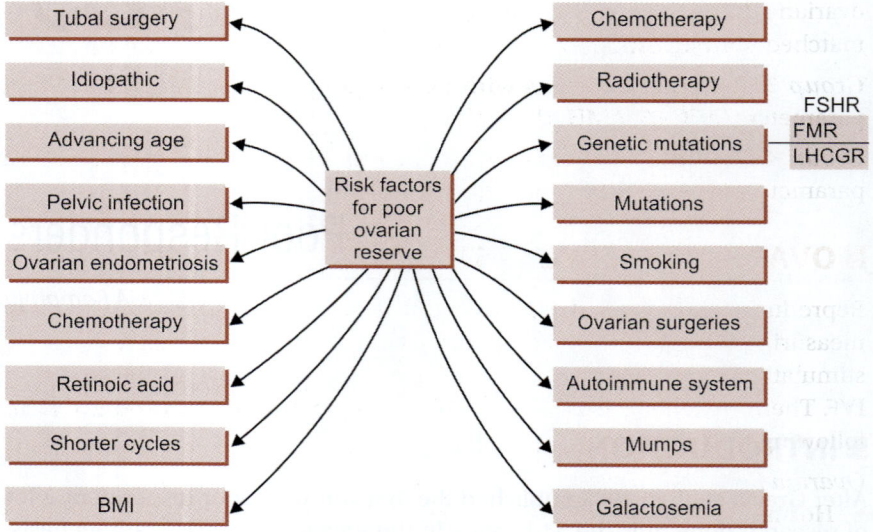

**Fig. 1:** Risk factors for poor ovarian reserve.

- Advanced maternal age (≥40 years) or any other risk factor for POR;
- A previous POR (≤3 oocytes with a conventional stimulation protocol);
- An abnormal ovarian reserve test [i.e. antral follicle count (AFC) <5–7 follicles or anti-Müllerian hormone (AMH) <0.5–1.1 ng/mL].

By definition, the term POR refers to the ovarian response and, therefore, one stimulated cycle is considered essential for the diagnosis of POR. However, patients over 40 years of age with an abnormal ORT may be classified as poor responders since both advanced age and an abnormal ORT may indicate reduced ovarian reserve and act as a surrogate of ovarian stimulation cycle. In this case, the patients should be more properly defined as expected PORs.

## POSEIDON CLASSIFICATION

*Group 1:* Patients < 35 years with sufficient prestimulation ovarian reserve parameters (AFC R5, AMH R1.2 ng/mL) and with an unexpected poor or suboptimal ovarian response. This group could be further divided into: subgroup 1a, constituted by patients with fewer than four oocytes; and subgroup 1b, constituted by patients with four to nine oocytes retrieved after standard ovarian stimulation, who, at any age, have a lower live birth rate than age-matched normal responders.

*Group 2:* Patients ≥35 years with sufficient prestimulation ovarian reserve parameters (AFC R5, AMH R1.2 ng/mL) and with an unexpected poor or suboptimal ovarian response. This group could be further divided into: subgroup 2a, constituted by patients with fewer than four oocytes; and subgroup 2b, constituted by patients with 4–9 oocytes retrieved after standard ovarian stimulation, who, at any age, have a lower live birth rate than age-matched normal responders.

*Group 3:* Patients <35 years with poor ovarian reserve prestimulation parameters (AFC <5, AMH <1.2 ng/mL).

*Group 4:* Patients ≥35 years with poor ovarian reserve prestimulation parameters (AFC <5, AMH <1.2 ng/mL).

## ■ OVARIAN RESERVE TESTING

Reproductive lifespan and ovarian response to stimulation were predicted by measuring of primordial follicle pool (Baird et al., 2005). Ovarian response to stimulation and number of oocytes retrieved has an impact on the success of IVF. There is a strong association between number of oocytes and live birth following IVF.[4]

*Ovarian Reserve Markers*
- Hormonal biomarkers—FSH, inhibin B, AMH
- Functional markers—AFC
- Genetic biomarkers—single nucleotide polymorphisms (SNPs) for FSHR, LH, LHR.

### Hormonal Biomarkers FSH, Inhibin B, AMH

Various reproductive hormones such as AMH are closely correlated with the ovarian reserve and the inevitable process of follicle depletion. AMH and FSH have a direct and indirect impact on follicle number respectively.

### Functional Markers

Antral follicle count is a regular procedure for the assessment of follicles. According to the recent findings the correlation of several hormonal markers and AFC with age of women, AFC and AHM parallel the decline of follicles with age noted in a histological ovarian specimen (Hansen et al., 2008). Whereas FSH shows an inverse relationship with AFC.

### Genetic Biomarkers (SNPs) FSHR, LH, LHR

Various polymorphisms were identified in the genes for reproductive hormones which indicate women at risk of a poor response to COS. Polymorphism study in reproductive hormones and their receptors in women before initiation of IVF treatment will help to identify those who need tailored treatment regimens.

This pharmacogenomics (Fig. 2) approach will allow us to match all women to the optimum COS protocol for each individual.

Our recent publication, "Role of Lh polymorphisms and r-hLh supplementation in GnRh agonist treated ART cycles: a cross-sectional study" (Fig. 3) where we found a consistent association between LHCGR N312S polymorphism and require a higher dosage of r-hLH for women homozygous and heterozygous for serine with a significant increase in clinical pregnancy rates.[5]

## DIFFERENTIATION BETWEEN POOR RESPONDER AND HYPORESPONDER

A patient, who has the potential to develop a required number of eggs, but due to inadequate dosage or Lh receptor polymorphism, she could not get the requisite number of eggs, is classified as hyporesponder. A poor responder can be classified as a woman for whom we cannot increase the number of eggs by any treatment/procedure.

### Older Poor Responder

The decline in infertility over 40 years happens by a combination of aneuploidy, cytoplasmic abnormalities. Live birth in this group depends on the number of oocytes obtained. The pregnancies rate in these group ranges from 3% to 13%. In these women an optimal stimulation protocol involves optimal dosage, Lh supplementation if needed and correction of comorbidities if present.

### Younger Poor Responders

The pregnancy rate of older poor responder lies ranging from 7.6% to 17.5% whereas for normal responders it is 25.9% to 36.7%. Thus the poor responders have a lower pregnancy rate ranging between 1.5% and 12.7% compared with the normal responder.

## ROLE OF LH HORMONE

In the process of follicular development, LH plays a vital role in regulating steroidogenesis. An adequate volume of LH is very important for oocyte maturation. According to recent findings, the effect of exogenous LH in patients with the suboptimal response or low baseline serum LH concentrations is more comprehensive in long agonist protocol. The Asia Pacific Fertility Advisory Group in 2011 strongly recommended the treatment with r-hLH and r-hFSH in patients with a history of poor response as in suboptimal response on day 6 in long agonist cycles—absence of more than 10 mm follicles, endometrial thickness of less than 6 mm, estradiol levels <200 pg/mL.

## GUIDELINES IN PLANNING A PROTOCOL

Segregation of young and older poor responders. Optimization of starting dose with importance to age, BMI, AFC, AMH, exclusion of health and metabolic disorders. The choice of protocol should take care that there is no excessive downregulations be it agonist or antagonist. Evaluation of receptor polymorphism to find who needs LH supplementation is the key.[5-7]

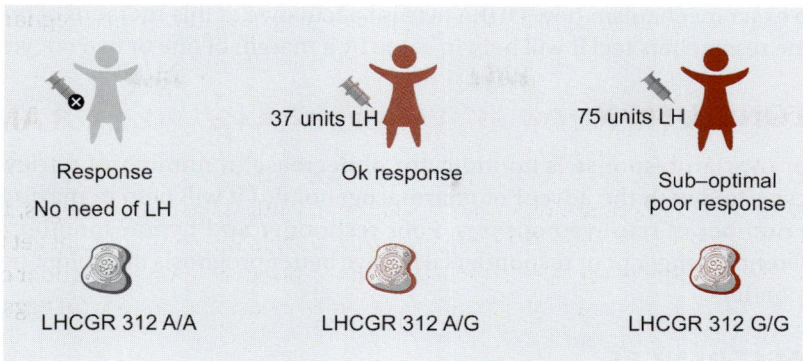

**Fig. 2:** Concept of pharmacogenomics.

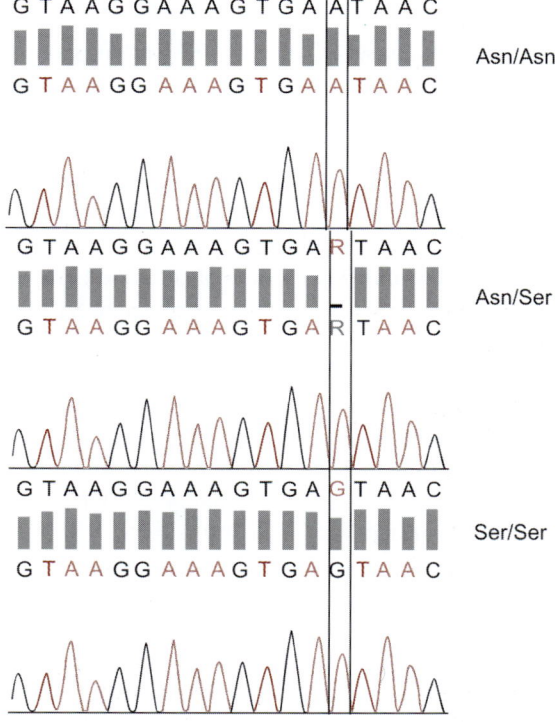

**Fig. 3:** Electropherogram of LHCGR N312S polymorphism.

## ■ ADJUVANT THERAPIES

There are many adjuvants in use for poor ovarian responder which include estradiol in luteal phase, growth hormone, aspirin, L-arginine for which there scanty evidence. Only for DHEAS as a pretreatment adjuvant at dose of 75 mg for a period of 2 months there some evidence which is of moderate quality.

The exact mechanism how DHEA acts is speculative at this moment of time. Some researchers feel it will help in some by a margin of one or two oocytes.[8]

## ■ CONCLUSION

Poor ovarian response is an indicator of decrease in number of retrieved oocytes and with the advent of pharmacogenomics it will help to maximize the number of retrieved oocytes. Poor responder and hyporesponder are different. Younger poor responders will have better prognosis than older poor responders.

## ■ REFERENCES

1. Garcia JE, Jones GS, Acosta AA, et al Human menopausal gonadotropin/human chorionic gonadotropin follicular maturation for oocyte aspiration: phase II, 1981. Fertil Steril. 1983;39(2):174-9.
2. Ferraretti A, La Marca A, Fauser BC, et al. ESHRE working group on Poor Ovarian Response Definition. ESHRE consensus on the definition of poor response to ovarian stimulation for in vitro fertilization: the Bologna criteria. Hum Reprod. 2011;26(7):1616-24.
3. Alviggi C, Andersen CY, Buehler K, et al. A new more detailed stratification of low responders to ovarian stimulation: from a poor ovarian response to a low prognosis concept. Fertil Steril. 2016;105(6):1452-3.
4. La Marca A, Sunkara SK. Individualization of controlled ovarian stimulation in IVF using ovarian reserve markers: from theory to practice. Hum Reprod Update. 2013;20(1):124-40.
5. Ramaraju GA, Cheemakurthi R, Prathigudupu K, et al. Role of Lh polymorphisms and r-hLh supplementation in GnRh agonist treated ART cycles: a cross sectional study. Eur J Obstet Gynecol Reprod Biol. 2018:119-25.
6. Wong PC, Qiao J, Ho C, et al. Current opinion on use of luteinizing hormone supplementation in assisted reproduction therapy: an Asian perspective. Reprod Biomed Online. 2011;23(1):81-90.
7. Raju GA, Chavan R, Deenadayal M, et al. Luteinizing hormone and follicle stimulating hormone synergy: a review of role in controlled ovarian hyperstimulation. J Hum Reprod Sci. 2013;6(4):227-34.
8. Rutkowski K, Sowa P, Rutkowska-Talipska J, et al. Dehydroepiandrosterone (DHEA): hypes and hopes. Drugs. 2014;74(11):1195-207.

# CHAPTER 30

# Poseidon Criteria

*Anuradha Chaudhary*

## ■ INTRODUCTION

The management of patient with an impaired ovarian reserve or poor ovarian response (POR) to exogenous gonadotropin stimulation has challenged reproductive specialists for decades.

Apart from limited understanding of the pathophysiology, wide heterogeneity exists in the definition of the poor responder patient as well as overall disappointing outcomes in assisted reproductive technology (ART).

Main points of debate and concern regarding Bologna criteria are:
1. Homogeneity of population
2. Cut-off values of age, number of retrieved oocytes, antral follicle count (AFC) and anti-Müllerian hormone (AMH)
3. Risk factor other than age
4. Oocyte quantity versus quality
5. Overdiagnosis
6. Large scale validation.

The *Poseidon criteria* (**P**atient **O**riented **S**trategies **E**ncompassing **I**ndividualize**D** **O**ocyte **N**umber) was recently established in 2016 by a group composed of reproductive endocrinologist and reproductive medicine specialist from seven countries to focus specifically on the diagnosis and management of low prognosis patients.

They proposed a new stratification to classify patients with reduced ovarian reserve (OR) or unexpected in appropriate ovarian response at exogenous gonadotropins.

The four Poseidon subgroups are based on quantitative and qualitative parameters:
1. Age and expected aneuploidy rate
2. Ovarian biomarkers, i.e. AFC and AMH
3. Ovarian response in previous stimulation cycle.

The Poseidon concept is based on:
- A better stratification of women with low prognosis in ART
- Individualized therapeutic approaches in each group having as end point the number of oocytes required to have at least one euploid embryo for transfer in the patient.

Clinician has to give importance to both quantity and quality of oocytes. Equally important is the age-related decrease in oocyte quality, which largely depends on chromosomal abnormalities occurring prior to meiosis–II. It should not be applied for retrospective analysis having live birth rate as end point, and only prospective approach can be made.

## ■ CLASSIFICATION

### Poseidon Group 1
- Young patient <35 years with adequate ovarian reserve parameters (AFC ≥1.2 ng/mL) and with an unexpected poor or suboptimal ovarian response
- Subgroup 1a: <4 oocytes
- Subgroup 1b: 4–9 oocytes retrieved
- After standard ovarian stimulation.

### Poseidon Group 2
- Older patient ≥ 35 years with adequate ovarian reserve parameters (AFC ≥1.2 ng/mL) and with an unexpected poor or suboptimal ovarian response
- Subgroup 2a: <4 oocytes
- Subgroup 2b: 4–9 oocytes retrieved
- After standard ovarian stimulation.

### Poseidon Group 3
Yong patient (<35 years) with poor ovarian reserve prestimulation parameters (AFC <5; AMH<1.2 ng/mL).

### Poseidon Group 4
Older patient ≥ 35 years with poor ovarian reserve prestimulation parameters (AFC <5; AMH <1.2 ng/mL).

## ■ MANAGEMENT

The proposed stratification will serve on a guide to personalize treatment protocol by:
- Using different gonadotropin-releasing hormone (GnRH) analog regimens
- Detecting polymorphism of gonadotropins and their receptors
- Tailoring the follicle-stimulating hormone (FSH) starting dose

- Personalizing gonadotropin doses [FSH monotherapy or addition of luteinizing hormone (LH)/LH containing drug]
- Evaluating special regimens including oocytes/embryo accumulation to maximize outcome.

## Management of Poseidon Group 1 (a) Young, Normal OR

I. Reassessment of ORT
II. Checking for genetic polymorphism
III. Checking stimulation protocol starting
IV. Tailoring FSH starting dose ↑
V. Adding r-hLH from beginning of stimulation with 75–150 IU/day.

## Poseidon Group 1 (b)

I. Tailoring FSH staring dose ↑
II. Checking for genetic polymorphism
III. Adding LH from beginning of stimulation with 75–150 IU/day.

## Poseidon Group 2 (a) Old with Normal OR

I. Changing stimulation protocol strategy
II. Adding r-LH from beginning of stimulation with 150 IU/day
III. Aneuploidy screening if required preimplantation genetic screening (PGS).

## Poseidon Group 2 (b) Old with Normal OR

I. Tailoring FSH staring dose
II. Adding LH from beginning of stimulation with 150 IU/day
III. Embryo accumulation.

## Poseidon Group 3—Young/Decreased OR

I. Follicular synchronization
II. Optimal FSH stimulation
III. Adding LH from 1st day of stimulation
IV. Dual stimulation
V. Oocytes accumulation.

## Poseidon Group 4—Individualization of Dosage, Type and Regimen

I. GnRH antagonist
II. Rec h-FSH 300 IU + Rec LH supplementation 150 IU/day
III. Adjuvants—GH, DHEA, testosterone
IV. Minimal stimulation
V. AccuVit (Duostim; PGS)
VI. Egg donation.

## KEY POINTS

- Hyporesponse (impaired response) and poor response are not same.
- Hyposensitivity to standard FSH dose is a polygenic trait and can cause expected poor suboptimal response.
- There is evidence that FSH-R Polymorphism Ser680 plays a crucial role in determining sensitivity to standard doses of FSH.
- Polymorphism of LH and LH-R also seems to be involved in determining hyporesponse.
- Type and dose of gonadotropins will not compensate when ovarian reserve is poor.
- LH rescue helps in hyposensitive ovaries with impaired (suboptimal and poor) response.

## FURTHER READING

1. Alviggi C, Andersen CY, Buehler K, et al. Poseidon Group (Patient-Oriented Strategies Encompassing IndividualizeD Oocyte Number). A new more detailed stratification of low responders to ovarian stimulation: from a poor ovarian response to a low prognosis concept. Fertil Steril. 2016;105(6):1452-3.
2. Ata B, Kaplan B, Danzer H, et al. Array CGH analysis shows that aneuploidy is not related to the number of embryos generated. Reprod Biomed Online. 2012;24(6):614-20.
3. Ferraretti AP, La Marca A, Fauser BC, et al. ESHRE consensus on the definition of poor response to ovarian stimulation for in vitro fertilization: the Bologna criteria. Hum Reprod. 2011;26(7):1616-24.
4. Nagels HE, Rishworth JR, Siristatidis CS, et al. Androgens (dehydroepiandrosterone or testosterone) for women undergoing assisted reproduction. Cochrane Database Syst Rev. 2015;26(11):CD009749.
5. Pandian Z, McTavish AR, Aucott L, et al. Interventions for poor responders to controlled ovarian hyperstimulation (COH) in in-vitro fertilisation (IVF). Cochrane Database Syst Rev. 2010;20(1):CD004379.
6. Papathanasiou A, Searle BJ, King NM, et al. Trends in poor responder research: lessons learned from RCTs in assisted conception. Hum Reprod Update. 2016;22(3):pii.
7. Patrizio P, Vaiarelli A, Setti L, et al. How to define, diagnose and treat poor responders? Responses from a worldwide survey of IVF clinics. Reprod Biomed Online. 2015;30(6):581-92.
8. Sakakibara Y, Hashimoto S, Nakaoka Y, et al. Bivalent separation into univalents precedes age-related meiosis I errors in oocytes. Nat Commun. 2015;6:7550.

# CHAPTER 31

# Ovum and Embryo Donation: First or Final Choice in Poor Responders?

*Nayana Patel*

## ■ INTRODUCTION

Poor ovarian response (POR) is a challenging situation as there is a lack of consensus on the definition of POR. A huge variation in treating women with previous POR exist amongst infertility specialist. However, the most common criterion to diagnose POR is retrieval of low number of oocytes despite adequate ovarian stimulation cycle.[1] The ESHRE working group on POR definition (the Bologna criteria) reached a consensus on the minimal criteria needed to define POR by the presence of two of the following three features: (1) Advanced maternal age (≥40 years) or any other risk factor for POR; (2) a previous characterized POR cycle (≤3 oocytes with a conventional stimulation protocol); (3) an abnormal ovarian reserve test [antral follicle count (AFC) <5–7 follicles or anti-Müllerian hormone (AMH) <0.5–1.1 ng/mL].[2] Two episodes of POR after maximum stimulation considered sufficient to define a patient as POR in the absence of other criteria. A POR occurs in 9–24% of all IVF cycles.[3] Reduced ovarian reserve is the primary reason underlying a POR, and basal follicle-stimulating hormone (FSH) levels, AMH levels, inhibin B levels, and AFC are used as predictive indicators of POR.

## ■ TREATMENT OPTIONS FOR POOR RESPONDERS

Discussion of treatment options for poor responders needs consideration of multiple factor and may range from aggressively trying to give the couple its own genetically linked to both, to utilization of donor egg or as a last resort donor embryo.

In today's era of advancing assisted reproductive technology (ART) and improved techniques, donor egg and donor embryo would remain the final and not the first choice, but in patients who need higher success rate, less number of trials and where cost is an issue, with need to decrease time to conception donor egg or embryo may be the first choice. Although as mentioned earlier the various factors to be taken into account before deciding are—

1. Age of the patient and other comorbidities.
2. The socioeconomic status of couple.
3. Religious beliefs.
4. Previously failed cycles.
5. Accessibility of all the treatment options available.
6. Legal norms of the country.

Certain important aspects and options currently considered in treatment of poor responders to get good egg and thereby genetically linked offspring are discussed here.

## Gonadotropin-releasing Hormone Antagonist Protocols

The use of a gonadotropin-releasing hormone antagonist (GnRHant) protocol was recommended for poor-response patients.[4] In contrast with the GnRH agonist protocol, the GnRH antagonist protocol does not include an initial downregulation of pituitary hormones and can prevent a premature luteinizing hormone (LH) peak without ovarian suppression during the critical early follicular phase, a characteristic that is particularly important for patients with reduced ovarian reserve. The GnRH antagonist protocol thereby provided the possibility of new treatment options for ART. However, meta-analysis of 12 trials by Xiao et al. (2013)[5] showed that there was no statistically significant difference in the clinical pregnancy rates between the GnRH antagonist group compared with the long-protocol GnRH agonist group. The results also showed that there was no statistically significant difference in the clinical pregnancy rates between the GnRH antagonist group compared with the short-protocol GnRH agonist group. The results of this analysis showed no statistically significant differences in the stimulation period between the GnRH antagonist group and the short GnRH agonist group. The results of this analysis indicated that statistically significantly fewer oocytes were retrieved in the GnRH antagonist group than in the short-protocol GnRH agonist group ($P = 0.02$).

GnRHa versus GnRHant for pituitary downregulation: Seventeen randomized controlled trials (RCTs) ($n = 1,696$) that met the criteria were subjected to meta-analysis in study by Jeve and Bhandari (2016).[6] The results suggested no significant difference in the number of oocytes retrieved (mean difference 0.09; 95% CI 0.53–0.36) and no difference in CPR with an OR of 1.24 (95% CI 0.88–1.73).

## Protocols using Luteinizing Hormone as an Adjuvant

Some authors suggested the addition of recombinant LH during gonadotropin stimulation in poor responder patients.[7] However, two meta-analyses[8,9] showed that the addition of recombinant LH does not increase the number of oocyte retrieved, the total dose of FSH, the cancellation rates, and the ongoing pregnancy rates in poor responder patients. On the other hand, in a very recent meta-analysis of 40 randomized controlled studies,[10] significantly more oocytes were retrieved and significantly higher clinical pregnancy rates were observed with r-hFSH plus r-hLH versus r-hFSH treatment in poor responders, suggesting that there is a relative increase in the clinical pregnancy rates of 30% in poor responders and that the addition of r-hLH to r-hFSH may be beneficial for women with poor ovarian response.

Meta-analysis by Jeve and Bhandari (2016),[7] LH aids maintain adequate concentrations of intraovarian androgens and promote steroidogenesis and follicular growth. It has been proposed that addition of LH to ovarian stimulation protocol may benefit poor responders. Meta-analysis of eight trials did not show significant improvement in CPR with use of recombinant LH.

## Protocols using Growth Hormone as an Adjuvant

Growth hormone-releasing hormones increase the sensitivity of ovaries to gonadotropin stimulation and enhance follicular development. It enhances oocyte quality by accelerating and coordinating cytoplasmic and nuclear maturation. There are some propositions that GH-releasing factor supplementation may improve pregnancy rates in poor responders. It is started concomitantly with gonadotropins. The dose ranges from 4 IU to 8 IU daily or 10 IU to 24 IU on alternate days. Till date available evidence shows that GH supplementation improves pregnancy and live birth rates in poor responders without any adverse effects. However, none of the studies had independently found any significant benefit with GH supplementation.

## Protocols using Transdermal Testosterone as an Adjuvant

The effect of testosterone on follicular response is mediated by increasing FSH receptor activity and by stimulating IGF-1. This improves number of follicles recruited, oocytes retrieved, implantation rate, clinical pregnancy rates and decrease in cycle cancellation rates. 10 mg of testosterone gel is applied on external side of thigh for 21 days starting from first day of menstruation prior to initiation of ovarian stimulation. However, routine use of testosterone in poor responders is a matter of debate.

## Protocols using Aromatase Inhibitors as an Adjuvant

In Meta-analysis by Jeve and Bhandari (2016),[6] aromatase inhibition was proposed to improve ovarian response to FSH in poor responders. Meta-analysis included four RCTs and failed to show any improvement in outcome with the use of aromatase inhibitors.

## Protocols using Dehydroepiandrosterone as an Adjuvant

Androgens, produced primarily by theca cells, play a critical role for an adequate follicular steroidogenesis and for a correct early follicular and granulosa cell development. They are the substrate for the aromatase activity of the granulosa cells, which converts the androgens to estrogens. About 48–50% of follicular fluid testosterone during ovarian stimulation comes from circulating dehydroepiandrosterone sulfate (DHEAS), and DHEA could therefore act as a precursor for testosterone in the follicular fluid. Moreover, androgens may increase FSH receptor expression in granulosa cells amplifying the effects of FSH and thus potentially enhance responsiveness of ovaries to FSH. It is proposed that DHEA changes the follicular microenvironment by reducing hypoxic inducible factor-1, thus improving the quality of oocytes. Based on these observations, Casson et al. first suggested that the oral administration of DHEA before ovarian stimulation with gonadotropin could improve the response in poor responder patients. 75 mg/day of DHEA causes improvement in AMH concentration, AFC, peak estradiol, number of oocytes retrieved, number of metaphase 2 oocytes and high quality embryos.[11]

A recent meta-analysis of four RCTs of adjuvant androgens (DHEA and testosterone) in poor responder patients showed a significantly higher ongoing pregnancy rate in the androgen supplementation group.[12] But, overall quality of the evidence is moderate to draw any conclusions about the safety of either androgen. Definitive conclusions regarding the clinical role of either androgen await evidence from further well-designed studies.[13]

Actually, there is a need of robust data from randomized controlled studies that could justify the widespread use of DHEA before ovarian stimulation in poor responders and it is time to evaluate the clinical cost effectiveness of DHEA with large multicenter RCTs.

## ■ NATURAL CYCLE

Natural cycles IVF with or without minimal stimulation can be considered as an easy and cheap approach in the management of poor responders with low risk of multiple pregnancies and most importantly eliminates the risk of ovarian hyperstimulation syndrome. Natural cycles IVF has the same chance in terms of pregnancy and implantation rates.[14] Schimberni et al.[15] evaluated the IVF outcome in a large group of poor responders (500 patients) reporting very encouraging results especially in younger woman (<35 years). In this group, pregnancy rate was 18% per started cycle, 29% per transfer, and 31% per patient. In contrast, a recent paper analyzed the effect of natural cycles IVF in women defined as poor responders according to the "Bologna criteria": unexpectedly the data showed that the cumulative live birth per patient does not exceed 8%.[16] Morgia et al.[17] randomized natural cycle IVF and microdose

GnRHa flare along with FSH. It was found that natural cycle IVF may be as effective as IVF using controlled ovarian hyperstimulation.

## Oocyte Cryopreservation

Different strategies are applicable for poor responder involving oocyte cryopreservation. Some authors have recently suggested obtaining a large cohort of oocytes in these patients by accumulating vitrified oocytes over several stimulation cycles creating a similar situation as in normal responder patients. According to the results presented in the study, it could be possible to obtain higher live birth rate per patient treated and potentially to reduce the dropout.[18] Moreover, oocyte cryopreservation can also be used to preserve the fertility of all those women at risk to lose their ovarian potential over the time.

## IVF Lite Protocol

Gandhi et al., in (2014),[19] came up with protocol consists of Minimal Stimulation IVF (msIVF) + Vitrification + Accumulation of Embryos + Remote Embryo Transfer (rET).

msIVF is the protocol with Clomiphene Citrate, Human Menopausal Gonadotropin (hMG) and GnRH Antagonist Cetrorelix.

Vitrification and accumulation of embryos include fertilization of eggs using either IVF or ICSI and to freeze embryo on day 3 using vitrification. Back to back cycles of msIVF followed by ACCU-VIT are performed till about six top grade get accumulated per patient. A remote embryo transfer is performed when adequate embryos are accumulated. The embryos are transferred on day 4, after preparing the endometrium with Estradiol Valerate tablets.

## Regenerative Medicine to Rejuvenate Ovaries

Ovarian rejuvenation is a relatively new concept in the field, but one that is helping fertility specialists to make great strides forward. Using newly developed techniques, women who are poor responders or who have suffered early menopause or other conditions which limit fertility may still conceive using their own eggs. Ovarian rejuvenation can be done by using platelet rich plasma or stem cells. The procedure of ovarian rejuvenation is relatively painless and may be worth an attempt before moving on to other treatments. Two live birth after Stem cell ovarian auto transplantation in *poor responder* women have been reported in clinical trial by Herraiz S, et al. (Trial registration number: NCT02240342).

The above listed methods require time, patience and can be costly. But the success gives genetically related child. The alternative to these treatment options are use of donated egg or embryo.

Ovum donation and embryo donation, along with sperm donation and surrogacy, are forms of third party or donor-assisted reproduction, a technique of assisted reproduction in which DNA or gestation is provided by a third party or donor other than the one or two parents who will raise the resulting child. This goes beyond the traditional father–mother model, and the third party's involvement is limited to the reproductive process and does not extend into the raising of the child.

## Ovum Donation

Ovum donation, like sperm donation, is sensitive to local culture and regulation. In many countries including US, if desired (and if the egg donor agrees), the couple can meet and get acquainted with the egg donor, her children and family members, but in India, directed donation is not allowed.

IVF with donor oocyte involves following steps:
- Recruitment and screening of donor
- Screening of recipient and her partner
- Stimulation of donor
- Synchronization of donor and recipient
- Endometrial preparation of recipient
- Embryo transfer
- Hormonal support of recipient and management of pregnancy.

## Embryo Donation

An alternative to egg donation in some couples, especially those in whom the male partner cannot provide viable sperm, is embryo donation. Embryo donation is a procedure that enables embryos that were created by couples undergoing fertility treatment to be transferred to infertile patients in order to achieve a pregnancy. The process of embryo donation requires that the recipient couple undergo the appropriate medical and psychological screening recommended for all gamete donor cycles. In addition, the female partner undergoes an evaluation of her uterine cavity and then her endometrium is prepared with estrogen and progesterone in anticipation of an embryo transfer. Embryo donation is more cost-effective than egg donation on a "per live birth" basis.

Embryo donation is a controversial process from both an ethical as well as a legal standpoint. Of paramount importance is that informed consent and counseling be provided to both the donors of the embryos and the recipient couple to address all of the potential issues embryo donation might raise. Embryo donation for research is also a debatable topic. In addition, due to the absence of explicit laws regarding embryo donation, couples should consult with legal counsel regarding the necessity of a predonation agreement as well as the necessity of seeking a judicial determination or recognition of parentage.

## CONCLUSION

Variants of controlled ovarian hyperstimulation protocols with use of recombinant injection, addition of adjuvants such as growth hormone (GH), transdermal testosterone, aromatase inhibitors, dehydroepiandrosterone (DHEA) have been explored. But none as of now has supported its use with compelling evidence.

Accu-Vit (Accumulation and Vitrification) protocol, IVF-lite, minimal stimulation, etc. have proved to be of value in difficult cases. Regenerative medicine like stem cells and platelet rich plasma are also being used to rejuvenate ovaries for retrieval of better quality of eggs from these women, but the success rate varies.

Ovum donation and embryo donation are the alternative treatment options available for poor responders. However, to choose these treatment options as a first or last resort depends on personal, religious and financial dynamics. With advancements in ART and regenerative medicine, a genetically related offspring remains the aim for both patient and doctor before considering ovum/embryo donation.

## REFERENCES

1. Patrizio P, Vaiarelli A, Levi Setti PE, et al. How to define, diagnose and treat poor responders? Responses from a worldwide survey of IVF clinics. Reprod Biomed Online. 2015;30:581-92.
2. Ferraretti AP, La Marca A, Fauser BC, et al. ESHRE consensus on the definition of 'poor response' to ovarian stimulation for in vitro fertilization: The Bologna criteria. Hum Reprod. 2011;26:1616-24.
3. Keay SD, Lenton EA, Cooke ID, et al. Low-dose dexamethasone augments the ovarian response to exogenous gonadotrophins leading to a reduction in cycle cancellation rate in a standard IVF programme. Hum Reprod. 2001;16:1861-5.
4. Kolibianakis E, Albano C, Zikopoulos K, et al. GnRH antagonists in poor responders. Acta Obstet Gynecol Scand. 2004;83:1216-7.
5. Xiao J, Chang S, Chen S. The effectiveness of gonadotropin-releasing hormone antagonist in poor ovarian responders undergoing in vitro fertilization: a systematic review and meta-analysis. Fertil Steril. 2013;100:6.
6. Jeve YB, Bhandari HM. Effective treatment protocol for poor ovarian response: A systematic review and meta-analysis. J Hum Reprod Sci. 2016;9(2):70-81.
7. Hill MJ, Levens ED, Levy G. The use of recombinant luteinizing hormone in patients undergoing assisted reproductive techniques with advanced reproductive age: a systematic review and meta-analysis. Fertil Steril. 2012;97(5):1108.el-1114.e1.
8. Bosdou JK, Venetis CA, Kolibianakis EM. The use of androgens or androgen-modulating agents in poor responders undergoing in vitro fertilization: a systematic review and meta-analysis. Hum Reprod Update. 2012;18(2):127-45.
9. Fan W, Li S, Chen Q, et al. Recombinant luteinizing hormone supplementation in poor responders undergoing IVF: a systematic review and meta-analysis. Gynecol Endocrinol. 2013;29(4):278-84.

10. Lehert P, Kolibianakis EM, Venetis CA, et al. Recombinant human follicle-stimulating hormone (r-hFSH) plus recombinant luteinizing hormone versus r-hFSH alone for ovarian stimulation during assisted reproductive technology: systematic review and meta-analysis. Reprod Bio Endocrin. 2014;12(17).
11. Casson PR, Santoro N, Elkind-Hirsch K. Postmenopausal dehydroepiandrosterone administration increases free insulin-like growth factor-I and decreases high-density lipoprotein: a six- month trial. Fertil Steril. 1998;70(1):107-10.
12. Sunkara SK, Coomarasamy A. Androgen pretreatment in poor responders undergoing controlled ovarian stimulation and in vitro fertilization treatment. Fertil Steril. 2011;95(8):e73-e75.
13. Nagels HE, Rishworth JR, Siristatidis CS, et al. Androgens (dehydroepiandrosterone or testosterone) for women undergoing assisted reproduction. Cochrane Database Syst Rev. 2015;(11):CD009749.
14. Ubaldi FM, Rienzi L, Ferrero S. Management of poor responders in IVF. Reprod Biomed Online. 2005;10(2):235–246.
15. Schimberni M, Morgia F, Colabianchi J. Natural-cycle in vitro fertilization in poor responder patients: a survey of 500 consecutive cycles. Fertil Steril. 2009;92(4):1297-301.
16. Polyzos NP, Blockeel C, Verpoest W. Live birth rates following natural cycle IVF in women with poor ovarian response according to the Bologna criteria. Hum Reprod. 2012;27(12):3481-6.
17. Morgia F, Sbracia M, Schimberni M, et al. A controlled trial of natural cycle versus microdose gonadotropin-releasing hormone analog flare cycles in poor responders undergoing in vitro fertilization. Fertil Steril. 2004;81:1542-7
18. Cobo A, Garrido N, Crespo J, et al. Accumulation of oocytes: a new strategy for managing low-responder patients. Reprod BioMed Online. 2012;24(4):424-32.
19. Gandhi G, Allahbadia G, Kagalwala S, et al. IVF Lite-a new strategy for managing poor ovarian responders. J Mini Stimulat. 2014;1(1);22-8.

CHAPTER
# 32

# Third Party Reproduction for ART

*Kanthi Bansal*

## ■ INTRODUCTION

After the birth of Louise Brown, new manipulation techniques have been developed to bring the gametes together, facilitating fertilization and the achievement of pregnancy. With the advent of new technologies, the role of a third party being involved in helping the infertile couple to achieve their goal became possible.

Involvement of a third party can be in the form of:
- Sperm donation
- Oocyte donation
- Embryo donation
- Surrogacy.

## ■ SPERM DONATION

Intrauterine insemination with donor sperms has been a routine clinical treatment for male infertility for many years.

But use of donor sperms in in-vitro fertilization (IVF) is mainly indicated when along with the male factor like nonobstructive azoospermia and risk of transmitting hereditary disease, the female partner has:
- Bilateral tubal block
- Severe endometriosis
- Advanced age
- Repeated failures with intrauterine insemination of donor sperms.

## ■ OOCYTE DONATION

Oocyte donation has now become feasible with the advent of IVF. Acceptance of gametes from another individual for procreation is understandably a difficult decision for any couple. However, situations do exist when this option should be considered and many clinical, scientific and ethical issues addressed.

In 1983, Trounson and colleagues reported the first pregnancy after transfer of a donated oocyte fertilized in vitro to a cyclic recipient. The world's first pregnancy resulting from the transfer of an in-vitro fertilized single embryo from a 42-year-old donor to a 39-year-old recipient resulted in a spontaneous abortion, but the same group subsequently achieved an in-vitro fertilized donor pregnancy reaching full term (Lutjen et al., 1984).

## Indications for Donor Oocyte

Patients who require donor oocyte occur in two main groups:

1. *Women with nonfunctioning ovaries:*
   a. Premature ovarian failure: Idiopathic, genetic like Turner's syndrome, immunological, autoimmune, iatrogenic including surgical oophorectomy, chemotherapy and radiotherapy.
   b. Ovarian agenesis.
   c. Menopause.
   d. Resistant ovary syndrome.
2. *Women with functioning ovaries:*
   a. Carriers of genetic disease or chromosomal abnormalities.
   b. Repeated IVF failures due to poor response to superovulation, failure of oocyte recovery, failure of fertilization due to poor oocyte quality and repeated implantation failure of apparently normal embryos.
   c. Inaccessible ovaries.
   d. Older women with reduced ovarian reserve or poor quality oocyte.

## Source of Oocyte Donors

A major challenge to oocyte donation program is to find an adequate number of women willing to donate eggs.
- *Known donors:* Some recipients seek their own donor, either a close friend or a relative.
- *Volunteers:* Some women are willing to undergo ovarian stimulation and egg donation altruistically to anonymous recipients.
- *Spare oocytes:* Some infertile patients undergoing IVF may volunteer to donate their excess eggs to anonymous recipient.
  – *Advantages*
    - Donor does not have to suffer additional risk
    - Egg sharing reduces the cost
  – *Disadvantages*
    - Donation from infertile women is less successful than from fertile women
    - When the best oocytes are used for the donor, the outcome for the recipient may be suboptimum.
- *Professional oocyte donors*: These donors give their oocytes for payment.

Alternative sources of donor oocytes need to be explored like:
- In-vitro maturation of eggs
- Cryopreservation of oocytes
- The use of cadaver ovaries, and fetal ovarian tissue
- Human embryo twinning.

## Selection and Screening of Recipient

- Upper age limit ideally should be 45 years, subject to the health of the recipient
- Detailed family history, medical history
- Pelvic examination and ultrasound scanning to exclude pelvic pathology and to assess the uterine size and endometrium
- Routine blood work-up
- Laboratory studies: Blood chemistry, blood grouping, hematological profile, thyroid profile, rubella antibody titer, screening for venereal diseases, HbsAg, human immunodeficiency virus (HIV), Pap smear and diabetes
- Office hysteroscopy to evaluate the endometrial cavity
- Mock endometrial preparation cycle to assess the endometrial adequacy
- Male partner should have a semen analysis and physical examination if indicated
- Proper counseling becomes the first step of the screening procedure. They should be given a detailed explanation of the procedure and legal, moral and ethical implications.

Thus, potential recipients should be evaluated by selection criteria that include appropriate medical indications for oocyte donation and ascertainment of the woman's ability to tolerate pregnancy, labor and delivery both physically and psychologically.

## Selection and Screening of Potential Oocyte Donor

- Age: 21–35 years
- Family history, medical history
- Endocrine profile: Follicle-stimulating hormone (FSH), luteinizing hormone (LH), estradiol, thyroid-stimulating hormone (TSH), prolactin, progesterone
- Ultrasound examination
- Complete blood count, blood sugar, blood group and Rh typing
- Exclude infectious diseases like HIV, hepatitis B, syphilis, chlamydia, and gonorrhea
- Written consent
- Counseling regarding the procedure
- It is advisable not to allow the donor to donate oocytes for more than 6 times.

## Cycle Management

Firstly the cycle of the donor and the recipient should be synchronized followed by stimulation of the donor and endometrial preparation of the recipient.

### Treatment of the Donor

The donor is stimulated with a combination of GnRh analog, FSH and hMG after a proper day 2/3 hormonal work-up and baseline ultrasound scanning.

The donor will be treated with a period of long downregulation with the GnRh analog, leuprolide or buserelin for up to 2 weeks, after which the serum levels of LH, progesterone and estradiol are measured.

Once the baseline stimulation been achieved, follicular stimulation with gonadotropins can begin. Recombinant FSH 150 IU or 225 IU daily is given. Monitoring starts after 5 days of stimulation and the stimulation is continued until two leading follicles reach at least 18 mm in mean diameter and serum estradiol level are commensurate with the number and size of follicles. Human chorionic gonadotropin (hCG) 10,000 IU is given 34–36 hours before the intended time of oocytes recovery.

Oocytes and sperms are incubated and embryos are kept frozen for a minimum of 3 months. During the last month, the host mother is further counseled, the genetic parents both have a further test for HIV and when the result is confirmed negative, the host's replacement cycle is started. Fresh embryos are transferred when the recipient wants it but with informed consent.

### Treatment of the Host Mother

Majority of the medical and psychological assessment is already done. If the host mother is on the oral contraceptive pill, then it is recommended that this be discontinued one or two cycle before the treatment cycle and barrier methods of contraception used.

The host may be treated with either frozen-thawed embryos or fresh embryos from "quarantined sperms".

### Replacement in a Natural Cycle

This method is suitable for women, who have been sterilized or whose husbands have had a vasectomy. The host is monitored daily from about day 8 of the cycle until natural LH is detected. Embryos are thawed after 24 hours and transferred after another 24 hours.

### Replacement in a Hormone Controlled Cycle

Control of the host's replacement cycle is recommended:
* If the menstrual cycle is irregular, anovulatory or if luteal phase insufficiencies is detected.
* If the host is fertile and has to rely on barrier contraception.

By downregulating the host and controlling the cycle with a gonadotropin releasing analog and then replacing estrogen in increasing doses, creating an artificial proliferative phase, the chance of implantation of the embryo is increased if the host tends to have inefficient cycles. Also, by taking control of the cycle, natural conception with the host's partner is prevented. This control is achieved by the administration of leuprolide or buserelin subcutaneously, from the previous cycle day 21 until day 2 of the next menstrual period, when serum LH, progesterone and estrogen are checked and development of the endometrium and ovaries is monitored by ultrasound. If downregulation has been achieved, oral estradiol valerate (Progynova) is given in increasing daily doses from 2 mg to 6 mg. Progesterone, in the form of natural micronized injectable 50 mg daily intramuscularly, is given from day 15. The embryos are replaced on day 17 of the artificial cycle. Progynova 6 mg orally daily and micronized vaginal pessary 400 mg twice daily or injectable progesterone 100 mg intramuscularly daily are continued, until the result of pregnancy test is known. If it is positive, then both are continued until 12–14 weeks gestation, by which time endogenous sources of both hormones are sufficient to maintain the pregnancy.

## Result of Oocyte Donation Treatment

- Pregnancy rates following oocyte donation are excellent in comparison with those achieved after the transfer of the patient's own oocytes.
- Transfer of fresh embryos has a higher pregnancy rate than that of frozen embryos.
- Neither the age of the recipient nor the diagnosis play a substantial role in the success of oocyte donation.
- The age of the donor is an important factor in achieving good pregnancy rate.
- Pregnancy rates are directly related to the number of embryos transferred.
- The risk of pregnancy for women increase considerably with increasing maternal age.
- There are no reports of increased risk of fetal abnormality following oocyte donation.
- Agonadal women have breastfed their infants normally after oocyte donation.
- Reasons for higher success rate are lack of hyperstimulation, no risk of hyperestrogenism, no specific cause for underlying infertility, no premature luteinization, and better control of window receptivity.

## ■ EMBRYO DONATION

Embryo donation is a well-established and successful form of assisted conception treatment where both partners are subfertile.

## Indications for Embryo Donation

- Menopausal and perimenopausal woman and subfertile partner
- Recurrent IVF failures
- Carriers of genetic disease or chromosomal abnormalities.

## Need for Embryo Donation

Whenever there are spare embryos in an IVF cycle, there are four choices of what to do with them—discard, donate to research, donate to infertile couples or cryopreserve for future use.

Couples, who have created embryos as part of their own IVF treatment, especially if they have completed their families, are often willing to donate excess embryos to infertile couples.

The advantages of embryo donation are good use of excess embryos—the recipient bears the child and hence the bonding with it is the advantage over adoption. This is relatively a simple procedure, cheaper treatment compared to oocyte donation or IVF and fewer medical complications.

- Selection, screening and counseling of embryo donors and recipients is essentially the same as oocyte and sperm donors.
- Data about the outcome of embryo donation is scarce. Asch reported 13 pregnancies in 17 embryo recipients (77% pregnancy rate per patient) which were higher than oocyte donation.

## ■ SURROGACY

Surrogacy has been an accepted form of treatment for certain group of infertile couples, yet not very prevalent in India.

Before the advent of modern assisted conception techniques, "natural surrogacy" was the only means of helping certain barren women to have children.

Later, artificial insemination became more acceptable than the natural way. When assisted conception methods such as IVF became available, it was a natural step to use the eggs of the woman wanting the baby, and with the sperm of her husband, to create their own embryos in vitro and transfer these to a suitable host.

The earliest mention is in the *Old Testament of Bible*. Ishmael was born to Abram and Sarai by the way of natural surrogacy, with the help of the maid.

## Definitions

- "Genetic Couple" or "Commissioning Couple" or "Intended Parent"—the couple who provide both sets of gametes.
- "Surrogate Host" or "Host"—the woman receiving the embryos created from the gametes of the genetic couple.

- "Natural Surrogacy" or "Traditional Surrogacy" or "Partial Surrogacy"—where the egg belongs to the female carrying the pregnancy, the intended host is inseminated with the semen of the husband of the genetic couple.
- "Gestational Surrogacy" or "IVF Surrogacy" or "Full Surrogacy"—a treatment by which the gametes of the genetic couple or intended parents in a surrogacy arrangement are used to produce embryos and these embryos are subsequently transferred to a woman who agrees to act as a host for these embryos.
- "Commercial Surrogacy" arrangements: This is when the surrogate is paid over and above the necessary medical expenses.
- "Altruistic Surrogacy" arrangements: This is when the surrogate is paid only the necessary pregnancy related expenses and at times nothing at all.

## Indications for Treatment

### Patients without Uterus

- Women with congenital absence of the uterus, Mullerian agenesis (Rokitansky–Kuster–Hauser syndrome).
- Women who have had hysterectomy for various reasons like uterine fibroids, carcinoma, antepartum or postpartum hemorrhage, uterine rupture, severe adenomyosis or ruptured uterus.

### Patients with Uterus

- Women who suffer repeated miscarriages.
- Repeated failures in IVF cycle—nonreceptive uterus.
- Women with certain medical conditions, which make pregnancy life reatening like severe heart disease or kidney disease.
- Women for whom the prospect of carrying a baby to term is deemed to be very remote.
- No women are considered for treatment by surrogacy who request it for career or social reasons.

## Patient Selection

The genetic couples are usually first seen alone and in-depth consultation and counseling of all the medical aspects of the treatment is conducted. If medically suitable for treatment, they are given some guidance on finding a host for themselves or take the help of a professional surrogate.

When the suitable host is found, she and her partner are interviewed and explained in detail of the implications of acting as a surrogate host.

## Screening of Surrogate

- Age <35 years (preferably).
- No severe medical disorders or personal habit like smoking, alcohol and drug abuse.

- See for hereditary disorders, infectious diseases, hemoglobinopathies.
- Psychological assessment especially possessiveness.

## Counseling

The role of counseling in surrogacy is to help and prepare all parties contemplating this last-resort treatment and to consider all the factors that will have an influence on the future lives of each of them. The counseling ensures that they be confident and comfortable with their decisions, and have trust in each other, so that no one party is felt to be taking advantage of the other.

Both the couples should be counseled regarding the failure of the treatment, as it could have a profound effect on them and their families.

## ■ CONCLUSION

Sperm donation oocyte donation, embryo donation and surrogacy are all the accepted form of assisted conception treatment.

In the past 3 decades, there has been a spectacular change in the field of reproductive technologies. Continuing research and advancement of the technology has given hope to many who are devastated when they cannot have children.

Assisted reproduction technologies involving a third party in the treatment of infertile patients have definitely helped to fulfill the dreams of many childless couples.

# CHAPTER 33

# Comparison of Growth of Newborn Babies Conceived Naturally with those Born following Assisted Reproduction Technology

*Saugata Acharyya, Kakoli Acharyya*

## ■ INTRODUCTION

A large number of newborn babies are born following conception by assisted reproductive technology (ART). Recent literature reviews have focused attention on the growth and long-term follow up of these babies. Many authors have suggested varying impact of ART on the growth and future development of these children. However, data from eastern India, about the growth of these neonates and their comparison with matched naturally conceived babies, are still lacking. Therefore, we intend to have a closer look at the current opinion and describe our experience regarding the babies we are following up.

## ■ COMPARISON OF ART AND NATURAL PREGNANCY

Assisted reproductive technologies like in vitro fertilization (IVF) and intracytoplasmic sperm injection (ICSI) are being used widely to treat infertility. Since the birth of the first child conceived by IVF in 1978, there has been a phenomenal growth in ART.[1,2] The various artificial procedures used during the ART often generate the concern to the parents and researchers—are these offsprings exposed to greater health risks than their naturally conceived counterparts? Apart from this, multiple embryo transfer during ART often increases the rate of multiple pregnancies. The later may be associated with a higher rate of prematurity and low birth weights and risk of increased morbidity in these children.[3,4] The effect on birth weight and growth of ART conceived newborn has been extensively studied. As mentioned earlier, these babies seem to be at a higher risk of lower birth weight, lower gestational age, perinatal morbidity and hospital admissions than their naturally conceived counterparts.[5] Multiple pregnancy is just one factor that is attributed to the poor perinatal outcome. However, only reducing the rate of multiple pregnancy will not likely to eliminate the risk of low birth weight and growth retardation. Studies have suggested that singletons born after ART are also at a higher risk of lower birth weight, younger gestational age, premature delivery, perinatal morbidity and hospital admission compared with naturally conceived singletons.[6] This may be explained by the poor fertility of the parents. The meta-analysis conducted by Bower and Hansen[6] found approximately two-fold increase in the risk of prenatal mortality, low birth weight and preterm birth, an approximate 50% increase in the risk of being small for gestational age, and a 30–35% increase in birth defects for singletons conceived via ART compared with NC singletons. A later study[7] with larger sample size found that the mean birth weight was 65 g [95% confidence interval (CI) 41–89] lower in all ART children compared with their NC siblings. In addition there was a higher risk of having a low birth weight [odds ratio (OR) 1.4, 95% CI 1.1–1.7] and a preterm birth (OR 1.3, 95% CI 1.1–1.6) in the ART conceived babies.

Keeping the above study observations in mind we have decided to enumerate our experience. To determine whether there was any significant change in the growth parameters at birth we had conducted an observational study based on the medical and birth records of 85 babies born following ART. All these babies were born between 2013 and 2015 by lower (uterine) segment cesarean section (LSCS) in tertiary referral center. To eliminate confounding factors we had only recruited those babies who were born after 36 completed weeks of gestation. They were all singleton pregnancies with maternal age between 30 years and 40 years. They were all born by elective LSCS with no evidence of maternal or fetal distress. Babies who required neonatal intensive care unit (NICU)/special care baby unit (SCBU) care following birth were excluded from the study. We had compared the anthropometric measurements [birth weight, length and occipitofrontal circumference (OFC)] of these babies with matched cohort of 85 naturally conceived babies born during the same period. Finally, we did follow up these two sets of babies till the age of 2 years. Only those babies whose complete medical records were available were recruited after obtaining necessary consent from their parents.

To begin with we had decided to concentrate on the physical growth parameters at birth of the two subsets (ART vs NC). As per our observation a significant increase in the number of babies weighing less than 3rd percentile (plotted in the Fentons gestational weight chart) in the assisted reproduction group compared to the natural conception group (18/85; 21.18% as opposed to 3/85; 3.53%, p<0.001) (Table 1). Similarly those weighing between 3rd and 10th percentile are also significantly more in the AR group compared to the NC group (17/85; 20% as opposed to 4/85; 4.71%, p<0.001). Hence, the proportion of intrauterine growth retardation (IUGR) in the AR group is significantly more than their naturally conceived counterparts (35/85; 41.18% as opposed to 7/85; 8.24%, p<0.001) (Table 3).

The lengths of the babies at birth were also significantly lower in the assisted reproduction group compared to the naturally conceived group (Table 2) as was the OFC (Table 4). The mean weight of the AR group (n = 85) was 2.3846 kg (SD 0.4017) compared to that of the NC group (n = 85; Mean weight 2.6227 kg, SD 0.2963) (Table 5). Hence, the mean weight of the assisted reproduction babies are significantly lower than the NC babies (p<0.001) (Table 6). These findings

**Table 1:** Weight centile comparison of babies born by the assisted reproduction group and the natural conception group.

| | | Group | | Total | p Value | Significance |
|---|---|---|---|---|---|---|
| | | Assisted reproduction | Natural conception | | | |
| Weight Centile | <3rd | 18 (21.18) | 3 (3.53) | 21 (12.35) | <0.001 | Significant |
| | 3rd–10th | 17 (20) | 4 (4.71) | 21 (12.35) | | |
| | 10th–50th | 24 (28.24) | 36 (42.35) | 60 (35.29) | | |
| | >50th | 26 (30.59) | 42 (49.41) | 68 (40) | | |
| Total | | 85 (100) | 85 (100) | 170 (100) | | |

**Table 2:** Length centile comparison of babies born by the assisted reproduction group and the natural conception group.

| | | Group | | Total | p Value | Significance |
|---|---|---|---|---|---|---|
| | | Assisted reproduction | Natural conception | | | |
| Length Centile | <3rd | 14 (16.47) | 3 (3.53) | 17 (10) | <0.001 | Significant |
| | 3rd–10th | 17 (20) | 2 (2.35) | 19 (11.18) | | |
| | 10th–50th | 24 (28.24) | 34 (40) | 58 (34.12) | | |
| | >50th | 30 (35.29) | 46 (54.12) | 76 (44.71) | | |
| Total | | 85 (100) | 85 (100) | 170 (100) | | |

**Table 3:** Comparison of intrauterine growth retardation (IUGR) of babies born by the assisted reproduction group and the natural conception group.

| | | Group | | Total | p Value | Significance |
|---|---|---|---|---|---|---|
| | | Assisted reproduction | Natural conception | | | |
| IUGR | No | 50 (58.82) | 78 (91.76) | 128 (75.29) | <0.001 | Significant |
| | Yes | 35 (41.18) | 7 (8.24) | 42 (24.71) | | |
| Total | | 85 (100) | 85 (100) | 170 (100) | | |

are consistent with those of other studies. Our observation also suggests that the growth parameter least affected in the AR group is the OFC (Tables 7 and 8). So the incidence of asymmetric IUGR is significantly more in the assisted reproduction group as compared to the naturally conceived group. These again tally with the observation in other studies.[6,7]

**Table 4:** Comparison of occipitofrontal circumference (OFC) of babies born by the assisted reproduction group and the natural conception group.

| | | Group | | Total | p Value | Significance |
|---|---|---|---|---|---|---|
| | | Assisted reproduction | Natural conception | | | |
| OFC Centile | <3rd | 0 (0) | 1 (1.18) | 1 (0.59) | 0.027 | Significant |
| | 3rd–10th | 6 (7.06) | 1 (1.18) | 7 (4.12) | | |
| | 10th–50th | 38 (44.71) | 27 (31.76) | 65 (38.24) | | |
| | >50th | 41 (48.24) | 56 (65.88) | 97 (57.06) | | |
| Total | | 85 (100) | 85 (100) | 170 (100) | | |

**Table 5:** Mean, standard error and 95% confidence interval difference in weight of babies born by the assisted reproduction and natural conception group

| | P value | Mean difference | Standard error difference | 95% confidence interval of the difference | |
|---|---|---|---|---|---|
| | | | | Lower | Upper |
| Weight (kg) | <0.001 | −0.238 | 0.054 | −0.345 | −0.131 |

**Table 6:** Mean weight comparison of babies born by the assisted reproduction group and the natural conception group.

| | Group | N | Mean | Standard deviation |
|---|---|---|---|---|
| Weight (kg) | Assisted reproduction | 85 | 2.3846 | 0.4017 |
| | Natural conception | 85 | 2.6227 | 0.2963 |

**Table 7:** Mean, standard error and 95% confidence interval difference in OFC of babies born by the assisted reproduction and natural conception group

| | p Value | Mean difference | Standard error difference | 95% confidence interval of the difference | |
|---|---|---|---|---|---|
| | | | | Lower | Upper |
| Length (cm) | 0.002 | −.599 | 0.505 | −2.596 | −0.601 |
| OFC (cm) | 0.038 | −0.584 | 0.278 | −1.133 | −0.034 |

(OFC: occipitofrontal circumference)

**Table 8:** Mean length and occipitofrontal circumference (OFC) comparison of babies born by the assisted reproduction group and the natural conception group.

| Group | | N | Mean | Standard deviation |
|---|---|---|---|---|
| Length (cm) | Assisted reproduction | 85 | 45.99 | 3.66 |
| | Natural conception | 85 | 47.59 | 2.88 |
| OFC (cm) | Assisted reproduction | 85 | 33.57 | 1.94 |
| | Natural conception | 85 | 34.15 | 1.68 |

## ■ CONCLUSION

Based on our observation, we can conclude that even the singleton babies born following ART are significantly growth retarded in comparison to their matched controls of similar gestational age, born to mothers of same age group. These findings are in conformity with larger studies worldwide reported by various other observers. Compared to conceptions via double embryo transfer (DET), single embryo transfer (SET) can improve neonatal outcome, leading to significantly fewer preterm births and low birth weight infants.[8]

## ■ REFERENCES

1. Nyboe Andersen N, Goossens V, Ferraretti AP, et al. Assisted reproductive technology in Europe, 2004: results generated from European registers by ESHRE. Hum Reprod. 2008;23(4):756-71.
2. de Mouzon J, Goossens V, Bhattacharya S, et al. Assisted reproductive technology in Europe, 2006: results generated from European registers by ESHRE. Hum Reprod. 2010;25(8):1851-62.
3. Alexander GR, Salihu HM. Perinatal Outcomes of Singleton and Multiple Births in the United States 1995–1998. In: Blickstein I, Keith LG (Eds). Multiple Pregnancy: Epidemiology, Gestation and Perinatal Outcome. Boca Raton: CRC Press; 2005. pp. 3-10.
4. Liu YC, Blair EM. Predicted birthweight for singletons and twins. Twin Res. 2002;5(6):529-37.
5. Källén B, Finnström O, Nygren KG, et al. In vitro fertilization in Sweden: child morbidity including cancer risk. Fertil Steril. 2005;84(3):605-10.
6. Bower C, Hansen M. Assisted reproductive technologies and birth outcomes: overview of recent systematic reviews. Reprod Fertil Dev. 2005;17(3):329-33.
7. Henningsen AK, Pinborg A, Lidegaard Ø, et al. Perinatal outcome of singleton siblings born after assisted reproductive technology and spontaneous conception: Danish national sibling-cohort study. Fertil Steril. 2011;95(3):959-63.
8. Kjellberg AT, Carlsson P, Bergh C. Randomized single versus double embryo transfer: obstetric and paediatric outcome and a cost-effectiveness analysis. Hum Reprod. 2006;21(1):210-6.

# CHAPTER 34

# Fertility Preservation in the Present Era

*J Tan, S Tannus, MH Dahan, R Youcef Khoudja, ZF Naz, S Kattera, P Chan, SL Tan*

## ■ INTRODUCTION

Over the past two decades, the concept of fertility preservation has emerged as a major portion of the field of reproductive health.[1] Initially, the concept of restoring or maintaining a couple's reproductive potential was developed to help individuals at risk of early menopause or sterilization, which include those undergoing gonadotoxic treatments such as chemotherapy or radiotherapy. However, the utility of fertility preservation has expanded to support individuals who suffer from a myriad of medical illnesses that adversely affect ovarian reserve and sperm production such as systemic lupus erythematosus, multiple sclerosis, and inflammatory bowel diseases.[2-5]

In addition, remarkable shifts in the social dynamics of childbearing have led to a rapid rise in the demand for social fertility preservation.[6] Social egg freezing is the process of cryopreserving reproductive cells on an elective basis for the purpose of delaying childbearing. While social trends have led to a dramatic increase in the average age of conception, particularly among women, the costs of delayed childbearing include a concomitant increased risk of infertility, miscarriage, and aneuploidy.[7] With advancements in cryopreservation techniques, however, social oocyte and embryo cryopreservation offer a safe and efficient option for couples to delay childbearing until such time that they are ready to have children without the aforementioned risks.

## ■ FERTILITY PRESERVATION IN WOMEN

There are several techniques that are employed in the process of female fertility preservation. Conceptually, the logical method to preserve fertility would be through ovarian cryopreservation and subsequent transplantation at a later point in life. Although preservation of an intact organ in its entirely has been previously demonstrated using a rat model,[8] it has been far more difficult to replicate such a procedure in human ovaries due to their much larger size. Therefore, at the present time, female fertility preservation is restricted to preserving embryos, ovarian tissue, or mature or immature oocytes derived from in vitro fertilization (IVF) or in vitro maturation (IVM) cycles.

## Embryo Cryopreservation

Embryo cryopreservation remains the oldest and most widely used procedure for female fertility preservation. In reproductive age women with an established partner (or those using donor sperm), it is often offered as the primary method of fertility preservation due to the well-established evidence supporting its safety and efficacy.[9,10] With regards to freezing techniques, both slow-freezing and vitrification have demonstrated efficient outcomes, particularly for blastocyst cryopreservation. The older slow-freezing technique tends to be more resource intensive. This is owing to the large amounts of liquid nitrogen and specialized controlled-rate freezers required for slow freezing. Conversely, vitrification, or ultra-rapid cooling eliminates mechanical injury from ice crystal formation. It is a technique that is less expensive than slow freezing and achieves superior survival rates.[11,12] Therefore, vitrification is becoming more widely accepted in fertility centers worldwide.[13]

It is important to note that embryo cryopreservation is limited to women who have gone through puberty and when sperm is available. Therefore, this technique may not be suitable for single women unless sperm donation is employed. Embryos are typically the joint property of the two individuals among established heterosexual couples. Hence, these legal elements must also be taken into account if and when these embryos are to be used. Finally, embryo cryopreservation requires that a woman complete controlled ovarian stimulation (COS), which may not be feasible among some cancer patients. This occurs when prompt cancer therapy is recommended, or when estradiol levels must be minimized due to risk of cancer advancement, such as in certain breast cancers. In these circumstances, IVM may be a superior alternative.[14] IVM is the process whereby immature oocytes are obtained from antral follicles without requiring ovarian stimulation.[15] Current studies have demonstrated no increase in fetal anomalies or adverse outcomes in pregnancy as compared to IVF.[16-18] However, the pregnancy rates observed are lower than traditional IVF; hence, further technological improvements are required before IVM oocyte vitrification can become a more well-established technique.[19,20]

## Oocyte Cryopreservation

Since the first reported human live birth from cryopreserved oocytes in 1986,[21] oocyte cryopreservation has evolved significantly with regards to technology and overall efficiency. Initial studies employed a slow-freezing technique similar to the established process for embryo cryopreservation. However, due to the high water content and low surface-area to volume ratio unique to oocytes, researchers noted lipid membrane and meiotic spindle damage due to the formation of ice crystals. This crystal formation resulted in an overall survival rate of only 50–60% after slow-freezing and an implantation rate of less than 5%.[22] Nonetheless, further research demonstrated that the meiotic spindle had a capacity for self-restoration after cryopreservation.[23,24] The advent of vitrification overcame these shortcomings by promoting an ice-free glass-like cryopreservation process. During the vitrification process either a closed cell storage system or an open system that places the cells in direct contact with liquid nitrogen can be employed and promotes more rapid and uniform freezing. Cao et al. showed a significantly higher survival and blastocyst rate using vitrification and an open system, the McGill cryoleaf, as compared to slow freezing.[25] Similarly, Antinori et al. used a similar open cryotop method and yielded an impressive 99% survival rate, 93% fertilization rate, and 33% pregnancy rate.[26] Since those seminal studies, similar results have been reproduced and the open direct systems has been shown to be the safest and most efficacious.[27] Cobo et al. reaffirmed the safety and efficacy of the vitrification technique by comparing 804 IVF pregnancies from vitrified oocytes compared with 1,224 fresh oocytes and demonstrate no differences in obstetric or perinatal outcomes.[28] As a result of these studies, the American Society for Reproductive Medicine (ASRM) removed the "experimental" designation on oocyte cryopreservation in 2012. Subsequently, the first clinical practice guideline for mature oocyte cryopreservation was published in 2013, thereby endorsing oocyte vitrification as a safe and efficacious tool for fertility preservation.[29]

A significant advantage of oocyte cryopreservation over more well-established embryo cryopreservation is the ability for women without an established partner to preserve their fertility after gonadotoxic cancer treatment or to delay childbearing for social reasons. Since reproductive age is the single most important predictor of conception potential and the rate of aneuploidy increases significantly with age, elective social oocyte cryopreservation allows women to preserve their fertility potential. However, the optimal age to undergo such a procedure and the appropriate number of oocytes to preserve is still a topic of significant debate.[30] Goldman et al. devised two equations to help guide how many cryopreserved oocytes may be needed. The first equation predicts the likelihood of a single cryopreserved oocyte to produce a viable blastocyst based on patient age, assuming that 95% of oocytes are viable after thawing: $p(blast) = 0.95 \times exp(2.8043 - 0.1112 \times Age)$. Using this model, a 37-year-old patient with eight mature oocytes would have two blastocysts.[31] Furthermore, a second equation was devised to predict the probability of a live birth assuming that approximately 60% of euploid blastocysts will result in a live birth and accounting for the fact that the probability of producing a euploid blastocyst decreases with increasing maternal age. Ultimately, these algorithms can aid in counseling by determining how estimating the number of mature oocytes a woman would need in order to attain a high likelihood of live birth at any given age. We introduced oocyte vitrification in Canada, and have had more than 300 women with a variety of cancer and other medical conditions have fertility preservation by IVF or IVM oocyte vitrification. We have also had more than 40 women who vitrified their own oocytes and then used them and had healthy livebirths. Finally, we achieved the first 4 IVM/IVF babies on the world.[32]

## Ovarian-tissue Cryopreservation

The first successful attempt at preserving an entire organ of any animal species was reported in 2002 when Wang et al. froze intact ovaries in the rat model and subsequently thawed and transplanted them successfully, with four of seven rats producing subsequent ovarian follicles.[8] However, because female ovaries are much larger, it has proven to be far more difficult to preserve a female ovary in its entirety.

Ovarian tissue freezing was first reported by Donnez et al.[33] and the first live birth achieved by orthotopic tissue transplantation in 2004. Approximately 30–41 babies have been born using this method to date, but it has not yielded widespread adoption due to the inherent difficulties of requiring surgical intervention for both acquiring and transplanting back ovarian tissue. Although, a technically feasible option for social fertility preservation, the logistic considerations make it a less popular option than cryopreservation of oocytes and embryos. Nonetheless, this technique continues to be relevant, particularly in the context of cancer patients, as it does not delay cancer treatment. It is also the only option currently available for prepubertal girls.[34]

Generally speaking, ovarian tissue that is surgically removed can be reimplanted to either an orthotopic site within the pelvic cavity or heterotopic such as the forearm or abdomen.[34] In general, orthotopic sites are thought to be more physiologically appropriate with regards to temperature, pressure, and blood supply.[35-37] However, heterotopic sites are more easily accessible if multiple reimplantations are anticipated.[37,38] Furthermore, the amount of ovarian cortex harvested also depends on a variety of factors including the pubertal status of the patient and type of gonadotoxic treatment anticipated. For young prepubertal patients and those at high risk of complete ovarian failure after treatment, a complete oophorectomy is typically recommended.[41] Conversely, fertile adults undergoing gonadotoxic treatment typically undergo ovarian cortical biopsy, with 4–5 tissue samples approximately 1 cm in length, 4–5 mm in width, and 1–1.5 mm in depth retrieved from a single ovary.[34,39-41] The contralateral ovary is typically left in place as a possible site for future orthotopic reimplantation.[38,41-43]

## ■ FERTILITY PRESERVATION IN MEN

Bunge et al. reported the first case of human spermatozoa cryopreservation in 1953.[44,45] Since then, reliable long-term data has emerged that supports the safety and efficacy of semen cryopreservation even after decades of storage.[44] As a result, several national and international guidelines are now well-established to support fertility preservation for fertile adolescent and adult males.[45] Though there is growing evidence confirming that sperm quantity decline with age, spermatogenesis is a robust physiological process that allows most men to reproduce in relative perpetuity compared to the age-related decline in fertility experienced by women, male fertility cryopreservation is most commonly employed to preserve fertility in cases of cancer that require gonadotoxic treatment among otherwise fertile individuals.[46]

## Sperm Cryopreservation

In the context of fertile adolescent and adult males, cryopreservation of semen is a safe and effective way of preserving fertility prior to exposure to gonadotoxic treatments that may lead to sterilization. Generally, sperm is retrieved from semen samples obtained at least 48 hours apart and incubated in a cryoprotectant solution of glycerol and Tris-TES egg yolk-citrate medium to minimize the mechanical stress induced by ice crystal formation while submerged in liquid nitrogen.[46] Seminal plasma is also included as it appears to additionally buffer spermatozoa from injury during the freezing process.[47]

Particularly for adult men with subfertility, such as those with subnormal semen parameters, the process of fertility preservation may be more challenging to obtain adequate amount of viable reproductive cells. Hence, if time permits, multiple depositions of ejaculated semen are encouraged prior to cancer therapies. It is important to note that men with certain malignancies such as testicular cancer often present with subfertility even prior to starting gonadotoxic therapies.[48] A recent systematic review found that among patients with testicular cancer, the majority of studies found mean semen analysis values consistent with oligospermia preorchiectomy.[48,49] In postadolescent azoospermic patients or those who fail to ejaculate, various techniques from penile vibratory stimulation, electroejaculation and testicular sperm extraction can be offered to obtain sperm for cryopreservation. Even in cases with testicular failure or nonobstructive azoospermia, sperm may still be retrieved via microsurgical testicular sperm extraction and successful fertilization after IVF and intracytoplasmic sperm injection (ICSI) has been reported. In fact, cryopreserved semen samples with normal parameters demonstrate relatively equivalent pregnancy outcomes compared to fresh samples.[50-54]

## Preservation of Spermatogonial Stem Cells in Testicular Tissue

Although semen cryopreservation remains the most well-established technique for preserving male fertility, testicular tissue cryopreservation currently represents the only potentially viable option for preserving the fertility potential of prepubertal boys at risk of sterilization. Since testicular tissue contains spermatogonial stem cells (SSCs), preservation of viable tissue allows for future SSC transplantation, testicular tissue grafting, or even in vitro spermatogenesis.[55] Unfortunately, the same challenges involved in ovarian tissue cryopreservation have also been observed in attempts to cryopreserve testicular tissue. Specifically, viable testicular tissue relies on the sophisticated interplay between multiple cell types that have varying cryobiological properties; unfortunately, the mechanical stress of cryopreservation often disrupts these cell-cell adhesions and often results in apoptosis and loss of tissue integrity.[56,57] Traditionally, slow-freezing protocols with dimethyl sulfoxide (DMSO) have demonstrated the most promising results for maintaining testicular tissue integrity, particularly over other cryoprotectant solutions such as ethylene glycol, glycerol, or 1,2-propanediol.[58,59] Furthermore, vitrification has also been demonstrated in both mouse and human models to successfully preserve the histology and proliferative capacity of testicular tissue; hence, this represents an avenue for further research.[55,60-63]

# ■ EMERGING TECHNOLOGIES

## Ovarian Stem Cells and the Artificial Ovary

The classical model of mammalian reproduction is predicated on the notion that female reproductive capacity is based on a finite germ cell pool that develops antenatally and ceases to proliferate after birth. However, the discovery of germ line oogonial stem cells in the mouse model has initiated an entirely novel avenue for future research.[64-66] By isolating and culturing either pluripotent embryonic or oogonial stem cells, it becomes possible to develop a multistep in vitro culture system that can regulate the maturation and differentiation of primordial cells into fertilization-competent oocytes.[67] This technology can thereby overcome the limitations of current technologies that rely on an existing pool of viable germ cells.[68]

Among the current limitations of this technology, it is important to note that oogonial stem cells constitute less than 0.02% of all cells. Therefore, isolating them remains a significant challenge.[67] Secondly, the process of maturation and differentiation of primordial follicles requires a complex set of activation, inhibition, and maintenance factors to produce viable mature reproductive cells. Replicating such a system in vitro requires a complex multistep culture system to support each of the transitional steps and the changing requirements of the developing oocyte and its surrounding granulosa cells.[69,70] Thirdly, significant concerns have been raised on whether an in-vitro system can adequately account for the complex influence of genomic and epigenetic stimuli that are also required for the development of fully competent oocytes.[71] Finally, it is clear that the viability of reproductive cells relies fundamentally on the unique vascular, hormonal, and structural environmental provided by the ovary.[72] Hence, a truly in vitro system of oocyte development and maturation would require a unique three-dimensional biomatrix scaffold to act as an artificial ovary. Vanacker et al.[73] used an alginate-matrigel matrix to successfully demonstrate the capacity of an artificial medium to support the grafting and ongoing maintenance of ovarian stem cells. However, the capacity of such a system to support the maturation and development of such cells into viable mature oocytes remains to be seen.

## Testicular Stem Cells and In Vitro Culture

Similarly, in vitro generation of spermatogonial stem cells represents a major avenue for future innovations in male fertility preservation. For instance, adult human germ line stem cells have been successfully derived from testicular spermatogonial cells[74-76] and even embryonic stem cells using the murine model.[77] Furthermore, Sato et al.[78] produced functional sperm cells from mouse testis tissue that were successfully used to generate healthy, fertile offspring. However, there are still significant safety issues to overcome before this technique can be considered for clinical use, particularly since male fertility preservation is often used to cryopreserve cells among men with testicular cancer and other types of malignancies. Indeed, the potential of reseeding malignant cells may predispose future offspring to a variety of pediatric malignancies and other unintended health consequences.[79] In fact, this adverse consequence has been demonstrated in the rat model with as few as 20 leukemic cells leading to recurrence of disease.[80] An obvious solution would be to isolate normal cells from those with malignant potential. However, the capacity of current methods of cell sorting in human studies are still in their infancy, limiting the current effectiveness of this separation.[81] Notwithstanding these limitations, it is indeed possible that future male fertility preservation strategies could involve harvesting and cryopreserving spermatogonial stem cells from prepubertal boys about to undergo gonadotoxic therapy and used to generate viable mature sperm at a later point.[82]

## ■ CONCLUSION

Cryopreservation of oocytes, embryos, and spermatozoa are all viable methods of fertility preservation for both social and medical reasons. For prepubertal children at risk of sterilization from gonadotoxic conditions or treatments, ovarian and testicular tissue cryopreservation are the only available methods but the safety and efficacy of such technologies are still currently under investigation. Experimental work on the in vitro generation of sperm and oocytes from harvested stem cells appears promising, yet there are still many scientific, technical, and ethical questions yet to be answered in the field of fertility preservation. Optimizing techniques and minimizing the risks of fertility preservation strategies represent the key challenges in the coming years.

## KEY POINTS

- Cryopreservation is a safe and reliable technique to preserve an individual's fertility for medical and social reasons.
- Current options for female fertility preservation include preserving embryos, ovarian tissue, or mature or immature oocytes derived from IVF or IVM cycles.
- Cryopreservation of sperm is a well-established technique of fertility preservation for fertile adolescent and adult males.
- For prepubertal children, ovarian and testicular tissue cryopreservation are the only available methods but the safety and efficacy of such technologies are still under investigation.
- Experimental work on the in-vitro generation of sperm and oocytes from harvested stem cells appears promising and forms a potential avenue for future research.

## REFERENCES

1. Stoop D, Cobo A, Silber S. Fertility preservation for age-related fertility decline. Lancet. 2014;384(9950):1311-9.
2. Gosden RG. Fertility preservation: definition, history, and prospect. Semin Reprod Med. 2009;27(6):433-7.
3. Gidoni Y, Holzer H, Tan SL, et al. Fertility preservation in non-oncologic patients. Reprod Biomed Online. 2008;16:792-800.
4. Elizur SE, Chian RC, Pineau CA, et al. Fertility preservation treatment for young women with automimmune disease facing treatment with gonadotoxic agents. Rheumatology. 2008;47:1506-9.
5. Huang JY, Tulandi T, Holzer H, et al. Cryopreservation of ovarian tissue and in vitro matured oocytes in a female with mosaic Turner syndrome: case report. Hum Reprod. 2008;23:336-9.
6. Donnez J, Dolmans M-M, Campion EW. Fertility preservation in women. N Engl J Med. 2018;378:399-401.
7. Ata B, Kaplan B, Danzer H, et al. Array CGH analysis shows that aneuploidy is not related to the number of embryos generated. Reprod Biomed Online. 2012;24:614-20.
8. Wang X, Chen H, Yin H, et al. Fertility after intact ovary transplantation. Nature. 2002;415(6870):385.
9. Bedoschi G, Oktay K. Current approach to fertility preservation by embryo cryopreservation. Fertil Steril. 2013;99(6):1496-502.
10. Cakmak H, Rosen MP. Ovarian stimulation in cancer patients. Fertil Steril. 2013;99(6):1476-84.
11. Richter KS, Ginsburg DK, Shipley SK, et al. Factors associated with birth outcomes from cryopreserved blastocysts: experience from 4,597 autologous transfers of 7,597 cryopreserved blastocysts. Fertil Steril. 2016;106(2):354-62.
12. Fernandez Gallardo E, Spiessens C, D'Hooghe T, et al. Effect of day 3 embryo morphometrics and morphokinetics on survival and implantation after slow

freezing-thawing and after vitrification-warming: a retrospective cohort study. Reprod Biol Endocrinol. 2017;15(1):79.
13. Roque M, Lattes K, Serra S, et al. Fresh embryo transfer versus frozen embryo transfer in in vitro fertilization cycles: a systematic review and meta-analysis. Fertil Steril. 2013;99(1):156-62.
14. Rao GD, Chian RC, Son WS, et al. Fertility preservation in women undergoing cancer treatment. Lancet. 2004;363:1829.
15. Huang JY, Chian RC, Gilbert L, et al. Retrieval of immature oocytes from unstimulated ovaries followed by in vitro maturation and vitrification: a novel strategy of fertility preservation for breast cancer patients. Am J Surg. 2010;200:177-83.
16. Zhang XY, Ata B, Son WY, et al. Chromosome abnormality rates in human embryos obtained from in-vitromaturation and IVF treatment cycles. Reprod Biomed Online. 2010;21:552-9.
17. Chian RC, Xu CL, Huang JY, et al. Obstetric outcomes and congenital abnormalities in infants conceived with oocytes matured in vitro. Facts Views Vis Obgyn. 2014;6(1):15-8.
18. Child TJ, Phillips SJ, Abdul-Jalil AK, et al. A comparison of in vitro maturation and in vitro fertilization for women with polycystic ovaries. Obstet Gynecol. 2002;100(4):665-70.
19. Moawad AR, Xu B, Tan SL, et al. L-carnitine supplementation during vitrification of mouse germinal vesicle stage–oocytes and their subsequent in vitro maturation improves meiotic spindle configuration and mitochondrial distribution in metaphase II oocytes. Hum Reprod. 2014;29:2256-68.
20. Moawad AR, Tan SL, Xu B, et al. L-carnitine supplementation during vitrification of mouse oocytes at the germinal vesicle stage improves preimplantation development following maturation and fertilization in vitro. Biol Reprod. 2013;88:104.
21. Chen C. Pregnancy after human oocyte cryopreservation. Lancet. 1986;327(8486):884-6.
22. Kuwayama M. Highly efficient vitrification for cryopreservation of human oocytes and embryos: the Cryotop method. Theriogenology. 2007;67(1):73-80.
23. Cobo A, Romero JL, Perez S, et al. Storage of human oocytes in the vapor phase of nitrogen. Fertil Steril. 2010;94(5):1903-7.
24. Cobo A, Remohi J, Chang CC, et al. Oocyte cryopreservation for donor egg banking. Reprod Biomed Online. 2011;23(3):341-6.
25. Cao YX, Xing Q, Li L, et al. Comparison of survival and embryonic development in human oocytes cryopreserved by slow-freezing and vitrification. Fertil Steril. 2009;92(4):1306-11.
26. Antinori M, Licata E, Dani G, et al. Cryotop vitrification of human oocytes results in high survival rate and healthy deliveries. Reprod Biomed Online. 2007;14(1):72-9.
27. Cobo A, Garcia-Velasco JA, Domingo J, et al. Is vitrification of oocytes useful for fertility preservation for age-related fertility decline and in cancer patients? Fertil Steril. 2013;99(6):1485-95.

28. Cobo A, Serra V, Garrido N, et al. Obstetric and perinatal outcome of babies born from vitrified oocytes. Fertil Steril. 2014;102(4):1006-15.e4.
29. Mature oocyte cryopreservation: a guideline. Fertil Steril. 2013;99(1):37-43.
30. Gunnala V, Schattman G. Oocyte vitrification for elective fertility preservation: the past, present, and future. Curr Opin Obstet Gynecol. 2017;29(1):59-63.
31. Goldman RH, Racowsky C, Farland LV, et al. Predicting the likelihood of live birth for elective oocyte cryopreservation: a counseling tool for physicians and patients. Hum Reprod. 2017;32(4):853-9.
32. Chian RC, Huang JYJ, Gilbert L, et al. Obstetric outcomes following vitrification of in vitro and in vivo matured oocytes. Fertil Steril. 2009;91:2391-8.
33. Donnez J, Dolmans MM, Demylle D, et al. Livebirth after orthotopic transplantation of cryopreserved ovarian tissue. Lancet. 2004;364(9443):1405-10.
34. Donnez J, Martinez-Madrid B, Jadoul P, et al. Ovarian tissue cryopreservation and transplantation: a review. Hum Reprod Update. 2006;12(5):519-35.
35. Kim SS. Assessment of long term endocrine function after transplantation of frozen-thawed human ovarian tissue to the heterotopic site: 10 year longitudinal follow-up study. J Assist Reprod Genet. 2012;29(6):489-93.
36. Rodriguez-Wallberg KA, Oktay K. Fertility preservation and pregnancy in women with and without BRCA mutation-positive breast cancer. Oncologist. 2012;17(11):1409-17.
37. Oktay K, Economos K, Kan M, et al. Endocrine Function and Oocyte Retrieval After Autologous Transplantation of Ovarian Cortical Strips to the Forearm. JAMA. 2017;286(12):1490-3.
38. Stern CJ, Gook D, Hale LG, et al. First reported clinical pregnancy following heterotopic grafting of cryopreserved ovarian tissue in a woman after a bilateral oophorectomy. Hum Reprod. 2013;28(11):2996-9.
39. Donnez J, Dolmans MM, Pellicer A, et al. Restoration of ovarian activity and pregnancy after transplantation of cryopreserved ovarian tissue: a review of 60 cases of reimplantation. Fertil Steril. 2013;99(6):1503-13.
40. Donnez J, Dolmans MM. Fertility preservation in women. Nat Rev Endocrinol. 2013;9(12):735.
41. Donnez J, Jadoul P, Squifflet J, et al. Ovarian tissue cryopreservation and transplantation in cancer patients. Best Pract Res Clin Obstet Gynaecol. 2010;24(1):87-100.
42. Donnez J, Silber S, Andersen CY, et al. Children born after autotransplantation of cryopreserved ovarian tissue. a review of 13 live births. Ann Med. 2011;43(6):437-50.
43. Bunge RG, Sherman JK. Fertilizing capacity of frozen human spermatozoa. Nature. 1953;172(4382):767-8.
44. Horne G, Atkinson A, Brison DR, et al. Achieving pregnancy against the odds: successful implantation of frozen-thawed embryos generated by ICSI using spermatozoa banked prior to chemo/radiotherapy for Hodgkin's disease and acute leukaemia. Hum Reprod. 2001;16(1):107-9.
45. Loren AW, Mangu PB, Beck LN, et al. Fertility preservation for patients with cancer: American Society of Clinical Oncology clinical practice guideline update. J Clin Oncol. 2013;31(19):2500-10.

46. Holoch P, Wald M. Current options for preservation of fertility in the male. Fertil Steril. 2011;96(2):286-90.
47. Anger JT, Gilbert BR, Goldstein M. Cryopreservation of sperm: indications, methods and results. J Urol. 2003;170(4 Pt 1):1079-84.
48. Meirow D, Schenker JG. Infertility: cancer and male infertility. Hum Reprod. 2017;10(8):2017-22.
49. Djaladat H, Burner E, Parikh PM, et al. The association between testis cancer and semen abnormalities before orchiectomy: a systematic review. J Adolesc Young Adult Oncol. 2014;3(4):153-9.
50. Nicopoullos JD, Gilling-Smith C, Almeida PA, et al. Use of surgical sperm retrieval in azoospermic men: a meta-analysis. Fertil Steril. 2004;82(3):691-701.
51. Baukloh V. Retrospective multicentre study on mechanical and enzymatic preparation of fresh and cryopreserved testicular biopsies. Hum Reprod. 2017;17(7):1788-94.
52. Giorgetti C, Chinchole JM, Hans E, et al. Crude cumulative delivery rate following ICSI using intentionally frozen–thawed testicular spermatozoa in 51 men with non-obstructive azoospermia. Reprod Biomed Online. 2005;11(3):319-24.
53. Friedler S, Raziel A, Soffer Y, et al. Intracytoplasmic injection of fresh and cryopreserved testicular spermatozoa in patients with nonobstructive azoospermia—a comparative study. Fertil Steril. 1997;68(5):892-7.
54. Verheyen G1, Vernaeve V, Van Landuyt L, et al. Should diagnostic testicular sperm retrieval followed by cryopreservation for later ICSI be the procedure of choice for all patients with non-obstructive azoospermia? Human Reprod. 2017;19(12):2822-30.
55. Onofre J, Baert Y, Faes K, et al. Cryopreservation of testicular tissue or testicular cell suspensions: a pivotal step in fertility preservation. Hum Reprod Update. 2016;22(6):744-61.
56. Klosky JL, Randolph ME, Navid F, et al. Sperm Cryopreservation practices among adolescent cancer patients at risk for infertility. Pediatr Hematol Oncol. 2009;26(4):252-60.
57. Williams DH. Sperm banking and the cancer patient. Ther Adv Urol. 2010;2(1):19-34.
58. Goossens E, Frederickx V, Geens M, et al. Cryosurvival and spermatogenesis after allografting prepubertal mouse tissue: comparison of two cryopreservation protocols. Fertil Steril. 2008;89(3):725-7.
59. Keros V, Rosenlund B, Hultenby K, et al. Optimizing cryopreservation of human testicular tissue: comparison of protocols with glycerol, propanediol and dimethylsulphoxide as cryoprotectants. Hum Reprod. 2005;20(6):1676-87.
60. Shaw JM, Jones GM. Terminology associated with vitrification and other cryopreservation procedures for oocytes and embryos. Hum Reprod Update. 2003;9(6):583-605.
61. Poels J, Abou-Ghannam G, Herman S, et al. In search of better spermatogonial preservation by supplementation of cryopreserved human immature testicular tissue xenografts with N-acetylcysteine and testosterone. Front Surg. 2014;1.

62. Radaelli M, Almodin CG, Minguetti-Câmara VC, et al. A comparison between a new vitrification protocol and the slowfreezing method in the cryopreservation of prepubertal testicular tissue. JBRA Assist Reprod. 2017;21(3):188-95.
63. Yango P, Altman E, Smith JF, et al. Optimizing cryopreservation of human spermatogonial stem cells: comparing the effectiveness of testicular tissue and single cell suspension cryopreservation. Fertil Steril. 2014;102(5):1491-8e1.
64. Albamonte MI, Albamonte MS, Stella I, et al. The infant and pubertal human ovary: Balbiani's body-associated VASA expression, immunohistochemical detection of apoptosis-related BCL2 and BAX proteins, and DNA fragmentation. Hum Reprod. 2013;28(3):698-706.
65. Tilly JL. Commuting the death sentence: how oocytes strive to survive. Nat Rev Mol Cell Biol. 2001;2(11):838-48.
66. Wallace WH, Anderson RA, Irvine DS. Fertility preservation for young patients with cancer: who is at risk and what can be offered? Lancet Oncol. 2005;6(4):209-18.
67. White YA, Woods DC, Takai Y, et al. Oocyte formation by mitotically active germ cells purified from ovaries of reproductive-age women. Nat Med. 2012;18(3):413-21.
68. Telfer EE, Albertini DF. The quest for human ovarian stem cells. Nat Med. 2012;18(3):353-4.
69. Nicholas CR, Chavez SL, Baker VL, et al. Instructing an embryonic stem cell-derived oocyte fate: lessons from endogenous oogenesis. Endo Rev. 2009;30(3):264-83.
70. Dunlop CE, Telfer EE, Anderson RA. Ovarian stem cells--potential roles in infertility treatment and fertility preservation. Maturitas. 2013;76(3):279-83.
71. Anckaert E, De Rycke M, Smitz J. Culture of oocytes and risk of imprinting defects. Hum Reprod Update. 2013;19(1):52-66.
72. Bhartiya D, Hinduja I, Patel H, et al. Making gametes from pluripotent stem cells--a promising role for very small embryonic-like stem cells. Reprod Biol Endocrinol. 2014;12:114.
73. Vanacker J, Luyckx V, Dolmans MM, et al. Transplantation of an alginate-matrigel matrix containing isolated ovarian cells: first step in developing a biodegradable scaffold to transplant isolated preantral follicles and ovarian cells. Biomaterials. 2012;33(26):6079-85.
74. Altman E, Yango P, Moustafa R, et al. Characterization of human spermatogonial stem cell markers in fetal, pediatric, and adult testicular tissues. Reproduction. 2014;148(4):417-27.
75. Conrad S, Renninger M, Hennenlotter J, et al. Generation of pluripotent stem cells from adult human testis. Nature. 2008;456(7220):344.
76. Golestaneh N, Kokkinaki M, Pant D, et al. Pluripotent stem cells derived from adult human testes. Stem Cells deve. 2009;18(8):1115-26.
77. West JA, Park IH, Daley GQ, et al. In vitro generation of germ cells from murine embryonic stem cells. Nat Prot. 2006;1(4):2026-36.
78. Sato T, Katagiri K, Gohbara A, et al. In vitro production of functional sperm in cultured neonatal mouse testes. Nature. 2011;471(7339):504-7.

79. Chessells JM, Veys P, Kempski H, et al. Long-term follow-up of relapsed childhood acute lymphoblastic leukaemia. Br J Haematol. 2003;123(3):396-405.
80. Jahnukainen K, Hou M, Petersen C, et al. Intratesticular transplantation of testicular cells from leukemic rats causes transmission of leukemia. Can Res. 2001;61(2):706-10.
81. Fujita K, Tsujimura A, Miyagawa Y, et al. Isolation of germ cells from leukemia and lymphoma cells in a human in vitro model: potential clinical application for restoring human fertility after anticancer therapy. Can Res. 2006;66(23):11166-71.
82. Tsurusawa M, Shimomura Y, Asami K, et al. Long-term results of the Japanese Childhood Cancer and Leukemia Study Group studies 811, 841, 874 and 911 on childhood acute lymphoblastic leukemia. Leukemia. 2009;24(2):335.

# CHAPTER 35

# Fertility Following Gynecological Cancer

*Biman Kumar Chakraborty, NR Mondal,
Rahul Roy Chowdhury, Tanmoy Chatterjee*

## ■ INTRODUCTION

Malignancies are on the rise throughout the world. Some cancers, like cancer of the uterine cervix, though have shown a decline, perhaps due to screening and early diagnosis. A variety of cancers are affecting young women. Though cancers of the vulva and vagina are extremely rare in the young population, concerns about their fertility following cancers are being raised. Conservative approaches are being explored, taking into consideration the potentials of future fertility. Contemporary research is being directed to address such a cause. The aim of this article is to focus on this issue.

## ■ FERTILITY FOLLOWING CERVICAL CANCER

Cervical cancer is the most common cause of death among women with cancer in developing countries. In India more than 85% of patients are found to be over 40 years of age, the peak age group being 55–59 years. 85% of patients present in advanced stage of the disease.

The goals of fertility sparing surgery are preservation of reproductive potential and preservation of hormonal function without compromising with curability. Traditionally, the treatment of cervical cancer in early cases is radical surgery or radical radiotherapy. Unfortunately, the fertility potential is lost after both these procedures.

In early localized cervical cancer, fertility preserving surgery is reserved for the following conditions: a strong desire for pregnancy, age below 40 years, no other cause of infertility and the stage of cancer is IA1, IA2 or IB1. The patient must be counseled about the risk of recurrence of cancer, complications of surgery and complications of pregnancy associated with the cancer. The need for regular and close follow-up must be stressed upon.

Preoperative investigations for correct staging include a thorough clinical and radiological imaging in the form of ultrasound, computed tomography (CT) scan, magnetic resonance imaging (MRI) or positron emission tomography-computed tomography (PET-CT) scan. MRI is regarded as the most adequate diagnostic option for assessment of stroma and parametrium involvement, while CT or PET-CT are best used to detect lymph node involvement. The value of a sentinel node frozen section biopsy, if possible, is stressed upon. Most surgeons agree that involvement of pelvic lymph node is a contraindication for conservative surgery. With reference to histological types, both squamous and adenocarcinomas have been treated by conservative surgery. Clear cell and neuroendocrine types are contraindications due to their aggressive nature.

Fertility-preserving surgical procedures include conization, radical trachelotomy, neoadjuvant chemotherapy followed by radical trachelectomy and total hysterectomy with ovarian transposition in stage IB1. Conization either by laser, loop electrosurgical excision (LEEP) or cold knife surgery is recommended in Stage IA, in cases without lymphovascular invasion, negative margins and a normal endocervical curettage. Results of conization by any of these methods are similar. Radical trachelectomy may be done abdominally or vaginally. Radical abdominal trachelectomy may be performed by laparotomy, laparoscopy or robotic surgery. Abdominal trachelectomy is indicated if the cancer is diagnosed in early pregnancy. Radical trachelectomy is recommended for stage IA2 and IB1. If lymphovascular involvement is present in Stage 1A1, radical trachelectomy is preferred to conization. Radical abdominal or vaginal trachelectomy both are equally effective. Clamping the uterine artery or the cervical branch selectively is the surgeon's choice. Care should be taken to leave behind at least 1 cm cervical tissue at the level of internal os. Permanent circlage is necessary to prevent mid abortion or preterm labor. There is no big series of laparoscopic or robotic radical trachelectomy to comment on the superiority of one over the other. Sufficient data regarding outcome is available with vaginal radical trachelectomy only. Radical vaginal trachelectomy has been more extensively used with comparable good result. Pelvic lymph nodes must be assessed laparoscopically prior to vaginal trachelectomy. Ideally pelvic lymph node involvement is a contraindication to radical trachelectomy, but some surgeons would proceed with complete pelvic lymphadenectomy in Stage 1A2 and IB1 cases. Common complications of radical trachelectomy include cervical stenosis, decreased cervical mucus, ascending infection and subclinical salpingitis, secondary hemorrhage, mid-trimester abortion, premature rupture of membranes, preterm labor and massive hemorrhage in early labor. Pareja R identified 485 patients with literature search from 1997–2012 who had radical trachelectomy, 413 (85%) were able to maintain fertility; 113 (36%) attempted pregnancy and 67 of them (59.3%) were able to conceive.[1] Kordak is in a reviewed article (2012) reported obstetric outcome of 805 radical vaginal trachelectomy a total of 359 pregnancies in 217 patients resulting in 229 births—67% over 36 weeks gestation.[2] Recently Kasuga Y (2016) reported 61 pregnancies after radical trachelectomy in single unit of which 42 were achieved by in vitro fertilization—embryo transfer (39 cases) and intrauterine insemination (3 cases).[3] Neo adjuvant chemotherapy to downstage stage IB2 cancer of the cervix followed by radical trachelectomy has been tried. Simple total hysterectomy with ovarian transposition are possibilities to consider regarding assisted reproduction procedures in future. Concerns regarding assisted reproduction techniques following conservative surgery may be limited to risks of multiple pregnancy and preterm labor, and difficulty in embryo transfer (a catheter may be placed in cervix during ovarian stimulation). Intraperitoneal insemination, intrafallopian transfer of gamete or zygote is a therapeutic option.

Fertility preservation in early cancer cervix is a viable alternative. Prerequisites must be satisfied. Strong desire for pregnancy and counseling is very important. The prospects of conservative surgery is limited in India, as 85% of cancer cervix cases are over 40 years of age and 85% present in advanced stage.

## PRESERVING FERTILITY IN PATIENTS WITH ENDOMETRIAL CARCINOMA

Endometrial carcinoma (EC) is the most common gynecologic malignancy in developed countries and affects mainly postmenopausal women. In India, the incidence rate is low. Conservative management of EC carries the risk of being unstaged and missing a synchronous ovarian cancer. Therefore, proper counseling and close follow-up is of paramount importance and definitive treatment after completion of childbearing is advised.

Early-stage EC, grade I, no myometrial invasion, young candidates highly motivated to maintain their reproductive potential, fully comprehend and are willing to accept the risk associated with deviation from the standard of care, agreeable to a close follow-up schedule, and thoroughly counseled on the oncologic risk associated with unstaged EC as well as the risk of synchronous ovarian cancer may be regarded as the ideal prerequisites of selection of candidates for fertility sparing treatment.

A thorough clinical examination is mandatory. Contrast-enhanced MRI is better than transvaginal sonography (TVS) and CT scan to assess myometrial invasion, lymph node status, cervical involvement and presence of any adnexal mass. A diagnostic dilatation and curettage is better than office endometrial sampling. Finally, evaluation should include assessment for Lynch syndrome.

Medical treatment may be classified as hormonal and nonhormonal. The two systemic progestins widely used are medroxyprogesterone acetate (MPA) 500–600 mg daily and megestrol acetate (MA) 160 mg daily, usually for 4–6 month, except in obese and ovulatory patients, who require longer treatment duration. An alternative to systemic progestins, levonorgestrel-intrauterine device (LNG-IUD), is well studied. Risks of thrombophlebitis, weight gain, headache, sleep disorders, mood and libido changes and leg cramps[4] must be counseled. Among the nonhormonal therapies, photodynamic therapy (PDT) is a novel treatment modality for early stage EC. It uses a nontoxic light-sensitive compound which upon selective exposure to light of a specific wavelength produces active oxygen species that are toxic to surrounding cancer cells.[5]

Hysteroscopic surgical excision of the localized lesion followed by progestin is an alternative conservative management approach in young women with EC.[6]

Documentation from tissue diagnosis by either dilatation and curettage or office endometrial biopsy at 3 month interval remains the standard criterion to assess response to treatment. The presence of simple hyperplasia and/or complex hyperplasia without atypia in follow-up biopsies is accepted as complete regression. Women achieving complete disease regression should be divided into two categories: those who promptly pursue fertility, if desired, should be referred to a reproductive endocrinologist and those who do not plan on an immediate pregnancy, should be placed on maintenance progestin therapy with low-dose cyclic progestin or an LNG-IUD. Women with disease progression or persistence after 9 months should undergo more definitive treatment.

Follow-up interval should be every 3–6 months after complete response. The methods of follow-up are thorough pelvic examination, endometrial biopsy, serum Ca 125 and imaging.[7]

Pregnancy itself is considered to be a natural, extremely high dose progesterone therapy. Assisted reproductive technology (ART) is associated with a higher live birth rate compared with spontaneous conception in young women with EC.[8] In summary, early referral to reproductive endocrinology should be considered in order to maximize the likelihood of a live birth and minimize the time between diagnosis and definitive EC treatment.

It is important to recognize that conservative treatment for EC although initially successful in the majority of women, is a temporary phenomenon. The risk of recurrence after completion of treatment is high, even among women who had a rapid complete response as well as among those on maintenance progestin therapy. EC recurrence rate varies from 24% to 40.6%, although most recurrence occurs within first 3 years. It can occur in as little as 2 months and upto 30 years after treatment.

Women who fail in conservative treatment due to either disease progression or lack of regression should undergo definitive treatment consisting of total abdominal hysterectomy with bilateral salpingo-oophorectomy and/or lymphadenectomy. This surgery should be done if no evidence of disease regression is observed within 6–9 month of treatment initiation. Once women who have been successfully treated with progestin have completed childbearing, they should also undergo surgery. Ovarian preservation affords an opportunity for fertility preservation in this setting of hysterectomy, given the potential for future oocyte retrieval and surrogacy.

Standard treatment for recurrence of EC is hysterectomy. However, a second-round progestin may be considered if the patient still wishes to maintain her reproductive potential after proper counseling regarding the risks involved.

Patients with EC should be carefully selected using strict selection criteria as mentioned before. Time to complete resolution of EC can vary from 3 months to more than 1 year. Therefore, a trial of 1 year of treatment with close follow-up is reasonable before abandoning medical treatment. Close follow-up is essential and definitive treatment after completion of childbearing is recommended.

## ▮ FERTILITY AFTER GESTATIONAL TROPHOBLASTIC DISEASE

Until about 70 years ago, a diagnosis of choriocarcinoma spelt doom. Treatment was limited to surgery with ablative intent. Since the disease arises from the placenta, the uterus was often sacrificed to save the life of the patient. The ovaries were also removed in certain circumstances under the belief that removal of the theca lutein cysts could be beneficial. Since gestational trophoblastic disease is primarily limited to the younger population, the woman had to sacrifice her prospects of fertility to save her life. Advances in chemotherapy with scientific and judicial use of ablative and mutilating surgery have changed the scenario.

Teratogenicity due to chemotherapeutic agents, however, remains a major cause of concern in the treatment of the patients of gestational trophoblastic disease. Methotrexate (MTX) remains the cornerstone in treating such patients. It may be used alone in low-risk cases or in combination with other drugs in high risk cases, as in the EMA-CO (Etoposide, MTX, Actinomycin D, Cyclophosphamide and Vincristine) or MAC (MTX, Actinomycin D and Cyclophosphamide) regimens. MTX is a methyl derivative of aminopterin. It inhibits the enzyme dihydrofolate reductase and thus affects DNA synthesis, leading to miscarriages, fetal chromosomal and congenital anomalies, and growth restrictions. A single high dose of MTX (50 mg/m$^2$) given before 8 weeks gestation causes abortion in over 95% of cases.[9] After administration, methotrexate is widely distributed in body tissues, the highest concentrations being in the kidneys, gallbladder, spleen, liver and skin. Its presence in the liver has been reported up to 116 days after exposure, although the amount of drug retained does not appear to be related to the dose received.[10] In order to allow for the persistence of MTX in tissues and to avoid potential chromosomal damage to the dividing follicle, a minimum delay of 12 months would seem logical. The neural tube closes at approximately day 29 of gestation, and weeks 4–7 are the most sensitive for limb development, hence exposure to teratogens such as MTX is unsafe for use in the first trimester. Exposure to teratogens after the first trimester tends to cause abnormalities in growth and brain development. It is not necessary for drugs to cross the placenta in order to exert a teratogenic effect, although MTX is known to pass to the fetus, even after maternal intrathecal administration. A large study looked at 2,308 offspring of survivors of child and adolescent cancer, 25% of whom were treated with chemotherapy. Details of the type of chemotherapy were not given, but no increased risk of cancer was seen, although follow-up was limited to the second decade of life.[11] Another study reported 243 conceptions, 169 term live births in 129 patients following full chemotherapy without any significant fetal abnormality.[12] However, the risks of recurrent moles must be borne in mind during counseling the patient who is desirous of fertility preservation and egg donation may be an alternative to be kept in mind. There has been a case report of six consecutive molar pregnancies.[13] Hysterectomy may have a role in patients with high and chemoresistant tumor burden; in such cases, artificial insemination with the patient's ova and surrogacy may offer a hope of fertility in such cases. Radiotherapy in modern day treatment of gestational trophoblastic neoplasia is limited to palliative intent in selective cases of cranial metastasis. New methods like selective uterine arterial embolization are now offered to women with massive uterine hemorrhage and a desire to maintain fertility in the future. Follow-up of these young patients, however, tend to be very poor as observed in a recent study.[14]

## ■ FERTILITY SPARING SURGERY IN OVARIAN CANCER

The International Agency for Research on Cancer, Lyon, France in its review in the year 2012, rates ovarian cancer as the fourth most common cancer in females across all age groups in India. The National Cancer Registry Programme (2012–2014) under the Indian Council of Medical Research puts the Age Adjusted Incidence Rate of ovarian cancer at 15 per 100,000 women, where Kolkata (8 per 100,000) and Mumbai fall in the top 10 metros on the list. That ovarian cancer is increasing in India is agreed to by all oncologists.

The majority of ovarian cancers in young adults are of the germ cell type, while epithelial ovarian cancers are more frequent in the age group of 40–50 years.

The goals of fertility sparing surgery are preservation of reproductive potential, preservation of hormonal function, preservation of healthy body image without compromise in curability. Therefore fertility sparing surgery must offer similar oncologic outcomes to standard therapy and favorable obstetric outcome. The benefits of the procedure must outweigh the risks and must have reduced morbidity.

### Epithelial Ovarian Cancers

It is recognized that in order to fully stage a patient with ovarian cancer a hysterectomy, removal of both ovaries, omentum, pelvic and para-aortic lymph nodes and collection of peritoneal washings and multiple random peritoneal biopsies are required. However in those that undergo fertility preservation the hysterectomy and removal of the normal ovary is not done. The risk of micrometastasis in the contralateral ovary is 2–3%. The European Society of Gynaecologic Oncology guidelines published in 2011 concluded that Stage IA grade 1 and possibly grade 2 tumors of mucinous, endometrioid or serous types were suitable for fertility sparing surgery. Grade 1 stage IC could also be considered. These women had a 10.3% chance of recurrence and 5.5% chance of death from disease.

## Borderline Ovarian Tumor

Borderline tumors of the ovary occur more commonly in younger women and have frequently been treated with conservative surgery. Borderline ovarian tumors are often diagnosed incidentally after ovarian cystectomies or unilateral oophorectomies in young women. An oophorectomy after a borderline tumor is diagnosed in a cystectomy specimen is not necessary. The risks of recurrence are 6% for an ipsilateral recurrence, 3% for a contralateral recurrence, and 3% for a bilateral recurrence. The survival rates are 95–97% at 5 years, although recurrences tend to occur late. Conservative surgery is normally offered in stage 1A disease but concern exists where disease has spread. For stage II or III disease the 5-year survival rates are 65–85% and as these are slow growing tumors, many more patients will eventually succumb to disease over a longer follow up duration. Although fertility sparing surgery has been used in advanced cases, there are no data to suggest this is safe and caution must be exercised.

## Germ Cell and Sex Cord Stromal Tumors of Ovary

These tumors are frequently limited to one ovary and almost always present at a very early stage without extraovarian spread. Surgery with staging is the mainstay of treatment but should not result in sterility. The uterus and normal contralateral ovary should be maintained, and chemotherapy should be used as indicated. Zanetta and colleagues[15] reported the largest experience of fertility-sparing procedures in young women with malignant germ cell tumors. Preservation of the uterus and contralateral ovary was possible in 138 (81%) of 169 patients. The survival rate of the patients treated conservatively (90–100%) was the same as that of the entire group (89–100%). Nearly 88% (28 of 32) of the patients who attempted to become pregnant were able to conceive whether they received adjuvant chemotherapy or not. 55 conceptions resulted in 38 (69%) full-term, normal infants.

## ■ CHEMOTHERAPY

Chemotherapy should be administered as indicated in patients with ovarian carcinoma. The development of premature ovarian failure after chemotherapy is always a concern and has been reported to be as high as 68%.

## KEY POINTS

- The patient must be counseled multidisciplinary team meetings between oncologists and fertility experts to chalk out a plan of management for all cancer patients where fertility preservation is planned.
- Patient must be counseled by all concerned to ensure that the expectations are realistic. Patients should be counseled regarding the principles of fertility sparing surgery, and that oncologic outcome always takes precedence over fertility preservation.
- Once fertility preservation is planned, oocyte collection, embryo preservation should be planned and executed meticulously so that treatment of cancer is not delayed.

## REFERENCES

1. Pareja R, Rendon GJ, Sanz-Lomara CM, et al. Surgical, oncological, and obstetrical outcomes after abdominal radical trachelectomy-a systematic literature review. Gynecol Oncol. 2013;131(1):77-82.
2. Kasuga Y, Nishio H, Miyakoshi K, et al. Uterine Papillary Serous Carcinoma. Int J Gynecol Cancer. 2016;26(1):163-8.
3. Kardakis S. Fertility-preserving surgery in patients with early stage cervical carcinoma. ISRN Oncology. 2012:2012:817065.
4. Montz FJ, Bristow RE, Bovicelli A, et al. Intrauterine progesterone treatment of early endometrial cancer. Am.J Obstet Gynecol. 2002;186:651-7.
5. Choi MC, Jung SG, Park H, et al. Fertility preservation via photodynamic therapy in young patients with early-stage uterine endometrial cancer, a long-term follow-up study. Int Gynecol Cancer. 2013;23;698-704.
6. Mazzon I, Corrado G, Morricone D, et al. Reproductive preservation for treatment of stage IA endometrial cancer in a young woman: hysteroscopic resection. Int J Gynecol Cancer. 2005;15:974-8.
7. Cade TJ, Quinn MA, Rome RM, et al. Progestogen treatment options for early endometrial cancer. BJOG. 2010;117:879-84.
8. Gallos ID, Gupta JK, Yap J, et al. Regression, relapse and live birth rates with fertility-sparing therapy for endometrial cancer and atypical complex endometrial hyperplasia; a systematic review and meta-analysis. Am J Obstet Gynecol. 2012;207(4):266.
9. Hausknecht RU. Methotrexate and misoprostol to terminate early pregnancy. N Engl J Med. 1995;333:537-40.
10. ASHP. AHFS Drug Information. Maryland: ASHP; 2016.
11. Mulivihill JJ, Connelly RR, Austin DE, et al. Cancer in offspring of long term survivors of childhood and adolescent cancer. Lancet. 1987;2:813-7.
12. Hideo M, Iitsuka Y, Suzuka K, et al. Outcome of subsequent pregnancy after treatment for persistent gestational trophoblastic tumour. Hum Reprod. 2002;17:469-72.

13. Al-Ghamdi AA. Recurrent hydatidiform mole: a case report of six consecutive molar pregnancies complicated by choriocarcinoma, and review of literature. J Fam Comm Med. 2011;18(3);159-61.
14. Chakrabarti B, Mondal NR, Chatterjee T, et al. Analysis of 58 cases of GTT from 2000-2013 at A Tertiary Cancer Center in India. BAOJ Gynaec. 2017;1(1):10.
15. Zanetta G, Bonazzi C, Cantu M, et al. Survival and reproductive function after treatment of malignant germ cell ovarian tumors. J Clin Oncol. 2001;19:1015-20.

CHAPTER
36

# Fertility Preservation in Oncological Patients (Oncofertility)

Rajan S Vaidya

## ■ OVERVIEW OF THE TOPIC

- Diagnosis of malignancy has a major impact on the life of any person
- Although cancer is commonly thought to be the disease of the elderly, nearly 20% of the cancer patients are diagnosed in their reproductive years that is, up to age of 45 years
- Some of the commonly occurring cancers in the young individuals are breast cancer, genital cancers, hematological cancers, etc.

## ■ NEED FOR FERTILITY PRESERVATION

- Remarkable breakthrough in the treatment of these cancers has made it possible for many young individuals with cancers to lead a long post-treatment survival
- Indeed, 5 year and 10 year survival rates for many patients are already around 75%
- However, all the modalities of cancer treatments like surgery, chemotherapy, or radiotherapy either very severely affect reproductive function or cause its total loss
- Chemotherapy and radiotherapy in the therapeutic doses cause serious damage to ovary and testis, rendering them incapable of producing healthy oocytes or sperms respectively, whereas radiotherapy causes damage to uterus too rendering it incapable of rearing a child to full term pregnancy
- Surgical treatment involves total removal reproductive organs in cases of genital malignancies
- Therefore, there is a need for fertility preservation to enable these young cancer survivors to procreate their progeny even after various cancer treatment options.

## ■ WHAT IS FERTILITY PRESERVATION?

- Fertility preservation in essence means preserving the ability of an individual or couple to start a family at a time of their choosing

- Oncofertility is a term coined for fertility preservation in cancer patients
- Improvement in cancer management and increasing survival rates has created a need for oncofertility
- Moreover, current data suggests that for most tumors post-treatment pregnancy does not increase the risk of cancer progression or adverse obstetric or neonatal outcome
- The emphasis, therefore has moved from providing life to providing quality of life.

## WHAT ARE THE VARIOUS METHODS OF FERTILITY PRESERVATION?

- With the advances in the assisted reproduction technology and cryopreservation techniques (freezing), it is now possible to freeze embryos, oocytes, sperms, ovarian tissue, and testicular tissue with great assurance
- Currently, embryo and mature oocyte cryopreservation following in vitro fertilization (IVF) and semen cryopreservation are the only techniques endorsed by the American Society of Reproductive Medicine (ASRM), and the other methods are still considered to be investigational or experimental
- Procedures like ovarian cortex or whole ovary freezing, and in vitro maturation of oocytes, are considered experimental although they hold a lot of promise and
- Procedures like ovarian suppression or transposition are found to be inadequate for fertility preservation.

## ALL THE FERTILITY PRESERVATION PROCEDURES HAVE TO OCCUR BEFORE INITIATION OF CANCER TREATMENTS

- In 2006, the American Society of Clinical Oncology first published recommendations on fertility preservation stating that, "as part of education and informed consent before cancer therapy, oncologists should address the possibility of infertility with patients treated during their reproductive years and be prepared to discuss possible fertility preservation options or refer patients to reproductive specialists"
- There is thus a need for a multidisciplinary collaboration between oncologists and reproductive specialists to improve awareness and availability of fertility preservation.

## IMPORTANCE OF PRETREATMENT OVARIAN RESERVE ASSESSMENT

- The number of oocytes retrieved and their quality are imperative factors predicting the potential efficacy of the fertility preservation procedure

- Consequently, information regarding the expected ovarian performance after controlled ovarian stimulation (COS) is crucial when consulting with the patient
- Therefore, the assessment of ovarian reserve with the use of antral follicle count (AFC) and/or anti-Müllerian hormone (AMH) before ovarian stimulation is necessary to provide more accurate prediction of ovarian response to COS and to determine the COS protocol and starting gonadotropin dose.

## SPECIAL CONSIDERATIONS FOR OVARIAN STIMULATION IN CANCER PATIENTS

- The patients referred for fertility preservation owing to a malignant disease do not represent the typical population of subfertile patients treated in IVF units
- Cancer may affect multiple tissues throughout the body and can result in a variety of complications during COS
- Determination of the COS protocol and gonadotropin dose for oocyte or embryo cryopreservation requires an individualized assessment
- To facilitate initiation of ovarian stimulation and avoid unnecessary delay, prompt consultation with a reproductive endocrinologist and coordination of care are:
  - In cancer patients, both the specific malignancy and the patient's multisystemic condition may have an impact on the response to ovarian stimulation
  - The increased catabolic state, malnutrition, and increased stress hormone levels associated with the malignancy may affect the hypothalamic-gonadal axis and decrease fertility
  - Possible adverse association between the presence of a neoplastic process and ovarian reserve or oocyte quality is also suggested
  - There are mixed reports about how cancer patients respond to the IVF stimulation protocols—some reporting no significant change and others demonstrating worse ovarian response in cancer patients compared with age-matched healthy women.
- In a recent meta-analysis conducted on seven retrospective studies, women with malignancies had lower numbers of total oocytes ($11.7 \pm 7.5$ vs $13.5 \pm 8.4$) and mature oocytes retrieved ($9.0 \pm 6.5$ vs $10.8 \pm 6.8$) after COS for fertility preservation compared with healthy age-matched patients
- Moreover, the relative risk of poor response leading to cycle cancellation was higher in cancer patients than in the control group (risk ratio 1.32, 95% confidence interval 0.78–2.17) although the observed difference did not reach statistical significance, possibly due to the small size of the groups
- *BRCA* genes play an essential role in double-strand DNA break repair, and their mutations are associated with an increased risk of breast and ovarian cancers
- In patients with *BRCA* mutations, oocytes may be more prone to DNA damage, clinically manifesting as diminished ovarian reserve or earlier menopause

Table 1: Comparison of antral follicle count (AFC) between cancer patients and healthy women in different age groups.

| Age (y) | Cancer patients | | | Healthy women | | | P value |
|---|---|---|---|---|---|---|---|
| | n | Median | Range | n | Median | Range | |
| 25–30 | 33 | 14 | 1–58 | 205 | 20 | 4–58 | <.001 |
| 31–35 | 47 | 11 | 0–54 | 216 | 15 | 5–48 | .004 |
| 36–40 | 49 | 7 | 0–40 | 227 | 12 | 0–52 | <.001 |
| 41–45 | 20 | 7 | 1–20 | 161 | 6 | 1–22 | .789 |

- In *BRCA* mutation, positive breast cancer patients, a low response to ovarian stimulation occurred more frequently than in patients without *BRCA* mutations (33.3% vs 3.3%) or in breast cancer patients not tested for their *BRCA* status (2.9%)
- Interestingly, all *BRCA* mutation—positive patients with a low response to ovarian stimulation and requiring higher doses of gonadotropins for their stimulation had *BRCA1* mutations, and a low response was not encountered in women who were positive for only a *BRCA2* mutation
- In a recent study, ovarian reserve assessed with AMH was found to be significantly lower in patients with lymphoma before chemotherapy compared with healthy control subjects
- Moreover, women with cancer before gonadotoxic therapy may have significantly lower AFC compared with healthy women aged 25–40 years (Table 1). This lower AFC in cancer patients may be explained by either accelerated follicle loss or a defect in recruitment of antral follicles owing to disease state
- Therefore, if lower oocyte and embryo numbers in patients with malignancy during an IVF cycle are true, this is not due to poor response to ovarian stimulation, but likely the result of decreased number of available antral follicles to be stimulated.

In conclusion, candidates for fertility preservation because of malignancy, especially *BRCA1* mutation carriers, should be informed that the expected number of oocytes retrieved after COS may be lower compared with healthy patients of similar age.

## GONADOTROPIN DOSE DURING OVARIAN STIMULATION

- Maximizing the number of embryos and oocytes cryopreserved during a fertility preservation cycle is extremely important, not only because the patient usually has a single cycle opportunity owing to time constraints, but also to increase the chance of future pregnancies
- Using higher doses of gonadotropins can be one of the strategies to increase the embryo and oocyte yield per cycle
- Higher doses of gonadotropins do not stimulate the recruitment of chromosomally abnormal or incompetent oocytes.

## OVARIAN STIMULATION PROTOCOLS

When stimulating cancer patients, several unique issues are important to consider:
- Avoidance of delays for cancer treatment—time delays can pose increased stress for the patient and oncologist, both and undue delay may mean that the patient may not be to go through treatment to preserve fertility
- *Consideration of additional safety issues:* Avoidance of high estrogenic state with certain cancers that are positive for estrogen receptors (for example, breast and uterine)
- Completely obviate ovarian hyperstimulation syndrome (OHSS)
- Understanding comorbid conditions that may either coexist or precipitate as a sequela from COS and/or oocyte retrieval procedure.

## CONVENTIONAL CONTROLLED OVARIAN STIMULATION

- Traditional ovarian preparation for IVF requires 9–14 days of ovarian stimulation with exogenous gonadotropins, preceded by ovarian suppression with gonadotropin-releasing hormone (GnRH) agonists for ~2 weeks to prevent premature ovulation
- Because GnRH agonist is initiated in the luteal phase of the previous cycle, this may add up to 3 additional weeks to the process, depending on when the patient presents for treatment
- The development of GnRH antagonists has significantly decreased the interval from patient presentation to embryo or oocyte cryopreservation
- In contrast to GnRH agonists, GnRH antagonists immediately suppress pituitary release of follicle stimulating hormone (FSH) and luteinizing hormone (LH) and do not require the 10–14 days of medication before gonadotropin initiation
- The GnRH antagonists are initiated to prevent premature LH surge when the size of the lead follicle reaches 12–14 mm at approximately day 6 of gonadotropin stimulation, which begins on day 2–3 of a menstrual cycle (Fig. 1A)
- This approach still requires awaiting menses before initiating gonadotropins, but it decreases the interval to oocyte retrieval compared to traditional IVF stimulation protocols
- Although multiple different COS protocols are used, the majority of patients are treated with a GnRH antagonist-based protocol, which likely allows the shortest deferral of the initiation of radio- or chemotherapy
- To date, there are no studies comparing agonist and antagonist protocols in women with cancer.

# NEWER CONCEPT OF FOLLICULAR RECRUITMENT IN OVARIAN PHYSIOLOGY

A newer concept of ovarian physiology indicates that there are multiple waves of follicle recruitment during each menstrual cycle.

# RANDOM-START CONTROLLED OVARIAN HYPERSTIMULATION

- Conventionally, ovarian stimulation for oocyte or embryo cryopreservation is initiated at the beginning of the follicular phase with the idea that this optimizes clinical outcomes
- It may require 2–6 weeks depending on the woman's menstrual cycle phase at the time of planning the treatment
- Adhering to this convention may result in either significant delay of cancer treatments or forgoing of fertility preservation owing to time constraints
- For cases not desirable to wait for the next menstrual period to start a stimulation protocol owing to the urgency of the cancer treatment. *"Random-start stimulation protocols"* have been proposed
- In a small prospective multicenter study (n = 40), a novel protocol for cancer patients that initiated ovarian stimulation during the luteal phase of the menstrual cycle was described.

Cancer patients in the luteal phase were started on GnRH antagonists to down-regulate LH and initiate luteolysis.

- Simultaneously, follicular stimulation was initiated with recombinant FSH only, thus avoiding exogenous LH activity, which might prevent luteolysis
- Compared with cancer patients stimulated during the follicular phase (n = 28) with either a short "flare-up" protocol or an antagonist protocol, the *luteal-phase* group (n = 12) had *similar* number of aspirated oocytes, number of MII oocytes, and fertilization rate
- A report of patients evaluated the effectiveness of initiating ovarian stimulation at the time of patient presentation (menstrual cycle days 11, 14, and 17) rather than waiting for spontaneous menses
- The GnRH antagonist was started to prevent premature LH surge when the lead follicle measured more than 13 mm
- The random-start ovarian stimulation resulted in a *reasonable ovarian response*, with 7–10 embryos cryopreserved per patient
- The recent report presenting clinical experience with random-start ovarian stimulation demonstrated that late follicular or luteal phase—start antagonist IVF cycles were as effective as conventional (i.e. early follicular) —start antagonist IVF cycles in cancer patients
- The late follicular phase was defined as after menstrual cycle day 7 with emergence of a dominant follicle (>13 mm) and/or progesterone level less

than 2 ng/mL. If the cancer patient presented in the late follicular phase, one of the following treatment plans can be deployed
- Ovarian stimulation started without GnRH antagonist, if the follicle cohort following the lead follicle was less than 12 mm and continued to be less than 12 mm before spontaneous LH surge (Fig. 1C)
  After the LH surge, GnRH antagonist started later in the cycle when the secondary follicle cohort reached 12 mm to prevent premature secondary LH surge. Or
- Ovulation was induced with human chorionic gonadotropin (hCG) or GnRH agonist and ovarian stimulation was started in 2–3 days in the luteal phase (Fig. 1E).
- If the cancer patient presented in the luteal phase or the ovulation was induced, ovarian stimulation was started without GnRh antagonist and similar to conventional COS, to prevent secondary LH surge, GnRH antagonist was added when secondary follicle cohort reached 12 mm and was continued until HCG or GnRH agonist trigger
- The numbers of total and mature oocytes retrieved, oocyte yield (i.e. number of MII oocytes or AFC), and fertilization rates were similar between groups (Table 2)
- However, the length of ovarian stimulation was ~2 days longer, and therefore, the total dose of gonadotropin used was significantly higher in late follicular and luteal phase—start groups compared with the conventional-start group (Table 2)
- In contrast to earlier belief, the presence of corpus luteum or luteal-phase progesterone levels did not adversely affect the follicular development, oocyte yield, or possibility of having secondary spontaneous LH surge in random-start patients
- Overall, this approach provides a *significant advantage* by decreasing total time for the IVF cycle, and in urgent settings, ovarian stimulation can be started at a random cycle date for the purpose of fertility preservation *without compromising oocyte yield and maturity*
- This is consistent with a *newer concept of ovarian physiology*, which indicates that there are multiple waves of follicle recruitment during each menstrual cycle
- With the advent of random-start ovarian stimulation protocols the "decision to retrieval" interval does not exceed 12 days.

## ■ CONTROLLED OVARIAN STIMULATION IN PATIENTS WITH "ESTROGEN-SENSITIVE CANCERS"

- During COS, there is a potential risk that the supraphysiologic $E_2$ levels resulting from ovarian stimulation with gonadotropins may promote the growth of estrogen-sensitive tumors, such as endometrial and estrogen receptor—positive breast cancers

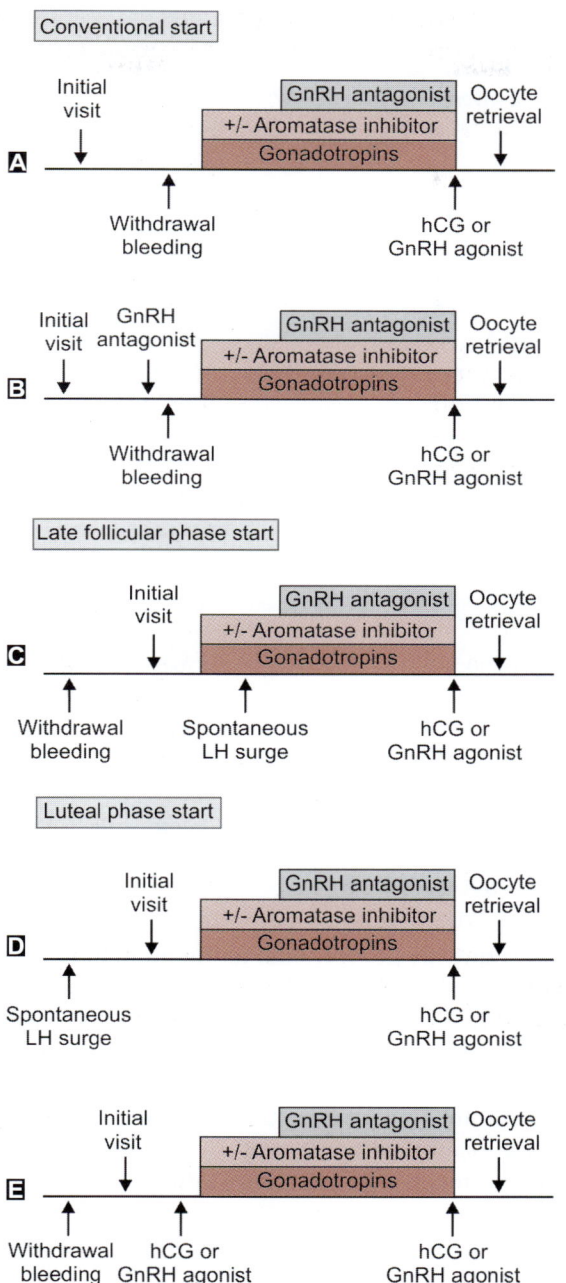

**Figs. 1A to E:** Conventional and random-start antagonist IVF protocols for cancer patients undergoing fertility preservation. COS can be started with spontaneous menses (A) or with menses following luteolysis induced by GnRH antagonist; (B) COS can also be initiated in the late follicular; (C) or luteal phase following spontaneous LH surge; (D) or after ovulation induction with hCG or GnRH agonist (E).
(IVF: in vitro fertilization, COS: controlled ovarian stimulation; GnRH: gonadotropin-releasing hormone; LH: luteinizing hormone; hCG: human chorionic gonadotropin)

**Table 2:** Comparison of characteristics and outcomes of conventional and random start antagonist IVF cycles in cancer patients.

|  | Conventional strat (n = 87; 101 cycles) | Random start (n = 24; 24 cycles) | P value |
|---|---|---|---|
| Age (y) | 33.9 ± 5.2 | 34.6 ± 5.0 | NS |
| AFC | 13 (9–19) | 11.5 (6–16) | NS |
| Days of ovarian stimulation | 9 (8–10) | 11 (10–12) | <.001 |
| Total dose of gonadotropins (IU) | 3,386 ± 1,085 | 4,201 + 1,147 | .001 |
| Follicles ≥ 13 mm | 12 (6–17) | 10 (8–15.5) | NS |
| Oocytes retrieved | 15 (9–23) | 12.5 (9–20.5) | NS |
| Mature oocytes (MII) retrieved | 11 (6–16) | 9 (5–14.5) | NS |
| Oocyte/AFC ratio | 1.1 (0.8–1.7) | 1.2 (0.9–1.7) | NS |
| Mature oocyte/AFC ratio | 0.8 (0.5–1.1) | 0.8 (0.6–1.2) | NS |
| Fertilization rate after ICSI (2PN/MII) | 0.77 ± 0.22 | 0.87 ± 0.15 | NS |

*Note:* Data are presented as mean ± SD or median (interquartile range).
(2PN: two pronuclei; AFC: antral follicle count; ICSI: intracytoplasmic sperm injection; MII: metaphase II; NS: not significant)

- The rise in $E_2$ is directly proportional to the number of follicles recruited to grow; therefore, alternative and potentially safer protocols have been introduced for fertility preservation for estrogen-sensitive cancer patients such as:
    – Natural-cycle IVF (without ovarian stimulation),
    – Stimulation protocols with tamoxifen alone or
    – Combined with gonadotropins, and
    – Stimulation protocols with aromatase inhibitors to reduce the estrogen production.
- *Natural-cycle IVF* gives only one or two oocytes or embryos per cycle and has a high rate of cycle cancellation
- Therefore, this technique would likely be ineffective and is not recommended, especially when a chemotherapy treatment is imminent and the patient does not have a chance for a second cycle of IVF treatment
- *Tamoxifen*, a nonsteroidal triphenylethylene compound related to clomiphene, has a well-known antiestrogenic action on breast tissue

# Fertility Preservation in Oncological Patients (Oncofertility)

with the inhibition of growth of breast tumors by *competitive antagonism* of estrogen at its receptor site, and it is accepted as the first-line drug in hormonal prevention and treatment of estrogen receptor—positive breast cancer
- Tamoxifen, besides its effect in the breast, also has an antagonist action in the estrogen receptors in the central nervous system similar to that of clomiphene
- The *selective antagonist action of tamoxifen* interferes with the negative feedback of the estrogen on the hypothalamic-pituitary axis, leading to an increase in GnRH secretion from the hypothalamus and a subsequent release of FSH from the pituitary-stimulating follicular development
- Tamoxifen can be used for COS alone starting on day 2–5 of the menstrual cycle in doses of 20–60 mg/d, or in combination with gonadotropins, similarly to the use of clomiphene
- Even though peak $E_2$ levels in ovarian stimulation with tamoxifen are not altered, owing to its antiestrogenic effect on breast tissue, it is desirable to be used in *estrogen receptor*—positive breast cancer patients
- Ovarian stimulation with the use of tamoxifen for fertility preservation in cancer patients was shown to increase the mature oocyte and embryo yield compared with natural-cycle IVF (1.6 vs 0.7 and 1.6 vs 0.6, respectively) and reduce cycle cancellations
- As expected, *combined protocol with tamoxifen and gonadotropins* further increased the number of cryopreserved oocytes and embryos (5.1 vs 1.5 and 3.8 vs 1.3, respectively)
- *Aromatase* is a cytochrome P450 enzyme complex that catalyzes the conversion of androstenedione and testosterone to their respective estrogenic products estrone and $E_2$
- *Aromatase inhibitors, such as letrozole*, markedly suppress plasma estrogen levels by competitively inhibiting the activity of the aromatase enzyme
- Aromatase inhibitors significantly reduce the risk of recurrence in postmenopausal women with hormone receptor—positive breast cancer owing to profound estrogen deprivation, especially with third-generation inhibitors (i.e. anastrozole and letrozole)
- Centrally, aromatase inhibitors release the hypothalamic-pituitary axis from estrogenic negative feedback, increase the secretion of FSH by the pituitary gland, stimulate follicle growth, and, thereby, can be used for ovulation induction
- In patients with estrogen-sensitive cancers, the main advantage of adding daily letrozole to gonadotropins in ovarian stimulation protocols is to decrease serum $E_2$ levels to be closer to that observed in natural cycles (i.e. $E_2$ <500 pg/mL) without affecting oocyte or embryo yield
- Stimulation protocols using letrozole alongside with gonadotropins are currently preferred over tamoxifen protocols as treatment with letrozole results in a higher number of oocytes obtained and fertilized when compared to tamoxifen protocols

- In a study comparing the efficacy of the letrozole plus gonadotropin protocol in breast cancer patients and the standard IVF protocol in age-matched noncancer patients with tubal-factor infertility, the breast cancer patients started to receive letrozole (5 mg/d) on menstrual cycle day 2 or 3, FSH (150–300 IU/d) was added 2 days later, all medications were discontinued on the day of hCG trigger, and letrozole was reinitiated after oocyte retrieval and continued until $E_2$ levels fell to less than 50 pg/mL
- This letrozole plus gonadotropin protocol resulted in similar number of total oocytes retrieved and length of ovarian stimulation compared with standard IVF protocol
- As expected, peak $E_2$ levels were significantly lower in the breast cancer patients receiving letrozole plus gonadotropin compared with the standard IVF group (483 ± 278.9 pg/mL vs 1,464.6 ± 644.9 pg/mL)
- The studies assessing the effect of letrozole on oocyte maturity and competence demonstrated that the addition of letrozole did not change numbers of mature oocytes retrieved and fertilization rates
- In addition, COS with aromatase inhibitors in combination with gonadotropins has been safely used for embryo cryopreservation in endometrial cancer patients
- Letrozole suppresses plasma $E_2$ levels significantly at doses of 0.1–10 mg/d
- Start letrozole at 2.5–5 mg/d, depending on the ovarian reserve of the patient, with the ovarian stimulation (Figs. 1A to E)
- Given the importance of keeping $E_2$ levels close to that observed in natural cycles in patients with estrogen-sensitive cancers, we check $E_2$ levels in every clinic visit and titrate letrozole dose up to 10 mg/d to keep $E_2$ levels less than 500 pg/mL
- These letrozole doses are well tolerated by the patients during ovarian stimulation without any side effects
- In addition, the mature oocyte or embryo yield after COS is not affected by letrozole at any dose used in clinical practice
- Continue letrozole after the oocyte retrieval if serum $E_2$ levels are still elevated (i.e. $E_2$ >500 pg/mL). In our experience, even if $E_2$ levels are more than 500 pg/mL before retrieval, only a minority of patients requires letrozole after retrieval
- Discontinuation of letrozole can either be at menses or with initiation of chemotherapy
- In contrast, anastrozole—another third-generation aromatase inhibitor—failed to adequately suppress $E_2$ levels during COS, despite gradually increasing the dose of anastrozole to a maximum of 10 mg/d, and therefore not recommend its use in fertility preservation cycles
- *In summary*, COS with letrozole plus gonadotropins in patients with estrogen-sensitive cancers undergoing fertility preservation is:
  - Safe,
  - Well-tolerated, and

- Yields similar number of oocytes and embryos compared with standard protocols while minimizing the risk of high-estrogen exposure and not increasing the recurrence of cancer in the short term.

## ■ PREVENTION OF OVARIAN HYPERSTIMULATION SYNDROME (OHSS) IN CANCER PATIENTS

- Ovarian hyperstimulation syndrome is the most serious complication of ovarian stimulation and can be associated with intravascular depletion, ascites, liver dysfunction, pulmonary edema, electrolyte imbalance, and thromboembolic events
- Although OHSS is often self-limited with spontaneous resolution within a few days, severe disease may require hospitalization and intensive care
- Selecting the appropriate ovarian stimulation regimen can be challenging in embryo or oocyte cryopreservation because it is important to balance the risk of OHSS and obtaining sufficient number of oocytes or embryos to maximize the chance of a successful pregnancy in the future
- The impact of OHSS can be profound in cancer patients because it may result in delaying or complicating planned life-saving cancer therapy
- Triggering the final oocyte maturation with hCG carries the well-known risk of inducing OHSS
- The GnRH agonist also induces this final oocyte maturation by promoting the release of endogenous gonadotropin stores from the hypophysis as long as the pituitary gonadotropin receptors are not down-regulated and can be used as an alternative to hCG
- The GnRH agonist trigger in GnRH antagonist-based protocols dramatically reduces the risk of OHSS, owing to the short half-life of GnRH agonist-induced endogenous LH surge
- Moreover, there was a significantly lower rate of moderate or severe OHSS in the GnRH agonist group compared with the patients receiving hCG trigger (3.7% vs 21.3%)
- The GnRH agonist trigger is particularly convenient in cancer patients pursuing oocyte or embryo banking, because luteal support is not needed to sustain a pregnancy
- In a study comparing GnRH agonist and hCG as the trigger for oocyte maturation in fertility preservation cycles, GnRH agonist trigger resulted in at least similar numbers of mature oocytes and cryopreserved embryos compared with hCG
- In addition, although hCG potentiates the endogenous production of estrogen during the luteal phase, GnRH agonist-induced endogenous LH may result in lower estrogen production owing to its longer half-life, which may be an advantage for patients with estrogen-sensitive cancers
- The number of follicles, more specifically the follicular pattern, in combination with serum $E_2$ levels predicts OHSS with high sensitivity and specificity

- However, one caveat is that cotreatment with aromatase inhibitors limits the use of $E_2$ level to help predict OHSS
- In this scenario, it is important to rely on the follicular pattern and the rate of $E_2$ rise rather than the absolute of serum $E_2$ levels. If the $E_2$ levels are rising rapidly while administering letrozole, especially in the presence of a high number of small follicles, the patient should be considered to be at risk for OHSS and GnRH agonist trigger should be used to lower that risk
- In conclusion, we recommend GnRH agonist trigger in GnRH antagonist-based fertility preservation
- The trigger must be confirmed the next morning by measuring serum LH level
- In the case of a GnRH agonist, trigger failure determined by low post-trigger LH (in our clinic, we use a cut off LH level of <12 mIU/mL), hCG (2,500–5,000 IU) trigger can be given on the same day.

## MEDICAL CONSIDERATIONS IN CANCER PATIENTS UNDERGOING CONTROLLED OVARIAN STIMULATION

- The patients referred for fertility preservation owing to a malignant disease do not represent the typical population of subfertile patients treated in IVF units
- Cancer may affect multiple tissues throughout the body and can result in variety of complications during COS
- Therefore, the goals during COS in cancer patients are to prevent these serious life-threatening complications with prophylaxis, and to recognize and manage them effectively when they occur.

## THROMBOPROPHYLAXIS

- Cancer patients undergoing COS are at increased risk of *thromboembolic events* because of a hypercoagulable state induced by their malignancy and supraphysiologic serum $E_2$ levels
- Therefore, these patients may require anticoagulation around the time of COS
- Currently, there are no guidelines for anticoagulation during COS
- Start prophylactic low-molecular-weight heparin with ovarian stimulation in high-risk patients and instruct the patient to take their last dose of medication 24 hours before the oocyte retrieval
- Low-molecular-weight heparin is reinitiated 12 hours after the retrieval and can be continued until $E_2$ returns to its baseline level
- The other strategy of preventing thromboembolic events is to use letrozole during COS to keep $E_2$ levels close to those observed in natural cycles. Letrozole at 2.5 or 5 mg/d can be started with ovarian stimulation, as in patients with estrogen-sensitive malignancies, and can be titrated up to 10 mg/d to keep $E_2$ levels less than 500 pg/mL

- Letrozole can also be continued after oocyte retrieval for up to a week depending on the $E_2$ level at the time of ovulation induction
- Malignancies with bone marrow infiltration or liver involvement may create a *tendency toward bleeding* during oocyte retrieval owing to thrombocytopenia, platelet dysfunction, or defective coagulation factor synthesis
- Therefore, *platelet count and coagulation panel* should be tested before COS in patients with hematologic malignancies or with malignancies involving the liver
- *Platelet or fresh frozen plasma transfusion* should be performed before oocyte retrieval to prevent excessive bleeding in these patients as needed
- *Higher risk of pelvic infection* after oocyte retrieval can be a problem especially in cancer patients with *neutropenia*
- Therefore, *absolute neutrophil count* should be evaluated before COS in cancer patients with possible bone marrow infiltration
- In the case of neutropenia, consultation from the patient's oncologist for the use of granulocyte colony-stimulating factor to increase the neutrophil count should be obtained, and prophylactic antibiotics should be given before oocyte retrieval to decrease the risk of infection
- Some of the cancer-related medical conditions, including respiratory dysfunctions due to tracheal compression, mediastinal mass, or large pleural effusion, and vascular disturbances, as in superior vena cava syndrome, may preclude safe administration of conscious sedation during oocyte retrieval
- Anesthesia consultation should be obtained in advance for the patients with these conditions. If safety and difficult intubation in an emergency situation are concerns, the oocyte retrieval should be performed either under general anesthesia with endotracheal intubation or only with local anesthesia
- The patients with recent mastectomies for breast cancer may have special needs during COS
- Owing to decreased mobility, they may need more assistance during office visits
- Intravenous line placements to the upper extremity on the same side of the axillary node dissection should be avoided, owing to concerns of lymphatic system damage and inadequate lymphatic flow
- In patients, who have had transverse rectus abdominis myocutaneous flap for breast reconstruction after mastectomy, abdominal distention, and therefore OHSS should be avoided to prevent wound dehiscence
- The medication list for all cancer patients should be reviewed before COS
- *Antiepileptic medications* should definitely be continued during COS in patients with brain tumor owing to increased risk of seizures
- The use of imatinib (Gleevec), a specific inhibitor of constitutively activated Bcr-Abl tyrosine kinase used in chronic myelogenous leukemia, should be temporarily stopped during COS owing to its adverse effect on ovarian hormone production and oocyte recovery.

## CONCLUSION

- Given the importance of reproduction for many young patients faced with cancer, counseling regarding fertility preservation is an essential part of comprehensive cancer care
- Embryo cryopreservation is the most established method for fertility preservation, and oocyte cryopreservation has gained efficacy and is now offered at many centers
- Determination of the COS protocol and gonadotropin dose for oocyte or embryo cryopreservation requires an individualized assessment
- Maximizing the number of embryos and oocytes cryopreserved during a fertility preservation cycle without causing OHSS is extremely important, because most patients have only a single cycle opportunity owing to time constraints before starting their oncologic treatment
- In urgent settings, random-start ovarian stimulation is emerging as a new technique for the purpose of fertility preservation without compromising oocyte yield and maturity
- Letrozole plus gonadotropin protocol is an effective method for safely inducing COS in patients with estrogen-sensitive cancers undergoing fertility preservation
- Newly developed protocols are efficient in inducing COS and obtaining appropriate number of oocytes or embryos.

## FURTHER READING

1. American Cancer Society. Cancer facts and figures 2012. [online] Available from: http://www.cancer.org/research/cancerfactsfigures/cancerfactsfigures/cancer-facts-figures-2012 [Accessed March, 2018]
2. Howlader N, Noone AM, Krapcho M, et al. (Eds.). SEER cancer statistics review, 1975–2009 (vintage 2009 populations). Bethesda, MD: National Cancer Institute. [online] Available from: http://seer.cancer.gov/csr/1975_2009_pops09/ [Accessed March, 2018.
3. Letourneau JM, Ebbel EE, Katz PP, et al. Pretreatment fertility counseling and fertility preservation improve quality of life in reproductive age women with cancer. Cancer. 2012;118:1710-7.
4. Letourneau JM, Melisko ME, Cedars MI, et al. A changing perspective: improving access to fertility preservation. Nat Rev Clin Oncol. 2011;8:56-60.
5. Rodriguez-Wallberg KA, Oktay K. Options on fertility preservation in female cancer patients. Cancer Treat Rev. 2012;38:354-61.
6. Sklar CA, Mertens AC, Mitby P, et al. Premature menopause in survivors of childhood cancer: a report from the childhood cancer survivor study. J Natl Cancer Inst. 2006;98:890-6.
7. Letourneau JM, Ebbel EE, Katz PP, et al. Acute ovarian failure underestimates age-specific reproductive impairment for young women undergoing chemotherapy for cancer. Cancer. 2012;118:1933-9.

8. Meirow D, Nugent D. The effects of radiotherapy and chemotherapy on female reproduction. Hum Reprod Update. 2001;7:535-43.
9. Hamilton BE, Martin JA, Ventura SJ. Births: preliminary data for 2011. Natl Vital Stat Rep. 2012;61(5):1-18.
10. Anderson RA, Wallace WH. Fertility preservation in girls and young women. Clin Endocrinol (Oxf). 2011;75:409-19.
11. Practice Committee of the American Society for Reproductive Medicine. Fertility preservation and reproduction in cancer patients. Fertil Steril. 2005;83:1622-8.
12. Practice Committee of the American Society for Reproductive Medicine. Mature oocyte cryopreservation: a guideline. Fertil Steril. 2013;99:37-43.
13. Reddy J, Oktay K. Ovarian stimulation and fertility preservation with the use of aromatase inhibitors in women with breast cancer. Fertil Steril. 2012;98:1363-9.
14. Agarwal A, Said TM. Implications of systemic malignancies on human fertility. Reprod Biomed Online. 2004;9:673-9.
15. Oktay K, Kim JY, Barad D, et al. Association of BRCA1 mutations with occult primary ovarian insufficiency: a possible explanation for the link between infertility and breast/ovarian cancer risks. J Clin Oncol. 2010;28:240-4.
16. Pal L, Leykin L, Schifren JL, et al. Malignancy may adversely influence the quality and behaviour of oocytes. Hum Reprod. 1998;13:1837-40.
17. Das M, Shehata F, Moria A, et al. Ovarian reserve, response to gonadotropins, and oocyte maturity in women with malignancy. Fertil Steril. 2011;96:122-5.
18. Maltaris T, Seufert R, Fischl F, et al. The effect of cancer treatment on female fertility and strategies for preserving fertility. Eur J Obstet Gynecol Reprod Biol. 2007;130:148-55.
19. Lee S, Ozkavukcu S, Heytens E, et al. Value of early referral to fertility preservation in young women with breast cancer. J Clin Oncol. 2010;28:4683-6.
20. Friedler S, Koc O, Gidoni Y, et al. Ovarian response to stimulation for fertility preservation in women with malignant disease: a systematic review and meta-analysis. Fertil Steril. 2012;97:125-33.

# CHAPTER 37

# Surrogacy: Present Position in India

*Shivani Sachdev, Sonali Kusum*

## ■ HISTORICAL ORIGIN AND BACKGROUND OF SURROGACY

### Surrogacy in Early Human Civilizations

Surrogacy has existed from the inception of human civilization since thousand years. The early human civilizations namely the Mediterranean, Mesopotamian, Roman, and Egyptian mention surrogacy as a well accepted cultural practice to ensure continuity of ancestral lineage, progeny. Surrogacy in Sumerian civilization—around 18th century BC, the Sumerian from Mesopotamia mention about the Codex Hammurabi or Hammurabi's Code named after the proponent King Hammurabi. This is the first authoritative legal document that regulated surrogacy by allowing surrogacy for producing male offspring. The Hammurabi Code states that "if a man takes a wife and she gives this man a maid servant and she bear him children and then this maid assume equality with the wife because she has born him children, her master shall not sell her for money but he may keep her as slave, reckoning her among the maid servants." This is hailed as one of the earliest sets of laws on surrogacy as a permissible practice.

Surrogacy in Mesopotamia civilization—among Nuzis community in Mesopotamian civilization, surrogacy is accepted as "copulation" wherein it is the obligation of the infertile wife to provide her husband with surrogate to bear child on behalf of her. This practice is documented in the old testament of Bible where in Rachel failing to conceive herself directed Jacob, her husband to her maid named Bilah to procreate children. Similarly Sarah failing to bear children, she offered her handmaid, Hagar to her husband Abraham to bear them a child.

### Surrogacy in Ancient India

The ancient India documents different forms of surrogacy it is evident from the mythological references. Around 4–5th century BC, as per the popular Indian religious epic Ramayana, the birth of lord Hanuman was possible through surrogacy involving donation of gametes.

The Lord Hanuman was born through the sperms of lord Shiva carried and stimulated through the assistance of Vayu, the God of wind implanted through the ear into the womb of Anjani, who and carried the fetus as gestational carrier or surrogate mother and delivered the child Hanuman. In this case, the Lord Shiva was the Genetic father, the Anjani was (both the egg donor or the genetic mother) the gestational carrier or the surrogate mother and delivered the baby boy Lord Hanuman as child born of surrogacy.

There is similar account of birth of Lord Rama as child born of surrogacy in the epic Ramayana. The king Dashratha of Ayodhya performed yagna or religious sacrament to have children, in the course of same, the God of fire, the Lord Agni offered his gametes in the form of sweet potion to be consumed by the Queen of Dashratha resulting in the birth of Lord Rama as a male surrogate child. Here, Lord Agni was the gamete donors or genetic or biological father, the Queen of Dashratha was both the gestational carrier and the egg donor and the Lord Rama is the surrogate male child.

In keeping with these, there is an old customary practice as *Niyoga* which allows widow to bear child for any closed relative infertile couples sharing the same blood line and this allows the widow to inherit property by widow if she bears a child for the infertile couples.

Advent of modern assisted reproductive technologies (ART) surrogacy in gestational form—around the late 1970s, there has been tremendous development in the field of reproductive technologies with the discovery of novel ART as artificial insemination, test tube baby method or in vitro fertilization technique (IVF) and a combination of these ART technologies has led to development of modern form of gestational surrogacy. The world's first IVF test tube baby Louise Joy Brown was born on 25th July 1978 at Oldham General Hospital, Oldham UK at the hands of Dr Robert Edwards through the IVF procedure. Dr Robert Edwards is credited with the development of IVF technology and he was awarded with British Nobel Prize medicine in 2010 year. In the year 1980, the first ever reported surrogacy took place in the US state of Illinois where a woman using the pseudonym as Elizabeth Kane age (37 years) who was both the genetic (egg donor) and gestational mother entered into surrogacy agreement with a US national in return for monetary compensation around $10,000 for gestation and delivery of surrogate child.

Contemporary landmark medical development on modern gestational and commercial Surrogacy in India—this was followed with another such scientific feat in the same year, as India's first IVF and world's second IVF baby Kanupriya Alias Durga was born in Kolkata on October 3, 1978 at the hands of Dr Subhash Mukhopadhyay, a Kolkata-based doctor is credited with the first ever successful delivery of India's first test tube baby and posthumously honored by the Indian Council of Medical Research (ICMR) India for the same. In 1986, India's second and Mumbai's first test tube baby named Harsha Shah, baby girl is born on August 16, 1986 at KEM Hospital in Mumbai at the hands of Dr Indira Hinduja and Dr Kusum Zaveri. In 1994, India's first gestational surrogacy took place in at GG Hospital Chennai at the hands of Dr Kamala Selvaraj. In 1997, a woman named Nirmala from Chandigarh acted as the gestational surrogate for monetary compensation around rupees 50,000 for an anonymous couples in order to meet medical expenses for her paralyzed husband. This was hailed as the first humanitarian gestational surrogacy and mostly reported as grandmother surrogacy.

## ■ DERIVATION AND DEFINITION, MEANING OF SURROGACY

### Meaning of Surrogacy

The word surrogacy is derived from the Latin word *surrogatus* which is past participle of *surrogate* meaning a substitute, that is, a person appointed to act in the place of another. Thus, a surrogate mother is a woman who bears a child on behalf of another woman, either from her own egg or from the implantation in her womb of a fertilized egg from other woman.

According to the Black's Law Dictionary, surrogacy means the process of carrying and delivering a child for another person.

## ■ DEFINITION OF SURROGACY IN INDIA AND FOREIGN NATIONS

In India "surrogacy", is defined as *"an arrangement* in which a woman agrees to a pregnancy, achieved through ART, in which neither of the gametes belong to her or her husband, with the intention to carry it and hand over the child to the person or persons for whom she is acting as a surrogate."

### Understanding on Surrogacy in India— Medicolegal Arrangement

Taking after the definition of surrogacy arising in the context of medical need, surrogacy is essentially a medical technological procedure involving extensive use of ART technology. Surrogacy is a substitutive or circumventive form of medicolegal arrangement where in conception (in vivo, i.e. inside the body) is taken outside the body and substituted through ART techniques in laboratory with the help of concerned stakeholders as the couples who seek such medical intervention, the same couples may donate gametes or may use gamete donors as necessary, a gestational carrier or surrogate mother is used for undertaking implantation of embryo, gestation and birthing for attaining procreation, child birth with or without genetic link for medically infertile or needy couples.

## Surrogacy Process—Stakeholders in Surrogacy Arrangement

Surrogacy involves a minimum of three to five stakeholders, primarily a surrogate mother or gestational carrier who is implanted through surgical ART techniques with the fetus in her uterus, as surrogate mother is the most integral, essential aspect of surrogacy, and the absence of surrogate mother in the ART procedure is short of surrogacy but merely an IVF or test tube baby procedure. No surrogacy is possible without the surrogate mother in the same.

Secondly, the intending couples including the intending father and the intending mother who intend to attain parenthood, to beget children after facing medical ailments, failing treatments there by initiate surrogacy. But for the intention of intending couple the surrogacy arrangement would not have been initiated.

Thirdly, the gamete donors including sperm and egg donors may be involved in the process, wherein either or both the couples could not produce gametes or their gametes may not be medically fit to be used for fertilization as necessary.

Fourthly, the surrogate child who is conceived using the gametes of the couples or gamete donors, then implanted in the surrogate mother for gestation and birthing and after birth the coupes receives the custody of child as parent to take care of the child.

Fifthly, the ART banks, ART clinics, National, State Advisory Bodies or the regulatory bodies under the draft bill.

These are other secondary stakeholders as well who are necessary part of this surrogacy arrangement play a significant role in conduct of surrogacy.

## ■ TYPES OF SURROGACY

Traditionally, there are three broad criteria for classification of types of surrogacy as follows:

## Surrogacy Classified on Monetary Payment— Altruistic, Commercial Surrogacy

- *Altruistic surrogacy:* It refers to such surrogacy arrangement in which the surrogate mother is not paid monetary returns or not financially compensated for her agreeing to be gestational carrier and for gestation, delivery, handing over the custody of child to couples rather the surrogate mother agrees to be gestational carrier for charitable or altruistic interest for helping the infertile couples to have child and form family.
- *Commercial surrogacy:* It refers to such surrogacy arrangement in which the surrogate mother is paid monetary returns or financially compensated for her agreeing to be gestational carrier and for implantation, gestation, delivery, handing over the custody of child to couples.

## Surrogacy Classified on Donation from Egg Donors—Traditional Straight Full Surrogacy and Host or Gestational, Partial Surrogacy

- *Traditional, straight, full surrogacy:* Where in the surrogate mother uses her own eggs therefore she is both the surrogate mother and the genetic mother using the artificial insemination technique thereby sharing biological relatedness between the surrogate child and the surrogate mother.
- *Host or gestational or partial surrogacy:* Where in the surrogate mother does not uses her own eggs rather donated eggs either from the anonymous donor or from the intending or commissioning couple using the IVF technique thereby no biological genetic connectedness between the surrogate mother and the surrogate child rather there is genetic connection with the intending parent.

In addition to the traditional classification, in the present context of global or cross border surrogacy regime, there has emerged three other modern form of surrogacy in the present world as follows:

## Contemporary Modern Forms of Surrogacy

- *Transnational, overseas international surrogacy:* It refers to surrogacy arrangements involving one or more of nationals of different countries in the surrogacy arrangement, export or import of gametes, traveling or conduct of surrogacy across borders in geographical locations.
- *Social surrogacy* is defined as surrogacy commissioned by intending couples for non-medical reasons rather as a life-style choice for women unwilling to undergo the nine months of gestation, pain of labor, delivery to prevent disfiguration/change of body in their day to day lives or to ensure careers or professional interests.
- *Single parent surrogacy*: Surrogacy commissioned by single individual either unmarried or widow or divorcee following death or desertion by spouse as an individual procreative or reproductive choice or right to family formation is hailed as single surrogacy.
- *Same sex surrogacy:* Same sex surrogacy is also referred to as gay or lesbian, gay, bisexual, and transgender (LGBT) surrogacy. Surrogacy commissioned by the members of homosexual community, sexual minorities as LGBT community along with their partners with or without civil union or such recognition for having a biologically related child to them.

## ■ SIGNIFICANCE OF SURROGACY

- *Surrogacy ensures genetically related child:* The most salient advantage of surrogacy is that it ensures "genetic connection" between the surrogate child and either of the couple, or both the couples by permitting use of their gametes. Surrogacy emphasizes on blood ties, genetic or biological connections, kinship ties and ensures descendance of genealogy by passing down intergenerational genetic similarity.

- *Surrogacy favorable over adoption:* As surrogacy ensures biogenetic connection surrogacy is preferred option over family formation through adoption in India as well as abroad.
- *Sociocultural religious reasons:* The most cardinal function of marriage toward society is child bearing, carry forward the ancestral, familial progeny, lineage, ensures line of successors or heirs of family line. In the Indian families, sociocultural context the biological, genetic connectedness, blood ties, the line of ancestry, purity of family clan, line of ascendency, inheritance or succession along the family line, the caste heritage, hold a very significant place. The religious texts Bible in the Old Testament refers to traditional surrogacy. The Hindu religious mythologies also documents instances of surrogacy.
- *Surrogacy is necessity for medical reasons:* "It is estimated that 15% of couples around the world are infertile. This implies that infertility is one of the most highly prevalent medical problems." In India there are over 20 million infertile couples. "Surrogacy may be necessary due to such medical condition that makes it impossible or dangerous to conceive, get pregnant and to give birth which may include absence or malformation of the womb, recurrent pregnancy loss, repeated IVF implantation failures." In addition to that, "surrogacy may be recommended in such medical conditions as recurrent miscarriage, premature menopause following cancer treatment, a hysterectomy, or an absent or abnormal uterus" as per the American Society of Assisted Reproduction. Surrogacy is particularly used in the couples who are facing medically identifiable or nonmedically nonidentifiable barriers to fertility, such as endometriosis, polycystic ovarian syndrome (PCOS), male factor infertility, irregular cycles, such other cases where the cause of infertility cannot be diagnosed or identified nor resolved, etc. In such conditions ART IVF surrogacy is used to circumvent infertility and facilitate child birth procreation by using either these or combination of techniques, technologies. It may be noted that in certain medical condition surrogacy is the only, the first and the last option to commission surrogacy, or the only means to have child with their own genetic connection.
- *Alternative family formation choice for certain groups:* For certain group of individuals namely the widows, single unmarried parent, widow, widower, same sex partners surrogacy is the sole or the only option for attainment of parenthood, begetting a child biologically related to them and family formation by allowing them to use their own reproductive gametes or of gametes their partners to be used in procreation, family formation, this would not have been possible but for surrogacy.
- *Surrogacy ensures reproductive or procreative freedom:* Surrogacy allows the reproductive freedom or choice to couples to choose the manner or means of using medical technology to attain parenthood by permitting

choice of using the gametes of either couples or both couples, and also by allowing the choice or freedom to securing choice of donor gametes from sperm or egg banks or collectively called ART banks after necessary medical screening of the gametes for same. It may be noted that the use of donor gametes, third party surrogate mother represents a reproductive choice or freedom of couples.

This is in compliance with the reproductive rights of couples guaranteed under right to life, personal liberty under Article 21 Indian Constitution and International Human Right conventions namely the International Conference on Population and Development (ICPD), Cairo 1994 expressly declared "the right to reproductive sexual or reproductive health as a human right" and integral part of right to privacy and right to life of individual.

## ■ DEVELOPMENTS ON SURROGACY IN INDIA

India is one of the first countries in the world to permit practice of commercial, overseas surrogacy as early as year 2002 under the medical tourism policy.

### Contemporary Developments on Regulating and Permitting Surrogacy in India

In India, the development on surrogacy has commenced since the early 1990s. The Indian Society for Promoting Assisted Reproduction (ISAR) was formed in 1991 with headquarters at Mumbai to create awareness and work on assisted reproductive technology (ART).

The first ever national level guideline on surrogacy is titled as "National Guidelines for Accreditation, Supervision and Regulation of ART Clinics in India" issued by ICMR nodal agency of Ministry of Health and Family Welfare Government of India in the year 2005. The Assisted Reproductive Technologies (Regulations) Bill 2008 is the first ever legislative draft on surrogacy formulated by the ICMR under the aegis of Ministry of Health and Family welfare Government of India modeled after ICMR Guidelines 2005 seeking to regulate surrogacy in India. The central feature of this ART 2008 Bill is the legal permit to gestational, commercial and overseas or foreign surrogacy under a surrogacy agreement to this effect which is enforceable in India. This draft ART Bill since its first ever formulation in year 2008 has been revised twice, once in the year 2010 and subsequently in the year 2014 with necessary modifications.

After these guidelines, the first ever formal legalization of commercial surrogacy in India is pronounced by the Indian supreme court (SC) in *Baby Yamanda Manji vs Union of India* involving the Japanese Intending couple (IP) who commissioned surrogacy in Anand, Gujarat in India with the help of an Indian surrogate mother for a fixed sum of monetary compensation to surrogate mother from the Japanese IP under a surrogacy agreement to this effect. In this case, the SC grants legitimacy to surrogacy by stating that surrogacy is the only available option for parents who wish to have a child that is biologically related to them and the SC mentions necessary medical reasons for the same. In this case, the SC defines "commercial surrogacy is a form of surrogacy in which a gestational carrier is paid to carry a child to maturity in her womb and is usually resorted to by well off infertile couples who can afford the cost involved or people who save and borrow in order to complete their dream of being parents." It may be noted that throughout the course of judgment SC raises no objection, no bar on overseas or foreign surrogacy. In the *Jan Bajaj vs Anand Muncipality* a German IP commissioned surrogacy in India with the help of an Indian surrogate mother resulting in birth of surrogate twins who is genetically connected to the German IP. The Gujarat high court reiterated and upheld the legalization of commercial surrogacy as pronounced by Supreme Court in this case. In this case, the Gujarat high court held "there is no law prohibiting artificial insemination, egg donation, lending a womb or surrogacy agreements. No civil or criminal penalties are also imposed on the same in India." "Commercial surrogacy is never considered to be illegal in India and few of the other foreign countries."

The Home Ministry Guidelines 2012 during the pendency of this draft ART Bill 2010, amidst the continuation of judicial proceedings, the Government of India, Ministry of Home Affairs (MHA), (Foreign Division) issued Guidelines regarding conditions for grant of visa to foreigners (including foreign nationals, foreign residents as NRI, OCI, PIO) intending to visit India for commissioning surrogacy. This MHA Guidelines permits surrogacy only to such "foreign heterosexual married couples" who are "married for more than 2 years" to secure "Medical visa S" for infertility treatment surrogacy not tourist visa for commissioning surrogacy in India.

*Jayashree Wad vs Union of India*, a public interest litigation (PIL) is filed in SC seeking necessary action from the SC for prohibition on commercial, transnational, foreigners or overseas surrogacy in India, to prohibit export or import of gametes, embryos in India for use by foreigners in commercial surrogacy in order to control exploitation of Indian surrogates, to control human trafficking in guise of overseas, commercial surrogacy and to seek enactment of stringent law controlling the same.

Ministry of Health and Family Welfare Government of India issues "Commissioning of surrogacy instruction to all ART clinics, Banks, infertility clinics offering surrogacy services, 2015. The ICMR under the aegis of the Health Ministry issued circular directing all ART centers, fertility clinics in India "to halt surrogacy for foreign couples for availing surrogacy services in India from the date of issue of the circular with immediate effect" and "not to initiate any surrogacy for foreign intending couples" and this "directed all ART centers, fertility clinics to provide surrogacy services only to Indian heterosexually married couples.

## Present Bill on Surrogacy in India

The proposed new legal regulations on surrogacy in India:
- *Surrogacy (Regulations) Bill 2016:* This is drafted by the Group of Ministers (GoM) constituted at the behest of the Prime Minister's Office. The surrogacy bill permits "altruistic surrogacy" where in the surrogate mother may be provided medical expenses and insurance related to surrogacy. This bill is silent on the permissibility of either gestational or traditional surrogacy. The surrogacy bill permits "only close relatives of couples to be surrogate" but does not define the term close relative.

The surrogacy bill permits "Indian nationals heterosexually married couples who have 5 years of substance of marriage, where in either of the couples is infertile, childless or having a child with mental disability" subject to such condition as prescribed under the bill to commission surrogacy in India. The Bill defines "surrogacy" means "a practice whereby one woman bears and gives birth to a child for an intending couple with the intention of handing over such child to the intending couple after the birth."

The surrogacy bill is "prohibitory" as it prohibits overseas or foreign intending couples from commissioning surrogacy in India, for the same reason, the bill prohibits inter country movement of human embryo or gametes for the purpose of surrogacy. The bill prohibits and penalizes commercial surrogacy and any such attempt of abetting or advertising for the same.

The bill is "exclusionary" as it excludes Indian national unmarried singles, Indian national ever married individuals as widow, divorcee, live in relation partners, NRI, OCI, PIO, same sex or homosexual partners from commissioning surrogacy in India. The surrogacy bill is restrictive as it imposes a series of arbitrary, restrictive preconditions to be complied by intending couples before commissioning surrogacy in India. The Surrogacy Bill 2016 does not mention about ever married Indian nationals individuals as divorcee, widow who are rendered single by death, desertion of spouse, they are excluded from commissioning surrogacy, though these ever married Indian nationals fulfill the requisite criteria of being Indian national, married heterosexually, with subsistence of 5 years of marriage, infertile, childless as prescribed under the bill.

The Surrogacy Bill 2016 directs the intending couples to secure "an order concerning the parentage, custody of the child" born through surrogacy from court of Magistrate of first class or above in order to establish parentage of the intending couples over the child born of surrogacy. The grounds for grant or denial of such order, minimum and maximum time duration to be required by the Magistrate in issuing such order are not stated. It is not provided if this order of the Magistrate court is final or there could be an appellate forum against the same. These gaps give rise to legal issues in establishing parentage of child born of surrogacy.

The surrogacy bill provides for legal recognition of surrogate child as biological child and entitlement to all the rights and privileges available to a natural child under any law for the time being in force. The surrogacy bill 2016 has no provision on the issue of birth certificate naming the intending couples who commissioned surrogacy as father, mother respectively for child born of surrogacy.

In keeping with these regulations, surrogacy in India is prohibited for foreign nationals and foreign residents. Though there is no binding legislation on surrogacy in India as the surrogacy bill 2016 is awaiting parliament approval and enactment.

It is contended by media and other reports that India is there is exploitation of Indian surrogate mothers by foreigners and there is misuse of the same. But there is lack of requisite data and evidence to substantiate the nexus between foreign or overseas surrogacy resulting in exploitation of surrogate mother and surrogate child in India. A RTI request to the ICMR, the regulatory body for ART Clinics, Banks in India, states "the ICMR has not received any complaint from surrogates about their exploitation by doctors and by intending couples or others."

A previous RTI reply from concerned Government Ministries and commissions at the national level revealed nil record on the total number of women registering as surrogate mothers annually in India for Indian national intending couples and for foreigner intending couples respectively, nil record on the total number of surrogate mothers incurring maternal mortality or organ loss or serious health risks during the course of surrogate pregnancy annually in India either for Indian nationals intending couples and for foreigners intending couples respectively, there is nil record on the total number of children born of surrogacy annually in India to Indian intending couples and to foreign intending couples respectively, there is nil record on the total number of children born of surrogacy in India but travelling to foreign countries with foreign intending couples annually from India. The dearth of such crucial data, it is difficult to demonstrate the actual number or percentage of surrogate mothers who are exploited (out of the total number of women registering as surrogate mother annually in India) either by Indian intending couples or by foreign intending couples respectively.

Some of other significant developments in surrogacy are the establishment of other regulatory bodies:

The National Registry of Assisted Reproductive Technology (ART) Clinics and Banks in India, (NRACBI) 2013–The NRACBI has been set up by the ICMR for creating a central database of ART clinics in the country by registering ART clinic offering infertility treatment using ART procedures as surrogacy.

The Indian Society for Third-Party Assisted Reproduction (INSTAR) 2013—The INSTAR is a group of doctors, social workers, lawyers who have formulated recommendations to protect the interest of surrogate mothers. INSTAR recommended for the first time a fixed, uniform sum of monetary compensation to be paid to all the surrogate mothers at the state and national level throughout India and additional fixed sum of monetary compensation in case of health eventualities or health risks arising out of surrogate pregnancy to be paid to the surrogate mothers.

## ■ END REMARKS

At the outset, there is a dire need to enact legislation and to give effect to the same on *Surrogacy in India*. However, the proposed legislation ought to be guided by rising need for infertility among Indian citizens, foreign nationals, residents and singles, same sex individuals subject to the permissibility under existing Indian laws. Surrogacy may be reconsidered as a form of family formation, procreative choice of individuals in cases of medical necessity as the sole option to have biologically related children. Besides there ought to be more safeguards incorporated in the bill for protection of interest of surrogate mother, intending couples children born of surrogacy, the misuses related to surrogacy may be stringently controlled.

Surrogacy needs more human consideration in lieu with this perspective in order to serve the greater interest of society rather than imposing a blanket ban on the same.

## ■ KEY POINTS

- Surrogacy is a medical necessity in cases of infertility and other severe medical conditions.
- Surrogacy is not novel but this has existed since human civilizations. The mentioning of Surrogacy is in religious texts and there are socially cultural practices as Niyoga which validate and this grants social acceptance to surrogacy.
- There is need for binding effective law on surrogacy but there is no statutory Act on Surrogacy. Surrogacy Bill 2016 is pending. Surrogacy is guided by the ICMR Guidelines 2005 at present and the directives form Ministry of Health and Family Welfare and Home Ministry from time to time.
- The Indian Supreme Court is adjudicating a public interest litigation on regulation of surrogacy the final verdict is awaited. In the former cases as Baby Yamnada Manji, Jan Balaz cases, the Supreme Court has raised no objection to permit of surrogacy for foreign nationals in the same.
- Though there is at present, suspension or on surrogacy for foreigners, NRI, PIO, there is need to revises this prohibition as all human beings have right to health and avail and access treatment including procreative or reproductive health surrogacy as an ART treatment to initiate family formation and have children.

## ■ FURTHER READING

1. Indian Society for Assisted Reproduction. Surrogacy. [online] Available from http://www.isarindia.net/Chapter VIII. [Accessed March, 2018]
2. Indian Council of Medical Research. Statement of Specific Principles for Assisted Reproductive Technologies, ICMR Ethical Guidelines for Biomedical Research. New Delhi: Indian Council of Medical Research; 2006.

3. Baby Manaji vs Yamanda. Union of India, (2008) 13 S.C.C. 518.
4. Jan Balaz vs Anand Municipality & Others. Letters Patent Appeal No. 2151 of 2009.
5. Indian Council of Medical Research. The Assisted Reproductive Technology (Regulation) Bill–2008 (Draft). New Delhi: Ministry of Health and Family Welfare, Government of India; 2008.
6. The Assisted Reproductive Technologies (Regulation) Bill-2010 (Draft). Ministry of Health & Family Welfare Govt. Of India. New Delhi: Indian Council of Medical Research; 2010.
7. The National Registry of Assisted Reproductive Technology (ART). Clinics and Banks in India, (NRACBI) 2013. New Delhi: ICMR; 2013.
8. Indian Society for Third party Reproduction. INSTAR Key Recommendation. Guwahati: INSTAR; 2013.
9. Government of India, Ministry of Health and Family Welfare (Department of Health Research). ART Bill 2014. [online] Available from http://www.prsindia.org/uploads/media/draft/Draft%20Assisted%20Reproductive%20Technology%20(Regulation)%20Bill,%202014.pdf. [Accessed March, 2018].
10. PRS India. Surrogacy (Regulations) Bill 2016. [online] Available at http://www.prsindia.org/uploads/media/Surrogacy/Surrogacy%20(Regulation)%20Bill,%202016.pdf. [Accessed March, 2018].
11. Department of Health Research, Ministry of Health and Family Welfare, Govt. of India. Commissioning of surrogacy instructions (Circular no .V.25011/119/250/HR). [online] Available from http://www.icmr.nic.in/icmrnews/art/DHR%20notification%20on%20Surrogacy.pdf. [Accessed March, 2018].
12. Jayashree Wad vs Union of India. Writ Petition civil no. 95 of 2015. (Last visited 8 March, 2017).
13. Sharma R. No complaint received about surrogate exploitation. New Delhi: Times News Network; 2016. Also available at http://timesofindia.indiatimes.com/city/ahmedabad/No-complaint-received-about-surrogate-exploitation/articleshow/53886097.cms.

# CHAPTER 38

# Stem Cell Therapy in Reproductive Medicine

*BN Chakravarty, Saeeda Wasim, Swarup Chakravarty*

## ■ INTRODUCTION

Application of stem cells in the field of reproductive medicine is a novel approach with initial promising results and many potential trials under initial phases. According to World Health Organization (WHO) 2010 estimates, infertility affects 15% of couples of reproductive age group.[1] Although with advent of assisted reproductive technologies, management of infertility has been revolutionized and many couples with previously presumed nontreatable infertility conditions have attained parenthood. Despite advances in in vitro fertilization (IVF) or intracytoplasmic sperm injection (ICSI), several conditions cannot be overcome by their application alone.

Successful fertilization essentially requires functional male and female gametes along with uterus and receptive endometrium. Whenever due to any reason either female or male partner fails to produce functional gametes, the only available treatment option is gamete donation. Gamete donation is not acceptable to many patients, primarily it entails no genetic linkage with the child and for some it is an unacceptable option due to religious reasons. Instances in which uterus is distorted, either anatomically or by disease process, or the endometrium is nonfunctional and is not corrected by either medical or surgical means, then the only recourse is surrogacy. Stem cells have been applied extensively in this area as well and initial reports are encouraging.

## ■ TYPES AND SOURCE OF STEM CELLS

Different stem cells have different level of plasticity and are termed according to their ability to differentiate in different lineage. Cells which can differentiate into cells of any lineage including extraembryonic tissue are termed as totipotent cells such as zygote, which is a totipotent cell. Pluripotent stem cells can differentiate into any cell type but not into extraembryonic tissue. The pluripotent cells are employed in many fields of stem cell research.[2]

Embryonic stem cells (ESCs) are derived from inner cell mass of the blastocyst; they have the ability to continuously grow in the culture keeping intact its developmental potential. The pluripotent ability of ESC and its unexhausting ability to divide make it an ideal candidate to study early embryonic development and is applied in cell-based therapy (Fig. 1).

The ESCs are derived from good blastocysts which are donated by couples who have completed their families via assisted reproduction. This has lots of ethical issues as many countries prohibit the use of healthy blastocysts for research purposes. The other sources of ESC are single blastomere biopsy (SBB), isolation of cells from poor quality embryos which are not considered for transfer, embryos which are rendered genetically aberrant by preimplantation genetic screening (PGS).[3]

Parthenogenesis is a condition where oocyte is stimulated to divide and develop into embryo without being fertilized. Somatic cell nuclear transfer (SCNT) is a technique in which nucleus of somatic cell of donor is introduced in the oocyte which has previously been enucleated. Transcription factor induced pluripotent stem cells (iPSCs) are yet another group of stem cells which if applied to human diseases have tremendous potential to cure several disorders

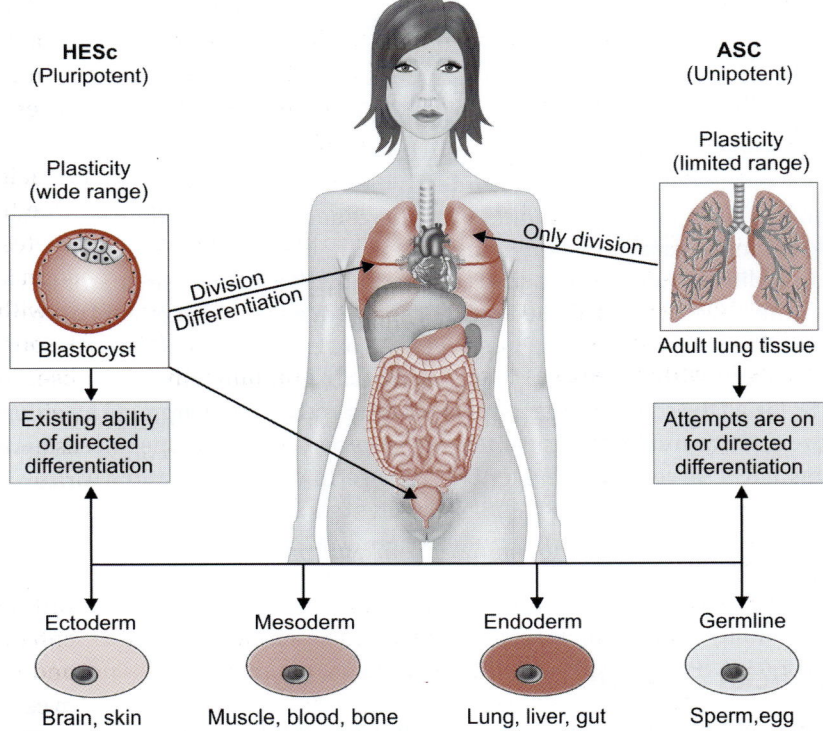

**Fig. 1:** Application of stem cell culture. (ASCs: adult stem cells; hESCs: human embryonic stem cells)

like type 1 diabetes, amyotrophic lateral sclerosis (ALS), long QT syndrome and others. These induced cells can be induced to reprogram to pluripotent stem cells by over expression of transcription factors like (Oct4, Sox2, Nanog, c-Myc, and Klf4).[4] Although these techniques have been successful to harvest ESC from mice, their application in humans is limited due to technical and ethical reasons.

## ■ ARTIFICIAL GAMETE

Gametes are specialized cells which are responsible for transmitting genetic and epigenetic information through generations.[5] Germ cells are differentiated from somatic cells very early during development when group of mesodermal cells separate from somatic cells during gastrulation, and acquire two basic properties, pluripotency and extensive epigenetic remodeling. Artificial gametes are mature germ cells (sperm and eggs) generated in vitro by specification and maturation of their natural diploid precursors, the primordial germ cells (PGCs), or by direct differentiation of pluripotent cells to the germ-cell lineage.

Functional gametes including a viable oocyte and a sperm are prerequisite for the process of fertilization. Conditions in which either of the partner are unable to produce viable gametes, have to resort to either gamete donation or adoption. For many couples either of the options is not acceptable due to either religious or personal reasons. Artificial gametes give these couples hope to have their own biological child. Patients of premature ovarian insufficiency, nonobstructive azoospermia, and cancer survivors in whom either of the germ cells have been destroyed by either chemotherapy or radiotherapy are contenders of such therapy. Patients with known genetic disorders who are at increased risk of passing the disorder to their offspring can also be benefited with artificial gametes, without losing the genetic linkage with the child and also having a disease-free offspring.

In addition to above mentioned couples, patients with same sex marriage, can have their own artificial gametes, either sperm or eggs, irrespective of their sex, giving chance to both partners to be genetic parents of the newborn. Similarly, postmenopausal women and single parents can also benefit from the same.

So far, all the studies on gametogenesis and embryo development have been done on mice model but as gamete development is species specific, artificial gamete will serve as an ideal tool to study germ cell biology and will provide intricate molecular and biochemical details of gametogenesis and fertilization. Moreover, availability of large number of artificial gametes may help to unravel many infertility issues which are not yet discovered and holds possibility of auto-correction of such issues at genetic level.

## Artificial Gametes Generation in In Vitro

Many adult tissues possess the ability of regeneration owing to the presence of adult stem cells (ASCs).[6] Presence of stem cells in the testis, termed as spermatogonial stem cells (SSCs), has been demonstrated by several studies.[7]

These stem cells occupy the basal layer of seminiferous tubule and are the source of continuous sperm production during the lifetime of males. Studies have suggested that these stem cells maintain their ability of self-renewal and differentiation to form sperms under the influence of a highly specialized environment maintained by Sertoli cells.

Human SSCs are obtained by using different membrane markers such as α6-integrin (CD49f) and β1-integrin, two laminin receptors,[8] CD9, a basal membrane cell attachment protein. Spermatogenesis have been attempted using SSC but due to difficulty in isolation and need for co-culture system with Sertoli cells, sperms obtained by this source have not shown in vitro fertilization and so far no live birth has been reported.[9] Presence of rare ovarian stem cells in mouse and human have been reported by some workers, giving a ray of hope of harvesting such cells in the future for generation of oocytes. Still, presence of oogonial stem cells is controversial and so far there is no concrete evidence for its presence, hence its use in infertile patients with no ovarian reserve is not yet applicable.

Human embryonic stem cells (hESCs) contain embryoid bodies, which spontaneously differentiate to form in vitro germ line cells.[10] For differentiation of hESCs into germ cells, certain markers should be expressed. Undifferentiated hESCs express markers such as C-kit and DAZL, which are responsible for early differentiation but not later markers such as VASA (a RNA helicase involved in germ cell maturation in both sexes) or SYCP3 (a structural protein of the synaptonemal complex critical for meiosis).

One of the requisites of gamete derivation from germ cells is the ability of these cells to undergo meiosis. Addition of several molecules like Bone morphogenetic protein (BMP) cytokines,[11] and retinoic acid (RA) to induce meiosis have not been very successful. However, meiotic progression is the most challenging step for the derivation of artificial gametes. In a recent study, pluripotent stem cells after being cultured in specific conditions and supplemented with BMPs, leukemia inhibitory factor (LIF), Rho kinase (ROCK) inhibitor and KnockOut serum replacement, have garnered large number of human artificial meiotic or sperm-like cells for use in research procedures.

As compared to males, comparatively fewer studies have been performed in female subjects, owing to the difficulties derived from the complexity of the oocyte cell. Still, oocyte-like cells, expressing oocyte-specific markers, have been developed from ESCs and iPSCs,[12] but the resultant product was far from being real and viable oocytes.

In gamete production, the challenge is to generate artificial gametes from opposite sex. This will be a breakthrough in providing genetically related offspring to same sex couples. However, it is a far-fetched goal and only few reports of incompetent sperm production from female cells have been reported.

In a nutshell, production of artificial gametes, although a promising option, yet it is far from being perfect for application in clinical setting. Any gamete obtained by artificial means should be safe in long-term use without any

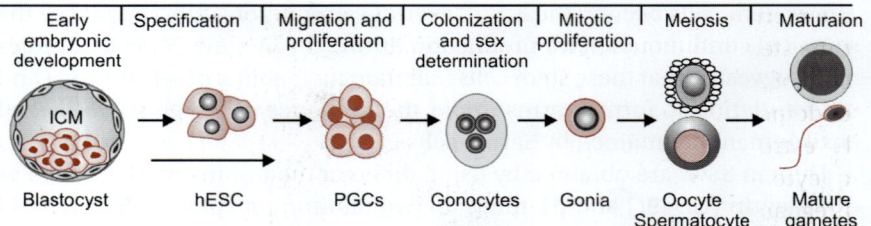

**Fig. 2:** Gametes generation from stem cells. (hESC: human embryonic stem cells; PGCs: primordial germ cells; ICM: inner cell mass)

predilection for imprinting disorders as reported in mice models, should be free from any tumorigenic potential and should be nonimmunogenic (Fig. 2).

## ROLE OF STEM CELLS IN ENDOMETRIAL PREPARATION

Human endometrium regenerates monthly throughout reproductive lifespan of a female under the influence of ovarian steroids. The cellular compartment of endometrium is replenished by ASCs and is essential for implantation and continuation of pregnancy.[13]

Embryo implantation is an essential event following fertilization which is governed by several maternal and embryonic factors, finally resulting in adhesion of blastocyst to endometrium.[14] For a short duration of time during the normal menstrual cycle, termed as window of implantation, endometrium is receptive for the implanting embryo. During the process of implantation, human endometrium undergoes complex changes, in response to circulating estrogen and progesterone resulting in receptive endometrium. These changes occur at morphological, biochemical, and molecular levels and any aberration at any of these factors results in failed implantation.[15]

In assisted reproduction for transfer of embryos, receptive endometrium is essential; however, method which can reliably predict endometrial receptivity is not yet established. Endometrium thickness is considered by many as the closest factor which can reliably predict endometrium receptivity. Poor endometrium thickness especially less than 4 mm is a difficult-to-treat entity and is responsible for many cases of implantation failure.

Different treatment modalities like extended estrogen administration, vaginal sildenafil, vitamin E, pentoxifylline and luteal phase GnRH-a supplementation have been tried in the treatment of thin endometrium but none have been proven to be effective.[16]

With limited success of medical treatment in the management of thin endometrium, many researches have been directed to the use of stem cells in endometrial preparation. In endometrial regeneration, in addition to local endometrial progenitor cells, hematopoietic and nonhematopoietic bone marrow-derived stem cells (BMDSCs) also play a significant role, these are recruited to the endometrium in response to injury. In 2011, for the first time stem cell therapy was applied in human endometrial regeneration in a case of Asherman's syndrome refractory to estradiol treatment.[17] Autologous endometrial angiogenic stem cells were infused into the uterine cavity followed by estrogen supplementation. At endometrial thickness of 7.1 mm, donor oocyte embryos were transferred resulting in a single viable intrauterine pregnancy. This was followed by a case series in which 6 patients with refractory Asherman's syndrome were treated with autologous mononuclear stem cells implantation.

Recently Santamaria and colleagues infused autologous CD133+ BMDSCs into the spiral arterioles of patients with refractory Asherman's syndrome and patients with refractory endometrial atrophy.[18] An increase in endometrial thickness lasting up to 6 months was noted in both set of patients, emphasizing the role of stem cell therapy in these patients. Peripheral blood stem cell transplant (PBSCT) has also been used for endometrial regeneration in mice models, but the results so far are not very promising. With existing knowledge, it appears that stem cells hold great promise for endometrial regeneration in women with scarred endometrium or in women with repeated failed endometrial preparation attempts but only large multicenter trials can validate its true efficacy.

## ROLE OF STEM CELLS IN VAGINAL RECONSTRUCTION

Vaginal functions can be impaired in variety of disorders, they may be congenital like Mayer-Rokitansky-Kuster-Hauser (MRKH) syndrome or androgen insensitivity syndrome; both these conditions are characterized by blind vagina. Apart from congenital disorders, infectious pathologies like warts or condyloma, vaginal prolapse, vaginal fistula, cancer and other types of trauma or surgeries can cause structural damage to vagina. Currently, surgery along with transplantation of synthetic or biological meshes is the only treatment option for vaginal reconstruction. However, these procedures are prone to infections and can lead to fibrosis further worsening the condition. Not only this, incorrect vascularization and graft rejection are also quite common.[19] Application of stem cells in vaginal reconstruction has been implied in mouse model with the use of muscle-derived stem cells (MDSC). MDSCs have been implicated in the treatment of muscular, cardiac and urological disorders. In mouse models, these cells have shown improvement in vaginal regeneration by epithelial tissue formation. Although it appears promising, relevant human studies are lacking and stem cell application in vaginal reconstruction is still in experimental stage.

## STEM CELLS IN SEXUAL DYSFUNCTION

Erectile dysfunction is on a rise in today's society keeping in pace with the rise in causative factors like diabetes, neuropathies, vascular diseases, postinflammatory disorders as in post chemotherapy and radiotherapy (Peyronie disease) or surgery.[20] Majority of studies involved stem cells injections derived from mesenchymal stem cell (MSC), neural crest stem cells, ESC, and endothelial progenitor cells in mouse models with modest improvements in symptoms owing to cytoprotective and antifibrotic properties of these agents. However, duration of beneficial effect is not ascertained. The only human study done so far has been use of intracavernosal injections of umbilical cord blood stem cells in diabetic patients suffering with erectile dysfunction. In this preclinical trial, patients reported enhanced penile rigidity and improvement in penile erection but the effects were short lasting and regressed over time. Current practice shows stem cell treatment as a promising tool in restoring normal erectile function but require further advances and their application.

## KEY POINTS

- Stem cell therapy in reproductive medicine is an expanding field with many clinical trials in their initial stages.
- Artificial gametes reproduced from stem cells, although a reality, yet their tumorigenic and immunogenic tendency renders them unsuitable for clinical use.
- Stem cell therapy in endometrial regeneration, erectile dysfunction and vaginal reconstruction holds a promise for wider application in future.
- Almost all research are based on murine or mouse models, so care should be taken in interpretation of these findings in human subjects.
- Till date, no stem cell therapy has been proven to be 100% effective and free from side effects, hence, it is prudent for both physicians and patients to make informed decision while opting for such therapy.

## REFERENCES

1. WHO. Mother or nothing: the agony of infertility. Bulletin of the World Health Organization. 2010;88(12):877-953.
2. Park TS, Galic Z, Conway AE, et al. Derivation of primordial germ cells from human embryonic and induced pluripotent stem cells is significantly improved by coculture with human fetal gonadal cells. Stem Cells 2009;27:783-95.
3. Kanatsu-Shinohara M, Ogonuki N, Inoue K, et al. Long-term proliferation in culture and germline transmission of mouse male germline stem cells. Biol Reprod 2003;69:612-6.
4. Lacham-Kaplan O, Chy H, Trounson A. Testicular cell conditioned medium supports differentiation of embryonic stem cells into ovarian structures containing oocytes. Stem Cells. 2006;24:266-73.
5. Rompolas P, Greco V. Stem cell dynamics in the hair follicle niche. Semin Cell Dev Biol. 2014;25-26:34-42.
6. Wabik A, Jones PH. Switching roles: the functional plasticity of adult tissue stem cells. EMBO J. 2015;34:1164-79.

7. Izadyar F, Wong J, Maki C, et al. Identification and characterization of repopulating spermatogonial stem cells from the adult human testis. Hum Reprod. 2011;26: 1296-306.
8. Conrad S, Renninger M, Hennenlotter J, et al. Generation of pluripotent stem cells from adult human testis. Nature. 2008;456:344-9.
9. Kanatsu-Shinohara M, Toyokuni S, Shinohara T. CD9 is a surface marker on mouse and rat male germline stem cells. Biol Reprod. 2004;70:70-5.
10. Clark AT, Bodnar MS, Fox M, et al. Spontaneous differentiation of germ cells from human embryonic stem cells in vitro. Hum Mol Genet. 2004;13:727-39.
11. White YA, Woods DC, Takai Y, et al. Oocyte formation by mitotically active germ cells purified from ovaries of reproductive-age women. Nat Med. 2012;18:413-21.
12. West FD, Machacek DW, Boyd NL, et al. Enrichment and differentiation of human germ-like cells mediated by feeder cells and basic fibroblast growth factor signaling. Stem Cells 2008;26:2768-76.
13. Cha J, Vilella F, Dey SK, et al. Molecular interplay in successful implantation. In: Sanders S (Ed.). Ten Critical Topics in Reproductive Medicine. Washington, DC: Science/AAA; 2013. pp. 44-8.
14. Paiva P, Hannan NJ, Hincks C, et al. Human chorionic gonadotrophin regulates FGF2 and other cytokines produced by human endometrial epithelial cells, providing a mechanism for enhancing endometrial receptivity. Hum Reprod. 2011;26:1153-62.
15. Paulson RJ. Hormonal induction of endometrial receptivity. Fertil Steril. 2011;96:530-5.
16. Senturk LM, Erel CT. Thin endometrium in assisted reproductive technology. Curr Opin Obstet Gynecol. 2008;3:221-8.
17. Nagori CB, Panchal SY, Patel H. Endometrial regeneration using autologous adult stem cells followed by conception by in vitro fertilization in a patient of severe Asherman's syndrome. J Hum Reprod Sci. 2011;4(1):43-8.
18. Santamaria X, Cabanillas S, Cervello I, et al. Autologous cell therapy with CD133+ bone marrow-derived stem cells from refractory Asherman's syndrome and endometrial atrophy: a pilot cohort study. Hum Reprod. 2016;31(5):1087-96.
19. Umoh UE, Arya LA. Surgery in urogynecology. Minerva Med. 2012;103:23-36.
20. Wespes E, Amar E, Hatzichristou D, et al. Guidelines on erectile dysfunction. Eur Urol. 2002;41:1-5.

# CHAPTER 39

# Past, Present and Future of ART

*BN Chakravarty, Ratna Chattopadhyay, Arup Kumar Majhi, Dibyendu Banerjee*

## ■ INTRODUCTION

The overall incidence of infertility globally has been estimated to be around 20%.[1] During last 20 years, incidence of infertility has increased. Based on the severity of the etiological factors, infertile couples may be classified into two groups: (1) easily manageable; which may be treated by a general gynecologist, and (2) the other group who requires specialized expertise and experience for rational management of their infertility problem. Majority of couples in the second group remained unmanageable till assisted reproductive technology (ART) was introduced in the management of infertility.

Since 1970s these unmanageable problems initiated exciting revolution in the treatment of infertility through three major "breakthroughs". The major breakthroughs were—(1) introduction of in vitro fertilization (IVF) and allied procedures (1978), (2) intracytoplasmic sperm injection (ICSI) (1993), which aimed at eradication of male factor infertility, and (3) regenerative medicine through stem cell culture (1998)—concentrating on tissue and organ engineering with the objective of preparing medical spare parts for repair and replace damaged organs and tissues of the body. Remarkable advancement and sensational outcomes have been achieved following these three breakthroughs in the later part of 20th century.

Assisted reproduction is the scientific discipline which has evolved faster during last four decades. Before the birth of the baby by IVF and ET in 1978 there was series of discoveries that enabled this miraculous success. The main reason of the success offered by ART is the association of different research areas of medical, biological and technological.

## ■ PREMODERN ERA

Little about physiology of reproduction was known till the discovery of sperm in 1678 by *Antonie van Leeuwenhoek*, a microscopist. Before that people have had a variety of vague ideas about how a baby is produced. Although the act of sexual intercourse had link in reproduction, and people understood that semen was somehow important, they at that time could not have the idea of the microscopic picture of gamete and internal process of conception, and sought to explain it in a variety of ways.

The Greek philosopher *Aristotle* believed that semen is composed of extremely small "seeds" of new humans, which grew in the "soil" of a woman's womb. Other ancient Greek philosophers argued that women produced semen internally, which mixed with the man's semen to somehow create the baby as babies resembled both parents.

Regarding production of semen there was difference of opinion. *Galen* believed that it came from the brain via his spinal cord. This belief was continued for more than a thousand years after Galen's death. Others argued that it was created from the extract of blood. Many believed that the semen contained small particles from each body part like heart, brain, arm, leg particles and so on. These particles assembled together to form the new human.

## ■ INTRODUCTION OF ARTIFICIAL INSEMINATION

Since the discovery of sperm under microscope, artificial insemination started on scientific basis, though deposition of semen artificially into the genital tract was known from as early as third century.

The first documented use of artificial insemination with husband's semen (AIH) was in 1770 by *John Hunter*, a Scottish surgeon who inseminated a woman using a quil with the semen of her husband who had hypospadias. This resulted in a successful pregnancy, and this is when the era of medically-assisted reproduction begun. It tooks nearly a century for a physician to report a pregnancy being successfully achieved through the use of donor sperm in artificial insemination because of the complex social issues.

## ■ INITIATION OF IN VITRO FERTILIZATION

The first IVF was attempted by Schenk, a Viennese scientist attempted IVF in 1879 with mammalian eggs in normal saline. Till 1970s and 80s, Ham F-10, Ham F-12, Menezo B2 and Earl's Media were very popular as culture media in IVF. In 1998, Gardner formulated IVF culture media closely approximated to human tubal fluid.

*Gregory Pincus* who synthesized Enovid, the first oral contraceptive pill in the market claimed to achieve IVF of rabbits in his Harvard laboratory in 1934. The first instance of in vitro fertilization of a human ovum was reported in 1944. *Robert Edwards*, a physiologist at Cambridge University was working on isolating hormones in mice since 1950. In 1965 Edwards successfully created a human embryo by adding his own semen to a human ovum in a Petri dish which he kept in secret due to fear of criticism. *Patrick Steptoe* was a gynecological surgeon practicing in Manchester, England. *Robert Edwards* and *Patrick Steptoe* jointly created the first human pregnancy through IVF on a couple John and Lesley Brown. Lesley's fallopian tubes were blocked. Dr Patrick Steptoe performed a Cesarean on Lesley Brown on July 25th, 1978 and the world's first test tube baby, Louise Joy Brown, was born weighing 5 pounds in Oldham, England. In the mid-1970s, the first pregnancy was reported; unfortunately, it ended in miscarriage. First test tube of India, Durga (Kanupriya Agarwal) was born in the same year as that of the baby of Steptoe and Edwards, in October 3, 1978 and was the second test tube baby of the world. Architect of first test tube baby of India is Dr Subhash Mukherjee who retrieved egg from the ovary, after pulling down it through posterior colpotomy, fertilized it outside and cryopreserved. He transferred the thawed embryo into the uterus in natural cycle. This was officially recognized much later in 2002 by the Indian Council of Medical Research (ICMR). The lead author of the present article was close associate of Dr Subhash Mukherjee and following the untimely sad demise of Dr Subhash Mukherjee he along with young generation pioneered the ART in India.

Development of sequential media by Gardner for blastocyst development in-vitro was major breakthrough in the history of culture media.

## ■ EARLIER DAYS OF ASSISTED REPRODUCTION

Due to increased demand of infertility treatment in post Second World War era there were improvements in two areas in infertility management. Firstly, the development of ovulation inducing drugs like clomiphene citrate and human menopausal gonadotropins from the urine of menopausal women and secondly introduction of laparoscopy in infertility evaluation and in management. Later, sonography has taken a great place in the procedure of assisted reproduction from evaluation of infertility to collection of oocytes and embryo transfer.

There were remarkable developments in basic and clinical research on folliculogenesis, preparation of media, in-vitro growth of human oocytes and clinical use of laparoscopy for diagnosis of pelvic pathology from mid-1960s to mid-1970s.

Before the wide use of ultrasound-guided oocyte pick up through vaginal approach, collection of oocyte was done through laparoscopic approach.

The ultrasound-guided oocyte recovery was first done by transvesical probe in 1982 (Lenz and Lauritsen). Transvaginal ultrasound-guided oocyte retrieval was first done by Wikland M in May, 1983.

For monitoring of ovulation and timing of ovulation trigger, specially for IUI, two very important clinical parameters were followed in *early and pre-IVF era*—(1) Insler's cervical mucus scoring; and (2) Basal body temperature chart (BBT) and other is infrequent use of urinary LH assay (by color change on paper strip) as sonographic folliculometry and day-to-day estimation of hormones was not widely available at that time.

Cervical mucus (Insler score) around periovulatory period is a biological mirror of rising E2 level in late follicular phase which was considered as guide for timing of hCG trigger followed by timed intercourse, intrauterine insemination or oocyte collection by laparoscopic method for IVF. It took decades longer to figure out the induction protocol, how to successfully fertilize the oocyte by sperm in vitro, support the fertilized egg and transfer the embryo to cause pregnancy.

## ■ INITIAL 25 YEARS AFTER SUCCESS OF IVF AND EMBRYO TRANFER

The initial 25 years after success of IVF and embryo transfer have been revolutionary. IVF and ICSI were the major areas of advancement in infertility management. But in early days pregnancies were few and far between. Every baby born was a cause for celebration. During this period there was a steady increase in the understanding of growth needs of embryos followed by refinements of stimulation regime and the medium in which the embryos were cultured (Fig. 1).

In addition, the various factors attributing to embryo stress in the culture laboratory and environment were realized and precautionary measures have been implemented. Recently monitoring of "volatile organic compounds (VOC)" level[2] and $O_2$ tension in the IVF laboratory is also an essential addition to improve laboratory quality control. With these modifications we reached a "peak", but after that we are in a "plateau" since last 10–15 years.

## Advances Achieved during Initial 25 Years

A remarkable advancement was possible in ART procedure through improvement in laboratory quality control. It was done by upgrading culture

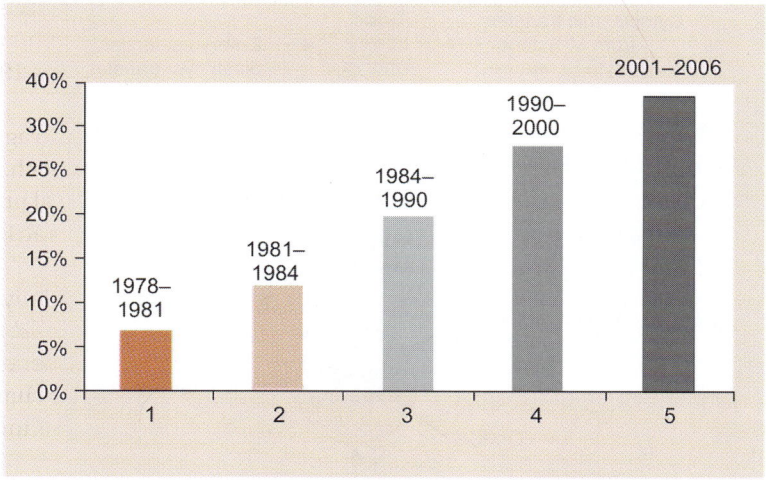

**Fig. 1:** Graph showing stagewise IVF success rate of modification of treatment strategies.

system with the development of HVAC system, Mini-incubator (MINC) and modified culture media optimized for IVF (Figs. 2A and B).

A revolutionary change in ovarian stimulation was possible following introduction of recombinant FSH and GnRH antagonist in 1998 by H Skovitz–Eldo ORJ, Kols et al.

Preimplantation genetic diagnosis (PGD) was introduced clinically by Alan Handyside in 1990.

Next generation sequencing (NGS) was a revolutionary invention in genetic diagnosis. This technique provides an unprecedented and accurate insight into pre-implantation 24 chromosome aneuploidy screening and monogenetic disorder diagnosis at a reduced cost.

Therefore, we are yet to achieve our anticipated expectations. The anticipated expectations are—(1) acceptable uniform success rate (60–80%), (2) simplification of the procedure, (3) reduction of cost; (4) elimination of associated hazards; and (4) prediction of outcome.

*And for these Improvements what does the Future Hold for ART?*

The following advancements are expected to improve the future prospect of ART management—(1) further refinements of stimulation protocol, individualization of stimulation regime; (2) development of cryobiology; (3) egg and embryo selection; (4) use of embryonic/adult stem cell for women with POF, male with azoospermia, and many others; (5) improvising health of children born of ART; (6) development of sperm biology; (7) further expansion

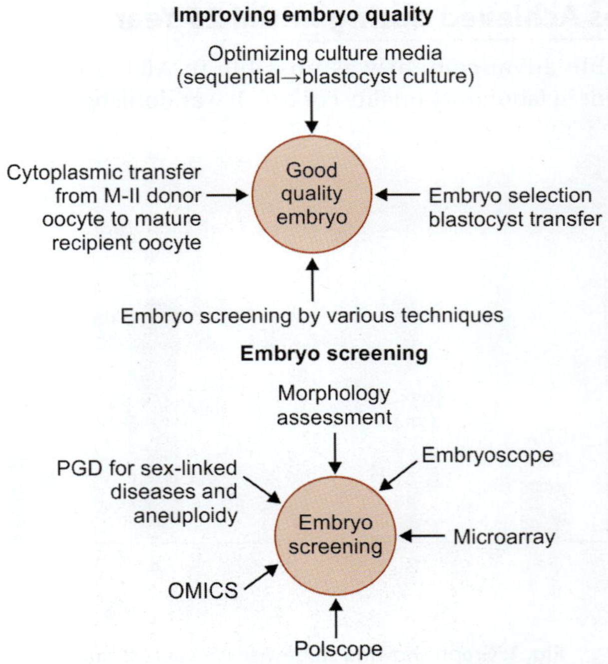

**Figs. 2A and B:** (A) Techniques to improve embryo quality; (B) Embryo screening.

of preimplantation genetic diagnosis; and (8) identification of predictive markers for IVF success/failure.

*Refinements of stimulation protocol:* Advances already made in the past decade through:
- Pen-style injection system
- Use of lower FSH doses
- Greater move toward use of GnRH antagonist downregulation protocol.

These advances have already become more patient friendly than before. Looking into near future, there is a trend toward further reduction of dose and greater uptake of antagonist regime. In addition, use of recombinant long-acting FSH (Corifollitropin); composition consists of recFSH + beta chain extension of hCG, the action of this compound; however, lasts for 7 days. But there is a concern about the use of long-acting FSH, increased risk of OHSS. Therefore this drug should be used cautiously in selected patients. But if introduced and proved to be safe it will be an attractive alternative because the protocol will consist of single injection instead of 7 doses in 7 days.

*Development of cryobiology*: First introduced in human IVF by Dr Subhash Mukherjee in 1978 (not accepted initially but subsequently confirmed by ICMR) (Fig. 3). Alan Trounson's team in Australia officially pioneered this, achieving viable pregnancy with transfer of frozen embryos (1981). Cryobiology currently is a central part of any modern ART program, providing approximately 30–35% of IVF births in well equipped ART units. In contrast, till recently, freezing of oocyte has a very low "success rate". However, a number of centers all over the world including India have used the technology with encouraging success rate slightly lower than that with cryopreserved embryos.

This technology will be of tremendous benefit for single women undergoing cancer treatment, a sort of "medical insurance".

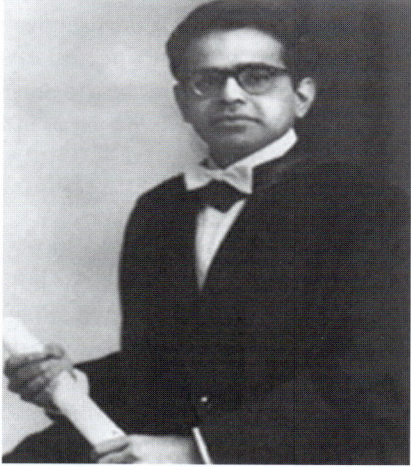

**Fig. 3:** Dr Subhash Mukherjee.

Outcome of "societal" egg freezing all over the world is variable. Experience of thawing (as opposed to freezing) of unfertilized oocyte is still limited. Eggs frozen at younger age may not yield anticipated outcome at older age when she is 38 or 40; "only future can say".

*Egg and embryo selection:* In late 1990s and early 2000s, there was a dramatic increase in IVF success rate. Further increase in success rate has been arrested possibly because of our poor understanding of unavoidable biological variations of gamete or embryonic genotype. Further improvement is expected by identification of the correct embryo for transfer. This may be possible by:
- Avoiding embryo "stress"
- Introduction of "microfluidics" and "time-lapse embryoscope" in culture technology
- Use of metabolic techniques to study waste products of developing embryos and thereby improving possibility of successful implantation
    - *Microfluidics:* This technique mimics in-vivo conditions of fertilization and embryo development. It provides dynamic flow of media (like in-vivo situation) in contrast to static pattern as in conventional culture. It is like sequential culture media supplemented with varying chemical treatments at prescribed time point. Qualities of embryos cultured in microfluidic device are superior to those grown in static system. The embryos are benefited from microfluidics. The benefit could be due to result of removal of harmful metabolic by-products like ammonia. This may be also due to gentle agitation of embryos which may activate intracellular signaling pathways and this physiologically mimics the action of ciliated epithelium. The process however is still in the learning stage.[3]
    - *Time lapse observation by embryoscope:* This procedure has the following advantages: (1) morphometry (diameter of oocyte and pronuclei) of oocyte and pronuclei can be easily assessed by embryoscope without alteration of culture environment; (2) oocyte activation can be measured by cytoplasmic waves in post-injected oocytes. Absence of cytoplasmic waves means non-activation which may be the cause of failed fertilization following ICSI. Early cleavage status which is an important criterion of embryo selection, can be assessed very precisely by time-lapse observation without exposure to outside environment or missing the step by conventional observation.[4]

This methodology of embryo selection is a revolutionary addition in the research field of ART. But there are limitations as well. Repeated exposure to light when digital images are obtained may have an after-effect. In practice until now no significant difference in pregnancy rate has been observed following the use of either time-lapse technology or conventional intermittent observation. Moreover, this is an expensive procedure without marked increase in success rate following ART.

## Use of Polscope

Use of imaging technique by Polscope to study the unfertilized egg, specially the spindle and morphologic features of developing embryo can improve selection of egg and embryos before ART or embryo transfer procedure. In addition, use of more sophisticated genetic techniques possibly involving microchips to predict genetic makeup of the embryo to be transferred is also in the process of research.[5]

Our observation of polscopic evaluation of oocyte before insemination:

We have observed the spindle characteristics, and the parameters evaluated were (Fig. 4):

- Length of meiotic spindle
- Angle between spindle and polar body
- Spindle retardance (birefringence)
- Zona thickness

Further improvement in embryo selection has been the use of comprehensive genomic hybridization (CGH) as against currently practiced technique of PGD to study expression of a single gene by PCR. The CGH technology will allow a more informative understanding of the future health of each embryo being cultured in the laboratory.

*Recently, in the IVF laboratory, monitoring of volatile organic compound (VOC) level is an essential addition to improve laboratory quality control.*

### Development in sperm biology:

Enormous advances have been achieved in our understanding of sperm biology. But these advances are yet to be translated into benefits in clinical practice. It is highly likely that developments in this area will significantly change the attitude of clinical practice of male infertility in next few years. Male may be responsible in recurrent fertilization, implantation failure and

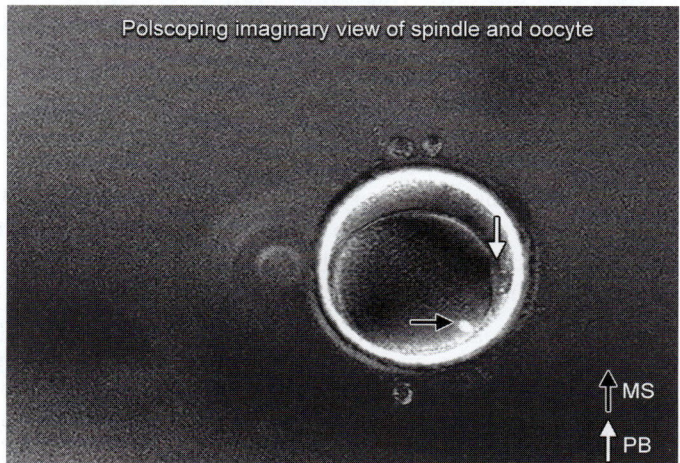

**Fig. 4:** Polscopic evaluation of oocyte.

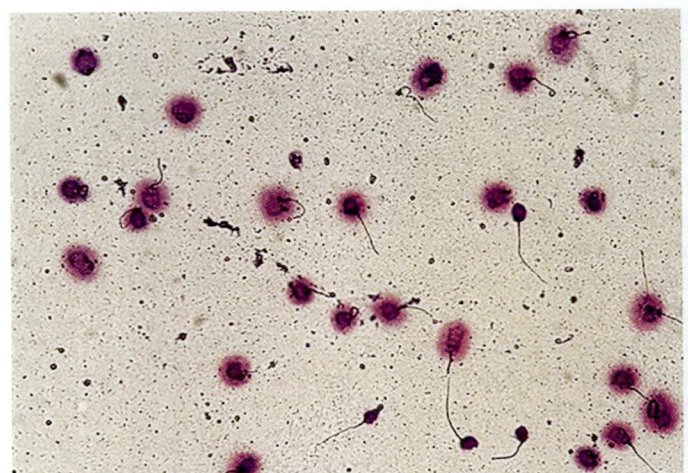

**Fig. 5:** Halosperm test for Sperm DNA fragmentation.

for recurrent pregnancy loss due to sperm DNA damage. Nowadays, DNA fragmentation index evaluation is essential by "TUNEL" assay or "HALOSPERM TEST" before ART procedure (Fig. 5).

*Improving health of children conceived after ART:* Excess perinatal mortality can be prevented by transfer of a single embryo. There is a growing concern about small increase in the incidence of congenital anomalies with ART conception. But those who need ART, are at a greater risk of having congenital anomalies rather than those who do not require ART process. Therefore, more research is needed to explore this area in next few years. Nowadays, precise sperm selection before ICSI like intracytoplasmic morphologically selected sperm injection (IMSI) and physiological intracytoplasmic sperm injection (PICSI) has become popular to improve success rate in severe male factor infertility.

*Embryonic stem cells (ESC):* Research in embryonic stem cells generated enormous interest with expectation to develop medical spare parts for diseased or damaged organs. We now realize that role of embryonic stem cells as opposed to adult stem cells, will be very limited. In future, induced pluripotent stem cell (iPSC) may be generated from adult somatic cell (may be from testis or from ovary) to create gamete through the process of somatic cell nuclear transfer (SCNT) (Fig. 6).

*Germ cell generation through stem cell culture:* Recently, attention has been focused on the generation of germ cells through stem cell culture. This will help in treating men with azoospermia and women with premature ovarian failure. Already experiments have been completed on animal model for application of stem cell culture in the treatment of infertility. The proposed ideas for derivation of human male and female germ cells have been based on animal experiments.

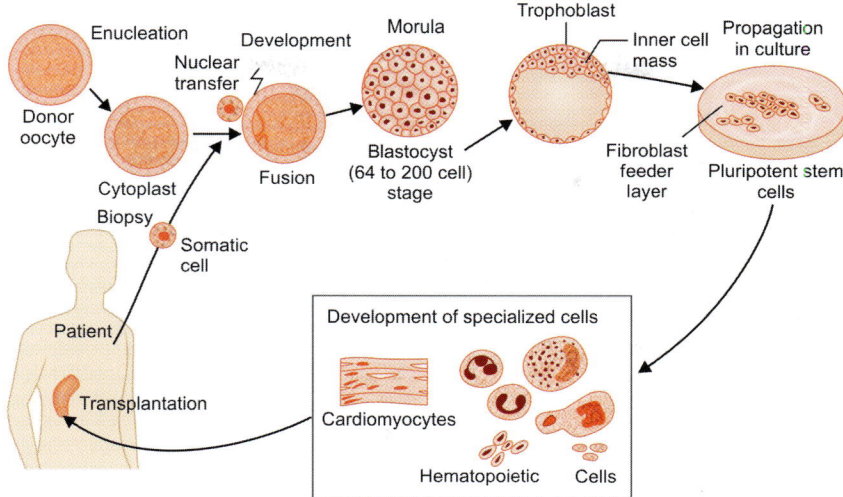

**Fig. 6:** Somatic cell nuclear transfer.

- From ES cells through embryoid bodies (Geijessen et al., 2004)
- From spermatogonial stem cells (adult stem cells) (Hiroshi Kubuta, 2001)
- From ovarian stem cells (adult stem cells) (Bokovsky et al., 2005).

The culture techniques used in these experiments are briefly described in Flowchart 1.

## What are Embryoid Bodies?

Embryoid bodies are aggregate of cells formed from differentiating embryonic stem cells in specialized suspension cultured with anti-differentiating agents

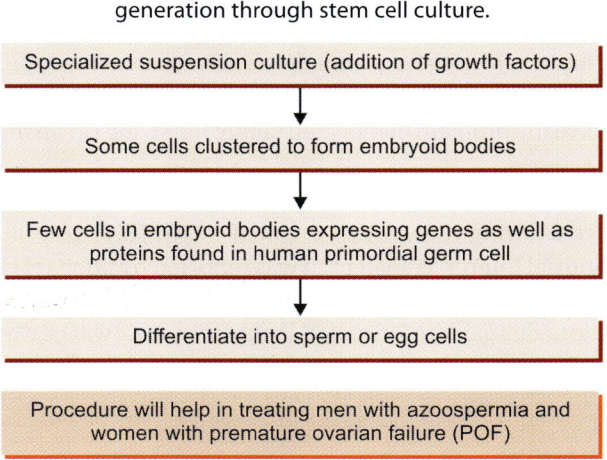

**Flowchart 1:** Culture techniques used for germ cell generation through stem cell culture.

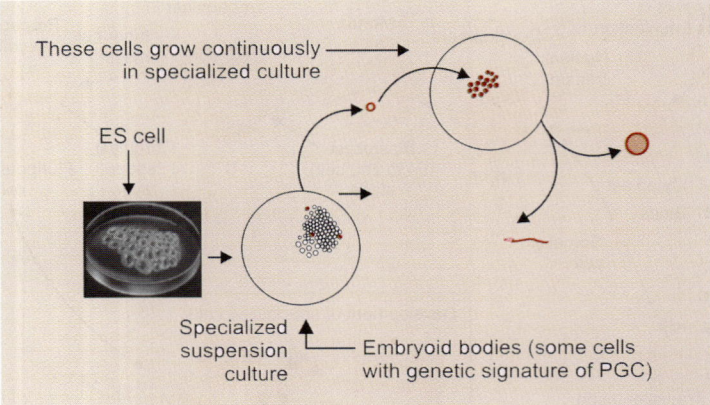

**Fig. 7:** Formation of embryoid bodies.

like leukemia inhibitory factor (LIF). The embryoid bodies consist of tissue lineages typical of early embryos (Fig. 7).

## ■ FUTURE ADVANCEMENT

The objectives of future advancements are to make ART procedure to make it more accessible and safe to the infertile couples. Mild stimulation, in-vitro maturation, less consumption of media, growth factor enriched and protein free media may make the treatment procedure less expensive and safer.

Cytoplasmic mitochondria can be defined as "battery for living". Mitochondrial dysfunction is one of the causes for repeated IVF failure in advanced maternal age. In advanced maternal age, there is reduced number and activity of mitochondria in oocytes leading to disruption of meiotic spindle. It results in misalignment of chromosomes, aneuploidy, poor embryo development and implantation, miscarriage and birth defects. Premature ovarian failure is observed in women with mitochondrial mutation. In future the donor cytoplasmic transfer, pronuclei transfer and meiotic spindle transfer has been suggested to prevent transmission of mitochondrial DNA disease. These may solve the problem of repeated failure following IVF in mitochondrial dysfunction.[6]

Autologous mitochondria from oogonial precursor cells can be injected into the oocytes during ICSI, which is called "AUGMENT (Autologous Germ cell Mitochondrial Energy Transfer)". It was reported by Michael H Fakih et al., that they may be another treatment option for repeated IVF failure in future.[7]

Last of all, artificial gamete formation in the laboratory will be a revolutionary advancement in future.

## KEY POINTS

- Incidence of infertility problem is increasing.
- Though there are "real" causes, yet "awareness" about availability of advanced technology of diagnosis and facilities of treatment of intractable infertility problems is a major reason for increased number of infertile couples approaching treatment.
- Categorization of infertile couples has a significant impact on treatment outcome.
- Infertility due to complex etiological factors should be treated in specialized centres with facilities of advanced technologies and expertise.
- In late 20th century ART including ICSI has made a major breakthrough in the management of complex infertility problems.
- The initial advances were revolutionary, while during last 15–20 years the research has not progressed to the desired expectation.
- The future challenges of infertility management include—fertility manipulation, fertility augmentation and fertility preservation.
- For fertility augmentation the objectives of ART in future are to achieve a steady improvement of results with minimum cost, discomfort and hazards. For this:
  - Individualization of stimulation protocol
  - Selection of right embryo for transfer
  - Identification of endometrial receptivity markers and treatment outcome
  - Artificial gamete formation are the areas of future research in infertility and ART practice.

## REFERENCES

1. Imhof M, Lackner J, Lipovac M, et al. Micronutrient supplementation increases sperm qality in the sub-fertile male. Eur Urol Rev. 2011;6(2):120-3.
2. Agarwal N, Chattopadhyay R, Ghosh S, et al. Volatile organic compounds and good laboratory practices in the in vitro fertilization laboratory: the important parameters for successful outcome in extended culture. J Assist Reprod Genet. 2017;34(8):999-1006.
3. Smith GD, Takayama S. Application of microfluidic technologies to human assisted reproduction. Mol Hum Reprod. 2017;23(4):257-68.
4. Desai N, Goldberg JM, Austin C, et al. Are cleavage anomalies, multinucleation, or specific cell cycle kinetics observed with time-lapse imaging predictive of embryo developmental capacity or ploidy? Fertil Steril. 2018:S0015-0282(17)32172-6.
5. González-Ortega C, Cancino-Villarreal P, Alonzo-Torres VE, et al. Polarized light microscopy for evaluation of oocytes as a prognostic factor in the evolution of a cycle in assisted reproduction. Ginecol Obstet Mex. 2016;84(4):217-27.
6. Craven L, Tuppen HA, Greggains GA, et al. Pronuclear transfer in human embryos to prevent transmission of mitochondrial DNA disease. Nature. 2010;465(7294):82-5.
7. Fakih MH, El Shmoury M, Szeptycki J, et al. The AUGMENT Treatment: Physician Reported Outcomes of the Initial Global Patient Experience. Reprod Med Genet. 2015.3:3.

# Index

Page numbers followed by, *f* refer to figure, *fc* refer to flow chart, and *t* refer to table.

## A

Abdomen 283
Abdominal discomfort 1, 184
Abdominal distension 184
    severe 50
Ablation therapy 73
Actinomycin 297
Adenomyoma 158
Adenomyosis 64, 109, 155, 156, 159, 161
    coexists 155
    degree of 162
    diagnosis of 155, 162
    features of 158, 158*t*
    impact of 157
    management for 159
    treatment of 158-160
Adenomyotic
    lesions, number of 162
    region 160
    tissue 159
    uterus 109*f*
Adhesion molecules 122
Adult respiratory distress syndrome 185
Adult stem cells 331*f*, 332
Albumin 48
    serum 132
Alfentanil 208
Alpha-2-macroglobulin 132
Amenorrhea, secondary 77
American and European Working Groups 86
American Society for Reproductive Medicine 135, 147, 148, 215, 227, 282, 303
Amino acid 34, 35
Amyotrophic lateral sclerosis 332
Analgesics 205
Androgen 104, 262
    insensitivity syndrome 335
    role of 177
    supplementation group 262
Anesthesia 213
    consultation 315
    general 60, 206, 208
    local 207
    regional 206, 207
    spinal 207
    use of 60
Anesthetic drugs 209
Aneuploidy 280
    risk of 179
Angiotensinogen converting enzyme 43
Anovulation 12, 135
Antiemetic agents 209
Antiepileptic medications 315
Antiestrogen clomiphene citrate 4
Anti-müllerian hormone 2, 86, 101, 102, 112, 148, 188, 189*t*, 191*f*, 192*t*, 225, 255, 259, 304
    basal 45
    importance of 190*f*
    serum 192*f*
    significance 189
Antioxidants 228
Antiphospholipid antibodies 47
Antitubercular drugs 205
Antral follicle
    count 45, 86, 108, 112, 112*f*, 189, 191*f*, 251, 255, 259, 305*t*
    use of 304
    small 188
Anuria 184, 185
Anxiety 24
Anxiolytics 205
Apoptosis 285
    premature 236
Arginine 79
Aromatase 311
    activity 101
    inhibitors 4, 265, 311
Arrhythmia 185
Arterial thrombosis 185
Artificial insemination, introduction of 339
Ascites, ultrasonographic evidence of 184
Asherman's syndrome 77, 217, 230
Assisted hatching, assessment of 178, 227
Assisted reproduction group 277*t*, 278*t*
Assisted reproductive technology 1, 21, 42, 62, 81, 83, 91, 100, 108, 135, 136, 138, 141, 142, 150, 155, 157, 164, 165, 173, 179, 183, 188, 190*f*, 199, 202, 203, 204, 213, 259, 275, 296, 324, 338
    anesthesia in 204
    complications of 118
    cycle
        agonist in 33, 36
        monitoring 104

future of 338
model 27f
modern 319
past of 338
pregnancies 82
present of 338
risk of 179
Autologous germ cell mitochondrial energy transfer 348
Azoospermia 222
   nonobstructive 332
   obstructive 17

## B

Benzodiazepines 208
Beta-human chorionic gonadotropin 67, 235
Biopsy guide 24
Birth
   defect, congenital 179
   weight, low 164
Bladder, distended 55
Blastocyst 178
   number of 193
   transfer 226
Blastomere biopsy 331
Bleeding 82
   antepartum 152
   intraperitoneal 167
   per vaginum 31
Blood
   flow, subendometrial 75, 129
   grouping 269
   investigations 24
   pressure, low 184
   supply, abnormal 222
Body
   mass index 141
   tissues 297
Bologna criteria 189, 249
Bone
   marrow stem cells 76, 334
   morphogenetic protein 333
Bowel perforation 168
Bromocriptine 166, 209
Bupivacaine 208
Buserelin 35, 270, 271

## C

Cabergoline 49, 166
   group 49
   use of 186
Cadaver ovaries, use of 269
Cancers
   genital 302
   hematological 302

Carbon dioxide 147
Cardiac
   defects 180
   disease 205
   disorders, treatment of 335
Catheter tip 63
Cavity, normal 110f
Cell adhesion molecule 145
Cellular adhesion molecule 128
Centers for Disease Control and Prevention 175
Central venous pressure 184
Cervical
   canal 59
   corporeal ratio 108
   dilatation 56
   dilation 65
   factor 12
      infertility 15
   fibroids 57
   issue scarring 14
   mucus 340
      presence of 68
   stenosis 55, 56
      presence of 56
   tenaculum 55
Cervicouterine angle 63
Cesarean section 152, 179
Chemoresistant tumor burden 298
Chemotherapy 299
Chloroprocaine 208
Chromosomal inversions, incidence of 222
Clamping uterine artery 294
Clamydia 73
Clomiphene citrate 4, 15, 103, 244, 263
Clonogenic multipotent stem cell 77
Comprehensive genomic hybridization 345
Corpus
   luteal function 1
   luteum 81, 82, 85
      cyst 111f
Cryobiology, development of 343
Cryocans 24
Cryopreservation 186
   options 98
   process 282
   program 32
   stress of 285
   techniques 303
   unit 32
Crystalloid infusion 200
Cumulus oophorus 115f
Cusco's speculum 67
Cycle cancellation rate 175
Cyclic guanosine monophosphate 75
Cyclophosfamide 297

# Index

Cyst
  endometriotic 201
  hemorrhagic 111*f*
  myometrial 158
Cystectomy, laparoscopic 149
Cytochrome p450 enzyme 311
Cytokines 122, 223, 333
Cytoplasmic mitochondria 348

## D

De novo mutations 180
Defective luteal phase 97
Dehydroepiandrosterone 141, 177, 262, 265
  role of 177
  sulfate 262
Dendritic cells 197
Dermoid cyst 111*f*
Deslorelin 35
Desynchronization, risk of 93
Dexmedetomidine 208
Diabetes 205, 335
  mellitus 199
    gestational 179, 185, 202
Diarrhea 184
Diethylstilbestrol, history of 57
Dimethyl sulfoxide 285
Diploid zygote 100
Donor
  assisted reproduction 263
  egg 259
  embryos 164
  oocyte 164
    cycles 178
    indications for 268
    pregnancy acts 179
  stimulation of 264
Dopamine agonist 49, 166, 209
Duchenne muscular dystrophy 180
Dydrogesterones 83
Dyslipidemia 136
Dysmenorrhea 155
Dyspareunia 155
Dyspnea
  mild 184
  severe 184

## E

Ectocervix 55
Ectopic pregnancy 76, 169, 201
  cause of 68
  risk of 169
Edema, pulmonary 313
Egg 332
  and embryo selection 344
  fertilization of 263
  in vitro maturation of 269
  multiple 69
Ejaculation, retrograde 13
Ejaculatory dysfunction 13
Elective social oocyte cryopreservation 282
Electrolyte imbalance 313
Embryo 204, 221, 228, 283, 310
  atraumatic
    delivery of 68
    placement of 64
  cleavage stage of 85
  cryopreservable 6
  cryopreservation 60, 230, 280, 281, 304, 307
  donation 259, 263, 264, 267, 271, 272
    indications for 272
  endometrium of 69
  expulsion, prevention of 68
  factors, evaluation of 225
  freezing of 166, 202, 303
  implantation 82, 101, 116, 334
  mechanism of 5
  quality 5, 6
  restricting number of 169
  screening 342*f*
  synchronization of 92
  transfer 28, 29, 54, 58, 60, 62, 65, 65*f*, 66, 67, 127, 147, 158, 159, 204, 264, 294, 341
    advantages of 69
    disadvantages of 69
    number of 1, 178
    procedures 66, 68
    single 92, 168
    techniques 231
    transabdominal ultrasound guided 59
    transmyometrial 57
    ultrasound image of 64*f*
  vitrification program 22
Embryoid bodies 347
  formation of 348*f*
Embryonic stem cells 331, 346
Embryoscope 27*f*
Empty follicle syndrome 235
Endocervical canal 58
Endocervix 65
Endocrinal factors 242
Endogenous progesterone secretion 88
Endometrial
  adequacy 269
  assessment 115
  biopsy 196
  blood flow 129
  carcinoma 295
  cavity 68, 108, 109, 269
  growth, stimulated 75
  injury 197, 230
  islands 158

markers 127
parameters 97
pattern 129
perfusion 230
pinopods 130
polyp 64, 110f, 229
preparation 91, 264, 334
    methods of 93
receptivity 6, 121, 127, 130, 145
    array 73, 121, 123, 131
    assessment of 128
    morphological assessment of 124
reconstruction 230
scratch 76, 196, 197
striae 158
subendometrial blood flow 130
thickness 72, 129
tissue, disadvantages of 123
vascularity 114, 116f
volume 115f
Endometrioid 299
Endometrioma 24, 111, 215
    management for 148, 149fc, 149t
    surgical treatment of 150, 150f
Endometriosis 15, 130, 145, 146f, 155, 242, 246
    effects of 145
    management for 147fc
    mild 150
    recurrent 151
    severe 267
Endometriotic cyst, rupture of 201
Endometrium 63, 72, 77, 96, 113, 131, 132, 197
    basalis layer of 77
    develops 74
    functional assessment of 122
    postreceptive 130
    synchronization of 92
    synchronized maturation of 129
    ultrastructural assessment of 122
Endomyometrial junction 108
    irregular 158
Epithelial
    estrogen receptor alpha 128
    ovarian cancers 298
Erectile dysfunction 335
*Escherichia coli* 73
Estradiol 45, 83, 100, 102
    estimation, serum 106
    level 48
        serum 48, 102, 103
    supplementation 85
    valerate 271
Estrogen 25, 73, 94
    administration 334
    dependent condition 146

    exogenous 96
    receptor 306, 311
    sensitive cancers 308, 311, 312, 313
Ethylene glycol 285
Etomidate 208
European Society of Human Reproduction and Embryology Guidelines 140
Extraembryonic tissue 330
Extraovarian spread 299

## F

Fallopian tube 111, 204
    patency of 111
Female pelvic anatomy, assessment of 108
Fentanyl 208
Fertility
    armamentarium of 128
    centers 180
    following cervical cancer 293
    following gynecological cancer 293
    loss of 173
    preservation 280, 283, 295, 302, 303, 305, 316
        methods of 303
    sparing procedures 299
    sparing surgery 298
    treatment 103
Fertilization
    rates 308
    recurrent 345
Fetal
    growth restriction 164
    ovarian tissue 269
Fibroids 214, 215, 222
    presence of 63
    submucous 110f, 222
Flow index 114
Follicle stimulating hormone 2, 33, 45, 100, 101, 112, 136, 137, 139, 188, 192f, 225, 306, 237, 256, 259
Follicular
    activity 94
    aspiration 168
    cells 81
    cohort, size of 103
    development 15, 308
        process of 252
    fluid 26, 117, 237
    growth 95, 236
        rate 93
    monitoring 108
    phase 36, 82, 94, 95, 307
        culminates 81
        late 4
    puncture 207
    rupture 245

stimulation 42
tracking 113
wall 240
Folliculogenesis 37, 236
Fragile ovary 167
Fresh frozen plasma transfusion 315
Frozen embryo 164
    transfer 3, 63, 72, 81, 85, 91, 91*f*, 92*f*, 93, 97, 130, 159, 166, 197
        cycles 95, 97
        natural cycle for 93
        over fresh embryo transfer, advantages of 97

# G

Gamete
    artificial 332
    donation 330
    functional 332
    generation 334*f*
    intrafallopian transfer 58, 204
Genetic
    biomarkers 251
    connection 322
    couple 272
Germ cell 285, 299
    generation 346, 347*fc*
    mature 332
    primordial 334*f*
    tumors, malignant 299
    type 298
Gestational age, large for 164
Gestational trophoblastic
    disease 297
    neoplasia 298
Gland, pituitary 33
Glycerol 285
Glycine 33, 34
Gonadotoxic
    cancer treatment 282
    therapy 305
Gonadotrope cell surface 34
Gonadotropin 1, 4, 25, 36, 96, 101, 311
    dose during ovarian stimulation 305
    exogenous 3
    high-dose 177
    releasing hormone 2, 24, 33, 35*t*, 73, 82, 136, 139, 146, 149, 159, 256, 306
        agonist 34, 36, 35*t*, 38*t*, 74, 83, 93-95, 138, 139, 159, 166, 313
        analog 4, 85, 270
        antagonist 49, 260, 306, 308
        molecule 34
        physiology 33
        structure 33*f*

requirements 137
stimulation, exogenous 255
therapy 137
total dose of 310
Goserelin 35
Granulocyte colony-stimulating factor 76, 224, 230
Granulosa cells 4, 188, 237, 285
    connection of 81
Granulosa lutein cells 43*f*
Growth hormone 141, 261, 265
    use of 177

# H

Halosperm test 346*f*
Hampers endometrial receptivity 223
Hematosalpinx 111
Hemoconcentration 42
Hemoglobin 166
Hemophilia A 180
Hemorrhage
    obstetric 162
    postpartum 72, 168
Heparin binding growth factor 128
Hepatitis B 31
Hexaethyl starch 166
Histidine 34
Histrelin 35
Homogeneous echogenic endometrium 57
Hormone
    analysis 101
    controlled cycle 270
    influence of 127
    replacement
        cycle 94
        therapy 72, 93, 160
Human
    albumin 166
    chorionic gonadotropin 3, 30*f*, 39, 43, 43*f*, 72, 74, 82-84, 93, 114, 139, 165, 183, 242, 270
        dosage 47
        low dose 74
        supplementation 87
    embryo twinning 269
    embryonic stem cells 331*f*, 333, 334*f*
    endometrium 127
        regenerates 334
    fertilization 175
    follicular fluid 43
    growth hormone, use of 177
    immunodeficiency virus 269
    menopausal gonadotropin 75, 263, 340
    oocytes, fertilization of 100
    ovum 339

Hydrosalpinges 169, 223, 231
　presence of 223
Hydrosalpinx 24, 111
　surgery for 214
Hydrothorax 184
　massive 185
Hydroxyethyl starch
　administration 200
　solution 49
Hydroxyprogesterone 100
Hyperandrogenemia 136
Hyperinsulinemia 138
Hyperplasia 155
Hyperprolactinemia 242
Hypertension
　pregnancy induced 179, 185
　uncontrolled 199
Hypertensive disorders 179
Hypoestrogenic side effects, risk of 95
Hypogonadism, hypogonadotropic 101
Hypospadias, anatomical problems like 13
Hypotension 165
Hypothalamopituitary axis 82
Hypothyroidism 103
Hypovolemia 201
Hypovolemic hyponatremic state 185
Hysterosalpingo-contrast-sonography 119
Hysterosalpingography 15
Hysteroscopic
　correction 56, 229
　examination 230
　metroplasty 217
　surgeries 213, 215
Hysteroscopy 64, 78, 124

# I

Imatinib, use of 315
Immature eggs, retrieval of 6
Immunoglobulin, intravenous 224
In vitro
　culture 286
　fertilization 1, 12, 13, 62, 100, 117, 121, 139, 141, 147, 149, 149$t$, 150, 157, 164, 184, 204, 213, 249, 267, 275, 281, 303, 330, 338, 339
　　batching of 21
　　complications of 164$t$
　　cycle 84
　　demerits of 21
　　initiation of 339
　　merits of 21
　　oocytes 174
　　process of 54
　　technique 319
　maturation 281
　oocyte maturation 47

In vivo follicular growth 6
Indian Council of Medical Research 298, 319
Indian Society for Promoting Assisted Reproduction 324
Indian Society for Third-Party Assisted Reproduction 327
Infertility 130, 145, 146$f$, 245
　and obstetric complications 216
　cause of 15, 204
　etiology of 62
　female factors of 108
　immunological 17
　management 18
　ovulatory factor 15
　risk of 280
　treatment 147, 180, 338
Inflammatory bowel diseases 280
Inhibin B 103, 193
Insulin resistance 136
　assessment of 138
Intensive luteal phase 87
Interleukins 223
Intra-abdominal pressure 50
Intracytoplasmic sperm injection 21, 81, 150, 151, 164, 164$t$, 213, 224, 228, 275, 284, 330, 338, 346
　physiological 346
Intramural fibroids 214, 222
　distorting uterine cavity 124
　effects of 215
Intraovarian vascularity 115
Intrauterine
　adhesions 229, 230
　growth
　　restriction 217
　　retardation 277$t$
　insemination 12, 64, 118, 147, 150, 164, 267
　　indications of 13$t$
　　results of 216
　pathology 124
　pregnancy 169
Intravascular volume depletion 42, 43

# J

Japanese intending couple 324

# K

Karyotyping 225
Ketamine 208

# L

Laminaria tents 56
L-arginine 76
Letrozole 4, 15, 311, 315
　plus gonadotropin protocol 312, 316

Leucine 34
Leukemia
    chronic myelogenous 315
    inhibitory factor 128, 333, 348
Leuprolide 35, 87, 270, 271
Leuprorelin 35
Levonorgestrel-intrauterine device 295
Limb defects 180
Liquid nitrogen 24, 284
Live birth rates 176
Liver dysfunction 165, 313
Local anesthetic agents 208
Loop electrosurgical excision 294
Low dose aspirin 75, 166, 230
Low molecular weight heparin 166, 224
Low ovarian reserve, evidence of 17
Lower embryo implantation 174
Luer lock fitting 57
Luminal epithelial cells 130
Luteal phase
    defect 82
    insufficiency 141
    protocols 86
    support 49, 83, 85, 141
        postanalog trigger 87
        progesterone for 84
Luteinized unruptured follicle 240, 243
    cycle 242
    syndrome 240, 241, 246
        diagnosis of 243
        diseases associated with 242
        etiopathogenesis of 242
        history of 241
        management of 244
        prevention of 244
        signs of 243
        symptoms of 243
    ultrasound of 241$f$
Luteinizing hormone 2, 33, 81, 100, 121, 137, 236, 240, 260
    baseline 136
    role of 252
    spontaneous 93

# M

Macromolecules, administration of 48
Male fertility 16, 284
Malecot catheter 56
Malignancy, diagnosis of 302
Mammalian reproduction, classical model of 285
Mayer-Rokitansky-Kuster-Hauser syndrome 335
Medical therapy 146
Medroxyprogesterone acetate 295
Megestrol acetate 295
Menopause 146, 173, 268
Menorrhagia 155
Menstrual
    blood serves 77
    cycle 241, 306
Mesenchymal stem cell 336
Metallic
    dilators 56
    stylet 55
Metformin 47, 165
Methotrexate 297
    single high dose of 297
Methylenetetrahydrofolate reductase 226
Metroplasty 217
Microarray technology, advent of 130
Microdose flare protocol 38
Microfluidics 344
Midazolam 208
Milder stimulation protocols, development of 2
Minimal stimulation 265
    protocols 40
Miscarriage 141, 157, 280
    rate 176
    risk of 179
    spontaneous 176
Mitochondria 348
Mock endometrial preparation cycle 269
Molar pregnancies 298
Monolateral disease 149
Mucin 1 128
Müllerian anomalies 109
    congenital 73
Müllerian inhibiting substance 102, 188
Multicenter trials, large 335
Multifetal reduction 168
Multifollicular development 13
Muscular disorders, treatment of 335
Myomectomy 64, 229
    aggressive 73
Myometrium 57, 108, 155
    posterior 57

# N

Nafarelin 35
Naphthylamine 34
National Cancer Registry Programme 298
National Institute for Health and Care Excellence 17, 140
National Registry of Assisted Reproductive Technology 327
Natural conception 278, 279
    group 277$t$, 278$t$
Natural cycle 3, 95, 96, 262, 270
    modified 93
    stimulation 3

Nausea 185
    mild 184
    postoperative 209
Neonatal intensive care unit 276
Neural tube defects 180
Neuromuscular electrical stimulation 79
Neutropenia 315
Neutrophil count, absolute 315
Next generation sequencing 342
Nitroglycerin 76
Nitrous oxide 209
Non-adenomyotic group 157
Nonhematopoietic stem cells 77
Nonsteroidal anti-inflammatory drugs 50, 209
Nonsteroidal triphenylethylene compound 310
Nucleotides regulating post-transcriptional gene 132

# O

Obesity 136, 137
    morbid 205
    visceral 136
Office hysteroscopy 217, 269
Oligoasthenozoospermia 222
Oligo-ovulation 135
Oligospermia 218
Oliguria 50, 184
Oncofertility 303
Oocyte 204, 228, 235, 236, 304, 307, 333
    aneuploidy, rate of 174
    cryopreservation 263, 269, 281-283, 313
    cumulus complex 26, 238
    donation 267
        treatment, result of 271
    donors
        professional 268
        source of 268
    fertilization, failed 103
    immature 281
    loss of 173
    number of 86
    pick-up 3, 86, 201
    polscopic evaluation of 345$f$
    poor quality of 174, 221
    quality 115, 208, 221, 255, 304
    quantity 255
    recovery 270, 315
    retrieval 108, 116, 117$f$, 206, 254, 260
        complications of 167
    unfertilized 344
Opioids 208
Oral contraceptive pills 25, 73
Ovarian
    abscesses 168, 201
    agenesis 268

biomarkers 255
cancer 298
    majority of 298
cyst 201, 213
    rupture of 201
failure, premature 268
follicle 114, 117, 235
    color Doppler evaluation of 114
function 146$fc$
    tests 225
hormone production 315
hyperstimulation 100, 121, 164, 213
    controlled 81, 138, 164, 188, 265
    presence of 97
hyperstimulation syndrome 1, 12, 42, 45, 69, 81, 91, 112, 118, 118$f$, 138, 139, 165, 183, 185, 188, 200, 306, 313
    classification of 44, 44$t$, 184
    critical 44$fc$, 50
    development of 49
    early 183
    management 46, 183, 184
    mechanisms of 46$f$
    mild 200
    moderate grade 200
    pathophysiology 183
    physiology of 183
    prevention of 200, 313
    preventive measures 185
    recognition of 200
    risk of 237
    severe 44$fc$, 50, 200
    treatment of 50
physiology 307
reserve 188, 214, 304
    markers 190, 191$f$
    normal 257
    test 3, 177, 190, 251
response 255
stem cells 285
    maintenance of 286
stimulation 42, 46, 137, 197, 200, 281, 304, 308, 310
    beginning of 166
    controlled 2, 100, 141, 147, 150, 191, 191$f$, 281, 308, 314
    conventional controlled 306
    days of 310
    mild 1-3, 5, 5$t$
    protocols 306
    standard 5$t$
    suboptimal 224
tissue cryopreservation 283, 285
torsion 167, 200
transposition 294

tumor 299
    borderline 299
  vascularity 113
  volume 112
Ovary 111
  artificial 285
  enlargement of 165, 184, 200
  hyperstimulated 167
  sex cord stromal tumors of 299
Ovulation 82
  induction 93
  leading 94
  trigger agent, modification of 48
  triggering 238
Ovum 259
  donation 263, 264, 265
  pick-up 2, 24, 26, 116, 238

# P

Pain, abdominal 67, 184
Paracentesis 50
  indications for 50
Paracervical block 207
Paternal leukocyte immunization 231
Patient controlled analgesia 207
Peak systolic velocity 113
Pelvic
  adhesions 59, 242, 245
  inflammatory disease 223, 242
Pentazocine 208
Pentoxifylline 75
Perinatal mortality 179
Periovarian adhesions 245
Peripheral blood stem cell transplant 335
Peritonitis 168
Personalized embryo transfer 123, 123*fc*, 131
Peyronie disease 336
Photodynamic therapy 296
Pinopodes-endometrial protrusions 128
Pituitary gonadotropes 34
Placental complications 152
Plasma
  androgens, measurement of 104
  expanders 166
  progesterone 105
Plasmin 237
Platelet-rich plasma
  autologous 78
  intrauterine infusion of 78
Polscope, use of 345
Polycystic ovarian
  disease 2, 7, 242
  syndrome 14, 102, 188

Polycystic ovary 31, 113*f*, 242
  syndrome 45, 95, 135, 136, 138, 139, 141, 142
    antagonist protocols in 139
    severe 36
Polyp 216
Poor ovarian
  reserve 250*f*
  response 189, 255, 259
Poseidon classification 249, 250
Poseidon concept 256
Poseidon criteria 255
  classification 256
  management 256
Poseidon group 256, 257
  management for 257
Poseidon subgroups 255
Positron emission tomography 294
Postembryo transfer 67, 88
Postinflammatory disorders 336
Preeclampsia 152, 202
Preembryo transfer procedure 63
Pregnancy 146
  clinical 18
  complication 168, 169, 179
    high rate of 199
  heterotopic 169
  multifetal 202
  multiple 6, 14, 168, 275
  outcomes 152
  rate 6, 39, 67, 96, 157, 271
    clinical 175
    higher 15
    prediction of 193
  spontaneous 183
Pretreatment ovarian reserve assessment,
    importance of 303
Progesterone 25, 67, 77, 83, 94, 96
  dose 95
  exogenous 88
  free luteal phase 88
  intramuscular 84
  oral micronized 83
  preparations 95
  supplementation 142
Progynova 271
Propofol 207, 208
  administration of 208
Prostaglandin 43, 122
  metabolism 131
  role of 242
Protein, alpha-induced 236
Prothrombotic disorder 230
Pulse frequency and amplitude 33
Pvarian hyperstimulation syndrome,
    pathogenesis of 43*f*

## Q

Quinagolide 166

## R

Radiotherapy 298
Randomized controlled trials 177, 181, 214
Random-start controlled ovarian hyperstimulation 307
Recombinant luteinizing hormone supplementation 88
Rectus abdominis myocutaneous flap 315
Recurrent implantation failure 31, 128, 178, 197, 221
    etiology of 221, 232
    evaluation and management 224
    management of 224*fc*, 226
    treatment of 224
Remifentanil 208
Renal disease, severe 205
Renal dysfunction 165
Reproductive
    health 280
    medicine 330
    surgery 204
Retrieved oocytes, number of 255
Rokitansky-Kuster-Hauser syndrome 273
Royal College of Obstetricians and Gynaecologists 44

## S

Saline infusion sonography 110*f*, 111
Salpingitis, subclinical 294
Secretomics 123
Selective estrogen receptor modulator 75
Selective serotonin reuptake inhibitors 205
Semen
    cryopreservation of 284, 303
    parameters 16
    samples 28*f*
        well-arranged 29*f*
Sepsis 185
Septoplasty 73
Sexual dysfunction 335
Sham embryo transfer 63
Sildenafil 79
    positive effect of 75
Sleep disorders 295
Small for gestational age 179
Smooth muscle myometrial cells 155
Somatic cell 332
    nuclear transfer 331, 346, 347*f*
Sonohysterography 225
Sperm 164, 332
    biology, development in 345
    capacitation of 100
    cryopreservation 284
    deoxyribonucleic acid
        fragmentation 346*f*
        integrity tests 225
    discovery of 339
    donation 263, 264, 267
    parameters, subnormal 13
    retrieval, surgical 204
    surgical retrieval of 229
    survival 16
Spermatogonial stem cells
    in vitro generation of 286
    preservation of 284
Staphylococcus 73
Stem cell 230, 334*f*, 335
    application of 330
    culture 346, 347*fc*
        application of 331*f*
    muscle-derived 335
    ovarian 263
    pluripotent 330, 331
    research 330
    role of 334, 335
    source of 330
    spermatogonial 284, 332
    therapy 77, 78, 330
        role of 335
    types of 330
Steroidogenesis 131
Steroids 100
Stimulation protocol 1
    mild 6
    protocol, refinements of 343
Strassman surgery 73
Streptococcus 73
Stromal fibroblast, source of 77
Subfertility 156, 245
Supraphysiological steroid hormone levels, secretion of 82
Surrogacy 263, 267, 272, 318, 320, 326
    altruistic 321, 326
    arrangement 321
    background of 318
    bisexual 322
    child born of 326
    commercial 321
    contemporary modern forms of 322
    counseling in 274
    developments on 324
    emphasizes 322
    favorable over adoption 323
    for medical reasons 323
    full 322
    gestational 273, 322

# Index

host 322
in ancient India 318
in early human civilizations 318
in India and foreign nations 320
in India medicolegal arrangement 320
in mesopotamia civilization 318
international 322
legal regulations on 326
natural 273
on monetary payment 321
overseas 322
partial 322
process 321
(regulations) Bill 2016 326
same sex 322
significance of 322
single parent 322
social 322
straight 322
traditional 273, 322
transgender 322
transnational 322
types of 321
Surrogate, screening of 273
Swiss cheese appearance 109
Syncope 184
Synechiae 217

## T

Tachycardia 50, 165
Tachyphylaxis, phenomenon of 35
Tailored gonadotropin regimen 165
Tamoxifen 75, 310, 311
    selective antagonist action of 311
Tenaculum 55, 58, 60
Tension ascites 200
Testicular
    failure 222
    sperm aspiration 25
    stem cells 286
    tissue 284, 303
        cryopreservation 284
        grafting 285
        integrity 285
        proliferative capacity of 285
        relies 285
Testosterone 100, 261
    gel 261
    transdermal 261, 265
Theca cells migrate 81
Thin endometrium 229
    causes of 73
    treatment of 73
Thromboembolism 166, 185

Thrombophilia 47
    evaluation of 226
    management for 230
Thrombophlebitis, risk of 295
Thromboprophylaxis 50, 314
Thyroid
    disorders 204
    dysfunction, assessment of 103
    function tests 100
    medications 205
    profile 269
Tissue
    function 130
    integrity 285
Titrate letrozole dose 312
Tocopherol 75, 79
Totipotent cell 330
Touching uterine fundus 67
Trachelectomy
    radical 294
        abdominal 294
        vaginal 294
Transcervical
    placement 56
    uterine instillation 77
Transcriptomic signature 130
Transvaginal
    ovum retrieval 204
    scan 164
    sonography 25, 108, 109, 109*f*, 111, 112, 116, 118, 156, 295
        role of 108
    ultrasonography 104, 108, 116, 124, 156, 223
Trapped egg syndrome 241
Trauma, myometrial 57
Trazodone 205
Trial embryo transfer 59, 63
Triptorelin 35, 48
T-shaped cavity 216
Tubal
    embryo transfer 58
    endometriosis 111
Tuberculosis 73
    genital 242
Tubo-adnexal mass 201
Tubo-ovarian masses, laparoscopic management of 24
Tumors, borderline 299
Tyrosine-glycine-leucine-arginine 33

## U

Ureaplasma urealyticum 73
Urological disorders, treatment of 335
Uterine 276
    anomalies, congenital 222

artery pulsatility index 129
biophysical profile 124
bleeding, abnormal 64
cavity 59, 64, 65
    functional 222
contraction 54, 59
dimensions 108
dysmorphism 216
factor 222, 229
    evaluation of 225
fibroids 64, 273
hemorrhage, massive 298
junctional zone contractions 55
malformations cervical stenosis 64
polyp 124
receptivity 118
relaxing substances 68
secretome 132
wall, anterior 57
Uterocervical
    axis 55
        acute anteflexion of 55
    canal 55
Uterus 108, 197
    anteverted 55
    hypoplastic 217
    normal 109*f*
    retroverted 55, 57

## V

Vaginal
    estrogen 74
    fornices 116
    functions 335
    micronized progesterone 84, 87
    progesterone 84
    reconstruction 335
    sildenafil 75, 76, 230, 334
Varicocelectomy 218
Vascular endothelial growth factor 43, 43*f*, 165, 183, 223
Vascularity flow index 114
Vasopressin injection technique 149
Vincristine 297
Vitamin E 334
Vomiting 184
    postoperative 209
Vulsellum 55, 58

## W

Wallace malleable stylet 58
Water-soluble progesterone, subcutaneous 84
Wilms tumor 180
World Health Organization 330

## Z

Zona hardening 222
Zygote 295